Critical Dementia Studies

This book puts the critical into dementia studies. It makes a timely and novel contribution to the field, offering a thought-provoking critique of current thinking and debate on dementia. Collectively the contributions gathered together in this text make a powerful case for a more politically engaged and critical treatment of dementia and the systems and structures that currently govern and frame it.

The book is inter-disciplinary and draws together leading dementia scholars alongside dementia activists from around the world. It frames dementia as first and foremost a political category. The book advances both theoretical and methodological thinking in the field as well as sharing learning from empirical research. Outlining the limits to existing efforts to frame and theorise the condition, it proposes a new critical movement for the field of dementia studies and practice.

The book will be of direct interest to researchers and scholars in the field of dementia studies and wider fields of health, disability and care. It will provide a novel resource for students and practitioners in the fields of dementia, health care and social care. The book also has implications for dementia policymaking, commissioning and community development.

Richard Ward is Senior Lecturer in Dementia Studies at the University of Stirling and Head of Division for Ageing and Dementia. He is a registered social worker who specialised in working with older people living with dementia. Richard's research interests include social care practice, the experience of living with dementia and how place-based experience can influence the lives of people with chronic and progressive conditions. Richard is part of a network of academics with a shared interest in studying the international development of dementia friendly communities. He is also the co-founder of the Critical Dementia Studies Network. His recently published book is Ward R, Clark A & Phillipson L (eds.) (2021) *Dementia and Place: Practices, Experiences and Connections.*

Linn J. Sandberg is Associate Professor in Gender Studies and Senior Lecturer in the School of Culture and Education, Södertörn University, Sweden. Sandberg's research interests are in the field of ageing, gender, sexuality, embodiment and dementia. Some of her most recent research interests include a qualitative interview study on sexual and intimate couple relationship after the onset of Alzheimer's disease. Currently she is the Principal Investigator of a project on LGBTQ people with dementia and Swedish dementia care, funded by the Swedish Research Council for Health, Working life and Welfare (FORTE). Sandberg is the co-founder of the Critical Dementia Studies Network, (https://memoryfriendly.org.uk/programmes/critical-dementia-network/) together with Richard Ward, and a co-managing editor of the book series Dementia in Critical Dialogue.

Dementia in Critical Dialogue

Series Editors:
Richard Ward (richard.ward1@stir.ac.uk)
Linn J. Sandberg (linn.sandberg@sh.se)
James Fletcher (james.fletcher@manchester.ac.uk)
Andrea Capstick (a.j.capstick@bradford.ac.uk)

If you wish to submit a book proposal for the series, please contact the Series Editors or Emily Briggs emily.briggs@tandf.co.uk

This series will bring together diverse and multidisciplinary commentators around key areas for development in the field of dementia studies. It will include, but not be restricted to edited collections and monographs that will embrace a dialogic and relational approach where writers from within the field of dementia studies engage in a critical exchange with those from other fields.

The series will offer a critical perspective on key and emerging issues for the field of dementia with relevance to research, policy and practice. It contains a reasonable mix of theoretical, policy-related, methodological and applied research contributions. We would like to encourage texts that incorporate transnational and majority world perspectives in the under-standing of dementia. The series editors will appoint a volume editor(s) and work closely with them to help bring together an appropriate mix of authors for each edition.

Critical Dementia Studies
An Introduction
Edited by Richard Ward and Linn J. Sandberg

For more information on the series please visit: https://www.routledge.com/Dementia-in-Critical-Dialogue/book-series/DCD

Critical Dementia Studies
An Introduction

Edited by
Richard Ward and
Linn J. Sandberg

Routledge
Taylor & Francis Group
LONDON AND NEW YORK

First published 2023
by Routledge
4 Park Square, Milton Park, Abingdon, Oxon OX14 4RN

and by Routledge
605 Third Avenue, New York, NY 10158

Routledge is an imprint of the Taylor & Francis Group, an informa business

© 2023 selection and editorial matter, Richard Ward and Linn J.
Sandberg; individual chapters, the contributors

The right of Richard Ward and Linn J. Sandberg to be identified
as the authors of the editorial material, and of the authors for their
individual chapters, has been asserted in accordance with sections
77 and 78 of the Copyright, Designs and Patents Act 1988.

British Library Cataloguing-in-Publication Data
A catalogue record for this book is available from the British Library

Library of Congress Cataloging-in-Publication Data
Names: Ward, Richard, editor. | Sandberg, Linn J., editor.
Title: Critical dementia studies : an introduction / Richard Ward,
Linn J. Sandberg.
Description: Abingdon, Oxon ; New York, NY : Routledge, 2023. |
Series: Dementia in critical dialogue | Includes bibliographical
references and index.
Identifiers: LCCN 2022054645 (print) | LCCN 2022054646 (ebook) |
ISBN 9781032118802 (hardback) | ISBN 9781032118833 (paperback) |
ISBN 9781003221982 (ebook)
Subjects: LCSH: Dementia—Research.
Classification: LCC RC521 .C755 2023 (print) | LCC RC521 (ebook) |
DDC 616.8/310072—dc23/eng/20230111
LC record available at https://lccn.loc.gov/2022054645
LC ebook record available at https://lccn.loc.gov/2022054646

ISBN: 978-1-032-11880-2 (hbk)
ISBN: 978-1-032-11883-3 (pbk)
ISBN: 978-1-003-22198-2 (ebk)

DOI: 10.4324/9781003221982

Typeset in Times New Roman
by codeMantra

Contents

Figures

Contributors

Ronald Amanze is the founder of the social prescribing Box of Smiles agenda and leads the Talk Dementia/music therapy radio programme. He is a Trustee with Arts 4 Dementia and an ambassador with the Alzheimer's Society and Stroke Association. Ronald had a stroke and sustained a brain injury before being diagnosed with dementia a couple of years later.

His background as a creative industries community worker and music producer has led him to be passionate about the role of creativity in improving the quality-of-life experiences for all those living with dementia through the arts.

Andrea Capstick is an Associate Professor in the Centre for Applied Dementia Studies at the University of Bradford, UK. She teaches the MSc in Advanced Dementia Studies. Her research interests centre on participatory visual methods, patient and public involvement, and arts-based approaches.

John Chatwin is a sociologist specialising in applied Conversation Analysis and Video Ethnography. He has a particular interest in the micro-level analysis of medical encounters. His current research is focused on developing ways to capture and analyse subliminal effects in naturalistic interaction.

Dáithí Clayton is an Irish human rights activist who advocates on behalf of older LGBTQI+ people. They are featured in numerous award-winning documentaries, including *Green On Thursdays* (US, 1993); *El Tiempo del Arco Iris* (Spain, 2017) and *Where Do All the Old Gays Go?* (Ireland, 2021). They currently live in the Flemish region of Belgium.

Patrick Ettenes is living with HIV and early-onset dementia. He is a speaker and writer involved with many groups and organisations to raise awareness around these conditions, particularly the needs of LGBT+ people affected by dementia. He is a long-running associate with Alzheimer's Society and does ongoing work with LGBT Foundation in the UK. As a key advisor to both these organisations he helped to launch an innovative programme called 'Bring Dementia Out', which since 2019, aimed to improve services for LGBT+ people affected by dementia. Patrick was awarded Positive Role Model of the Year in 2019 at the National Diversity Awards and in 2021, he was one of ten everyday LGBTQ heroes honoured at the Attitude Pride Awards. Patrick lives in Manchester in the UK and is originally from Barbados.

Richard Fleming is an Honorary Professor in the University of Wollongong, Australia. He began his career as a clinical psychologist specialising in the care of the elderly, especially those with dementia. He pioneered the use of small-scale residential units to replace admission to a psychiatric hospital for people living with dementia in Australia and built on this experience by developing organisations that delivered national educational and consultancy services in the Australian aged care sector. He specialises in assisting architects, designers, and aged and healthcare providers to understand the principles of designing well for people living with dementia.

Amanda Grenier is a Professor and the Norman and Honey Schipper Chair in Gerontological Social Work at the Factor-Inwentash Faculty of Social Work and Baycrest Hospital. Dr Grenier is an inter-disciplinary scholar and critical gerontologist focused on the interface of public policies, organisational practices and older people's lived experience, with a particular focus on ageing and inequality. She currently leads a SSHRC Insight Grant on Precarious Aging. Her books include *Late life homelessness*, *Precarity and Aging* and *Late Life Transitions*.

Birkby Griffith was born in Barbados and migrated to England to complete a General Nursing Diploma. While there, he met his future wife, who is from Jamaica. The couple soon married, had a daughter and migrated to Canada, where Birkby worked for the Manitoba government as Rehabilitation Counsellor/Nurse. There Birkby furthered his education with a Diploma in Psychiatric Nursing and the couple had their second daughter (Marsha). The young family settled in Victoria, British Columbia (BC) in 1972 and Birkby became a staff nurse for Glendale Lodge Society and then later a manager of their care home for children with developmental disabilities. In 1989, he transitioned to the Ministry of Health to serve as a Quality Assurance Consultant/Hospital Inspector. Towards the end of his career, Birkby went to Bermuda to experience health care in a different socio-cultural context and spent six years working in the developmental disabilities sector there before a final year in the island's first Substance Abuse program. Birkby returned to Victoria, BC in 2007 and was diagnosed with Alzheimer's disease in 2011. He continues to live at home with his family where he enjoys music and dancing.

Marsha Griffith has a BA in Linguistics from Carleton University. She taught English and travelled throughout Asia for many years, before returning to Canada in 2014. More recently, she has balanced caring for her father, Birkby, with working as a background performer in television series and movies. Marsha recently formed Sisters of Caribbean Ancestry (SOCA) to connect with other women in Victoria, BC whose parents migrated from the Caribbean and celebrate their shared cultural origins. While she has been her father's main care partner since 2014, Marsha only recently started sharing her experiences along with the videos and photographs she has taken with her papa, documenting their everyday activities and special occasions and/or outings.

Wendy Hulko is a Professor in the Faculty of Education and Social Work at Thompson Rivers University in Kamloops, British Columbia, Canada, who has worked with older adults for nearly 30 years as a care aide, hospital social worker, government policy advisor, educator and researcher. She holds a BAHon in Sociology and Spanish (Trent University), a Master of Social Work (University of Toronto) and a PhD in Sociology and Social Policy (University of Stirling). She is affiliated with the Centre for Research on Personhood in Dementia at the University of British Columbia and the Critical Dementia Studies Network. As an activist-academic and settler accomplice, Wendy conducts inter-disciplinary research on ageing, dementia and health care with equity-denied groups, including Secwepemc Elders, racialised older adults, sexual and gender minorities, and rural residents, and often works in partnership with practitioners and decision-makers from the local health authority. She has published extensively in peer-reviewed journals and edited books. She is a co-editor of *Indigenous Peoples and Dementia: New Understandings of Memory Loss and Memory Care*, published by UBC Press in 2019, and a co-author of the 2020 Routledge Press book *Gerontological Social Work in Action: Anti-oppressive Practice with Older Adults, Their Families, and Communities.*

Nick Jenkins is a Senior Lecturer in Sociology at the University of the West of Scotland. Since 2014, he has been exploring posthumanist, multi-species and post-qualitative approaches to understanding dementia. Alongside his colleagues, Dr Anna Jack Waugh and Dr Louise Ritchie, Nick convenes the *Multi-Species Dementia International Research Network* (https://multispeciesdementia.org/). Established in October 2019, the network seeks to advance more-than-human ways of responding to dementia. Nick is the lead editor for a book to be published by Bristol University Policy Press in 2023, entitled *Multi-Species Dementia Studies: Towards an Interdisciplinary Approach.*

Stephen Katz is Professor (Emeritus) of Sociology at Trent University, Canada. He is a founding member of the Trent Centre for Aging and Society; recipient of Trent's Distinguished Research Award; and author of several books and articles on ageing bodies, critical gerontology, sexuality, musical biography, cognitive impairment, design and health technologies. Currently he is working on a book collection, *Mind, Self and Body in Later Life*.

Andrew King is Professor of Sociology at the University of Surrey, UK, where he is also a co-director of the *Centre for Research on Ageing and Generations* and the *Sex, Gender and Sexualities Research Group*. His research mainly focuses on LGBT+ ageing and life course inequalities. His books include *Older Lesbian, Gay and Bisexual Adults: Identities, Intersections and Institutions* (Routledge, 2016), *Older LGBT People: Minding the Knowledge Gaps* (Routledge, 2018) and '*Intersections of Ageing, Gender and Sexualities*' (Policy Press, 2019). He recently led the project 'CILIA-LGBTQI+', which explored life course inequalities faced by LGBTQI+ people in four European countries. Much of Andrew's work engages with and critiques Queer Theory.

Annette Leibing is a medical anthropologist (PhD, U Hamburg, Germany), who had her first academic position at the Institute of Psychiatry of the Federal U Rio de Janeiro. There she founded and directed, during five years, the CDA – a multidisciplinary centre for mental health and ageing, with a special focus on dementia. After a post-doctoral fellowship at McGill University (Department of Social Studies of Medicine), she is now full professor at the Nursing faculty of Université de Montréal. Her research focuses on issues related to ageing, by studying – as an anthropologist – Alzheimer's and Parkinson's disease, ageing and psychiatry, pharmaceuticals, elder care and stem cells for the body in decline, among others. At the moment, her research focuses mainly on the prevention of dementia in different national and social contexts – undertaken in Canada, Germany and Switzerland (and, part of a different project, also in Brazil). This project focuses on digital biomarkers and preventive technologies.

Linda Örulv, PhD in Health and Society at Linköping University, is a communication ethnographer within the field of dementia studies. Her thesis focused on how residents in dementia care facilities actively and creatively used their remaining linguistic and cognitive resources in social interaction to make sense of their situations, their surroundings and their lives. As a team member of the Center for Dementia Research (CEDER), she partook in studies on the participation of people with dementia in a variety of situations and with varying resources and needs, especially in the context of mutual support and self-advocacy. After 19 years of research and teaching in that area, she nowadays works with advocacy and (mutual) support for autistic people.

Chris Phillipson is Professor of Sociology and Social Gerontology at the University of Manchester. He is a co-director of the Manchester Institute for Collaborative Research into Ageing. He has carried out a number of projects relating to social exclusion in later life, work and retirement, and the impact of social inequality. He has written extensively on issues relating to critical gerontology. His books include *Precarity and Ageing* (co-edited) and *COVID-19, Inequality and Older People: Everyday Life during the Pandemic* (co-authored).

Lyn Phillipson, Associate Professor, is a public health academic who engages in research and action to promote aged and dementia friendly communities. She is known for her community-engaged approach to undertaking research with impact. She uses qualitative and participatory methods to work with older people and people with dementia to promote the understanding and change in the social, physical and service environments that contribute to their well-being.

Hamish Robertson is a health and medical geographer in the Faculty of Health at the Queensland University of Technology with 25 years' experience in health, ageing and disability work. He conducts research in several areas, including health, ageing, disability, patient safety, big data sociology, cultural diversity and cultural heritage. His PhD research was on the geography of Alzheimer's disease, and he is interested in spatial science applications in the health, ageing and disability sectors, including spatial visualisation as a tool for collaborative research and analysis. He works with colleagues on a variety of projects relating to ageing, disability, including disability and dementia, human rights and Aboriginal health.

Helga Rohra is a German dementia activist and campaigner for raising dementia awareness. She is diagnosed with Lewy Body Dementia and Alzheimer's disease. Rohra is a writer who has published four books and has been a presenter in numerous Alzheimer and Neurology conferences. She has been involved in the Patient Council of the German Centre for Neurological Diseases, in the position of Chair, and has been appointed as an expert in the WHO Brain Health Unit's focus group. Rohra runs an international mixed group of people with dementia and professionals entitled 'TrotzDementia' (despite dementia) (www.trotzDEM.org). Rohra has a professional background as a translator in the field of neurology. She has also been working as a university professor teaching medical students.

Linda Steele, Associate Professor, is a socio-legal scholar whose research focuses on the role of law, human rights and transitional justice in perpetration, redress and repair of violence and institutionalisation experienced by disabled people and older people. Her recent projects include reparations for harm to people living with dementia in residential aged care and former disability institutions as sites of conscience.

Kate Swaffer, MSc, is an independent researcher with a focus in her work on human rights, disability rights, and desegregation and deinstitutionalisation of people in residential care homes. Kate is an author and a campaigner for dementia to be managed as a disability, and for the rights of all people with dementia and older persons. She is an Honorary Associate Fellow at the Faculty of Science, Medicine & Health of the University of Wollongong; and a co-founder and human rights advisor at Dementia Alliance International.

Joanne Travaglia is the Head of the School of Public Health and Social Work in the Faculty of Health at the Queensland University of Technology. Her research and teaching focuses on leadership and management, the social epidemiology of patient safety, vulnerability and precarity in health and social care, organisational development and improvement, and workforce development in health and social (aged and disability) care. She has a life-long commitment to improving the quality and safety of care for vulnerable individuals and groups. Over the last two decades, she has received multiple evaluation and research grants, including contracts with federal and state governments and instrumentalities across Australia.

Sadie Wearing is Associate Professor in Gender Theory, Culture and Film in the Department of Gender Studies at the London School of Economic and Political Science. Her research explores the cultural politics of film, literature and media practices. She has published widely on representations of aging in contemporary culture and on the critical questions posed by narratives of dementia. She is currently working on a manuscript (with Yvonne Tasker) on the socialist feminist Jill Craigie entitled *Jill Craigie: Film and Feminism in Postwar Britain*.

Hailee M. Yoshizaki-Gibbons is an Assistant Professor in Biomedical Humanities at Hiram College in Hiram, Ohio. She received her PhD in Disability Studies with a Concentration in Gender and Women's Studies from the University of Illinois at Chicago. Hailee's research employs an intersectional lens to examine the ways gender, race, class and immigration status mediate the lives of old and disabled people and those who care for them. As a scholar activist, Hailee is passionate about disability justice and abolition of sites of care and confinement. Her current project analyses how temporality influences the care relationships between old women with dementia and the immigrant women of colour employed to care for them in dementia units of nursing homes.

Maria Zubair is a sociologist, currently working within the Social Science, Applied Healthcare and Improvement Research (SAPPHIRE) group at the University of Leicester, UK. Following a PhD in Sociology, Maria began her post-doctoral research journey in social gerontology working within an ESRC-funded New Dynamics of Ageing project. Maria's research has focused primarily in the fields of ageing, dementia, health and care, and ethnicity. Her current research interests fall broadly within the areas of social identities, diversities and inequalities in old age.

This includes a particular focus on social constructions of old age, age-ing and health; ageing and later life among racialised/ minoritised ethnic groups; 'race'/racialisation within public health discourses; intersection-ality, negotiation and performativity of social identities; social relation-ships and support networks in old age; health and social care provision for older populations; and gendered experiences of ageing, later life, and health and well-being.

Acknowledgements

Richard Ward and Linn Sandberg jointly developed this book project, building upon a series of face-to-face and online workshops of the Critical Dementia Studies Network. The network was supported through funding secured by Sandberg from *Forte: The Swedish Research Council for Health, Working Life and Welfare* (Grant nr Dnr. F18-1231-1). The editors wish to thank the funders and all the members of the Critical Dementia Studies for making the workshops such stimulating and educative events. An equal editorial contribution to this book was made by the editors. Furthermore, Sandberg secured funding from *Riksbankens jubileumsfond* (Grant nr SAB20-0045) to make this book open access, and the editors wish to thank them for their generous support, enabling us to reach a much broader readership as a result.

Introduction

Why *critical* dementia studies and why now?

Linn J. Sandberg and Richard Ward

Who do we not save?

In May 2021, a series of texts and images leaked to the press gave an insight into the behind-the-scenes 'frenzied planning' that took place within UK central government in the early months of the coronavirus pandemic (Schraer, 2021). Of particular note was the image of a whiteboard covered in scribbled handwriting from a strategy meeting held on March 13, 2020. The meeting involved the then Prime Minister Boris Johnson, his chief scientific and medical advisers as well as government aids and data scientists. Towards the bottom of the board the question had been posed: 'Who do we not save?'

With the dubious benefit of hindsight, we now know the answer to that question. In the UK, as in many other parts of the world, people with dementia were disproportionately represented in the death toll from the pandemic. Many more faced serious privations as part of the human cost of COVID-19. What we saw, even in the earliest stages of this global health crisis, were efforts to sub-divide an amorphous 'public', to categorise and hierarchise so-called citizens in ways that made it very clear that the interests of some were being pitted against those of others. The pandemic is then a useful place for us to start arguing for the timeliness of a book that advocates for critical dementia studies.

As a number of chapters in this book observe, long-term aged care came to play a prominent role in the narrative of the pandemic, in part because it served as a site for the concentration of people with dementia. In many countries people were transferred from hospital to care home without prior screening for COVID. As the pandemic continued to evolve, the emerging dominance of a biomedical framing overshadowed any form of social response or consideration. Care homes remained locked down with visitors barred even as restrictions were lifted for other parts of the population. Older and disabled people and those with existing conditions were deprived of a voice and made visible only anonymously by a daily count of deaths and infections due to the virus. No official occasions or spaces were created to mourn the lives lost, sending a message that these lives were not to

DOI: 10.4324/9781003221982-1

be grieved. In the UK, bereaved relatives eventually began painting small red hearts on a wall in central London with a short memorialising message to their loved one. Over time, tens (eventually hundreds) of thousands of hearts appeared as grief and protest began to coalesce and bereavement turned into resistance. Meanwhile, government ministers bullishly claimed that they had 'got all the big calls right' both during and in the aftermath of the pandemic. While the scale of the tragedy in the UK was greater than for most other European nations, the pattern whereby vulnerable groups and individuals were often the *most* likely to be placed at risk was mirrored globally. All over the world, people with dementia were failed by state government and its institutions. This book makes clear – if we leave these events unanalysed, we risk normalising those conditions.

Defining dementia – The need for change

Commonly, dementia is understood as a disease category, or more specifically a syndrome, chronic and progressive in nature, that leads to deterioration in cognitive function. Like most biomedical constructs it is cast as value-free, a medical fact that supposedly transcends time and place. A history of dementia has been posed largely as a linear story of progress from the negative treatment of older people as senile, to the subsequent discovery of dementia as a disease, mostly 'in' but not necessarily 'of' old age. This historical narrative has done little to resolve the practical marginalising and de-valuing of people with dementia. Cure remains the dominant goal, not care. Discursively and materially, dementia has been ring-fenced as a 'health responsibility' and consequently been left out of broader analyses of disability and ageing. The canons of disability studies and social gerontology (arguably for rather different reasons) have been built largely through exclusion of dementia. There remains an unspoken anxiety that opening up to dementia might risk 're-medicalising' the hard-fought territory of sociological understandings of later life built up through discourses of successful and positive ageing. Despite the status of dementia as a cognitive disability, the field of disability studies has often struggled to acknowledge ageing or the problems that may come with it.

Conceptually, while dementia sits at the intersection of ageing, disability and mental health, dementia studies have been slow to embrace or benefit from the ideas and political resources developed within these related fields of scholarship. Culturally, the prospect of dementia encapsulates widespread fears about ageing and the loss of self. These are often amplified through mainstream media and popular cultural representations. Collectively, as we have outlined above, those living with dementia are frequently set apart from society; their care now and into the future is often depicted as a grave threat to economic and social stability. Policy outputs related to the condition routinely employ alarmist demography to this effect, formulated in terms of 'burden' or 'epidemic'. In this context, all too often the mantra of 'family and community' is offered as the only alternative.

To paraphrase Marcus and Fischer (1999) it sometimes seems that the field of dementia studies has an experimental edge but a vast conservative hinterland. As we argue in the final chapter of this book, this has a lot to do with the way that a biomedical paradigm continues to cast a long shadow over the field, while disciplines such as social gerontology appear to have ceded dementia to a pathological model. This means dementia scholarship has become siloed, only loosely intersecting with a wider academic debate, and is consequently often marked by insularity both theoretically and politically. However, as people with dementia around the world begin to mobilise, challenging the paternalistic, disempowering excesses of service provision coupled with gradual erosion of formal care through policies of fiscal consolidation (i.e. austerity), the time is right for a more radical rethinking of dementia.

What is *'Critical'* in critical dementia studies?

In this book, our focus is upon dementia as a political category, socially produced, with a history as well as an array of potential futures. We argue for more than just enhanced criticality (after all, what self-respecting researcher doesn't consider their work to be critical?). Rather, we seek to instil a commitment to *critical* studies that situate dementia according to its intersections with a broader political movement. By this, we are not proposing any uniform understanding of the *critical*. The theoretical and political genealogies of this book are manifold and sometimes in tension. The chapter authors write from within different ontological and epistemological framings, from the more materialist (including a focus on political economy) to post-structuralist and post-materialist. To borrow from Stephen Katz's characterisation of critical gerontology, we might similarly think of critical dementia studies as 'nomadic forms of thought' (Katz, 2003, p. 201).

At the heart of critical theory and practice is a commitment to *social justice*. Each branch or iteration opposes oppression and participates in a politics of coalition as it works for change. This includes throwing into question assimilationist arguments advanced by liberal-humanist and social citizenship scholarship that rest upon the belief in an essentially benign state. From this standpoint the state, and by extension its many institutions, including the health and welfare systems, are routinely assumed to be fair and just. Such a consensus worldview has long argued for the inclusion of people with dementia but without a critique of the conditions into which people are supposedly being included. Increasingly, critical scholarship also employs an intersectional lens, mistrustful of what Jackson (2013) describes as 'single liberatory strategies'. It rejects earlier reliance upon fixed and essentialised notions of identity that supposedly persist through continuous time. Crucially, a shared belief is that knowledge is socially constructed and historically contingent, and that this provides opportunities and openings for transformative action.

In many cases, critical scholarship adopts a contestatory stance in relation to more mainstream perspectives within its field (Hall, 2019). This entails critiquing what Grant (2016) has called 'power-silent' accounts of people's experience, and the overall failure to connect such accounts to broader power networks. We need to pause and consider the ways in which both research and practice depoliticise dementia. This has led to locating it as a question of individual struggle, formulated in terms of stigma and individual insensitivity and cruelty, rather than as a matter of systemic and structural inequity and oppression. On this point, Kafer (2013) has argued for looking beyond often biomedically constituted categories of illness and disability to seek out collective affinities. Such affinities can lead to building alliances and ultimately a politics of coalition. The challenge of turning dementia studies *critical* is then an open-ended endeavour.

Overview of the book

With the challenge issued by critical dementia studies outlined above, we have organised this book into four sections. Here, we briefly explain the thinking behind this structure while giving a flavour of what each chapter has to offer.

Reclaiming and recasting

'What does a person with dementia look like?' This question is explicitly raised in Chapter 3 by Patrick Ettenes, where he/she discusses not becoming intelligible as a person with dementia. Ettenes' question resonates with a wider issue explored in this volume: *who is 'the person with dementia'?* We need to *recast* just who is collectively envisaged as 'the person with dementia' and rethink the elliptical category 'people with dementia'. There remains an evident lack of intersectional analyses in current dementia research and a silence surrounding what this means for our understanding of the lived experience of the condition. Contributions to this first part of the book thus provide a living breathing account of what it means to 'fit into lots of categories' as Ettenes describes him/herself. From Helga Rohra (Chapter 4), Dáithí Clayton (Chapter 1) and Ettenes, we further hear about efforts to police the boundaries of dementia as a diagnostic category and the scepticism they have faced for not fitting into unspoken but normative constructions of the person with dementia. The homogenising ambition to 'treat everyone the same' is, as Clayton suggests in their chapter, effectively erasing differences and the specific life histories of marginalised groups. Clayton's contribution to this book underscores the value of learning drawn from a life lived along less normative or hegemonic lines. Their own refusal of conformity hints at the wealth of experience routinely obscured by efforts to compress people into categories for the expediency of policy or practice.

We have drawn together first-hand accounts by five people who live with and navigate dementia and cognitive ableism (i.e. disablement associated with cognitive impairment), but who also confront racism, misogyny, homo- and trans-phobia as well as other forms of ableism and health-ism. Such experiences of multiple forms of marginalisation and oppression are absolutely central to understanding what critical dementia studies is about, disrupting the homogenising impulse behind much existing research and practice. These first-hand contributions complicate the discourses of 'living well with dementia', pointing to how gender, sexuality, dis/ability, health, ethnicity and race pose particular kinds of vulnerabilities. Thus, Ettenes in his/her chapter tells of struggles with loneliness and mental health and Ronald Amanze (Chapter 2), through poetry, expresses frustrations at being unheard and discriminated against within the care system. Speaking as a dementia activist, Rohra (Chapter 4) shares her experience of how women with dementia are far more readily challenged when speaking publicly of their experience.

Yet, the chapters in this part also reflect various everyday joys, such as music, dancing and friendship, as well as significant forms of resistance, both in terms of organised activism and advocacy and through everyday resistance. This includes resistance against controlling care, 'I don't want to be drugged into submission' as Clayton phrases it. It also involves resistance to having one's identity erased as a queer person, and how this defiance could be expressed through simple things such as painting one's nails and wearing 'a fucking dress', as Ettenes puts it. As such the writers are not only *reclaiming* their voices but also *recasting* the narrative beyond binaries of tragedy or living well, proposing different possibilities for *liveable* lives that encompass vulnerability and struggles as well as happiness.

Reclaiming also concerns one's history, background and culture. Through an almost real-time poetic online diary Amanze has pursued his desire to connect with Black history, often through cultural intersections of words and music. Or, as Ettenes describes, returning to a place one has migrated from may bring back memories and sustain you through difficult times. The chapters also point to the significance of one's communities and relationships. Rohra describes the importance of peer support and the mentorship received from other dementia activists in order to become an activist herself. The photo essay with/by Birkby Griffith and his daughter Marsha portrays the role of intimate relationships, and how Marsha enables Birkby's identity as a runner and dancer. Supported by Wendy Hulko, the Griffiths share images from a photo-diary with the aim of making visible the lived experience of someone who no longer communicates verbally.

While this book starts with the 'voices' and experiences of people with dementia, this is not to suggest that critical dementia studies is a matter of simply adding more voices. Indeed, we would question the drive for 'authentic voices' in some existing dementia research (see further discussion in Chapter 19). Instead, we need to, in the words of Maria Matsuda (1991), 'ask the other question': how does the framing of 'the person with dementia' make some positions visible and intelligible while others are rendered invisible or unintelligible?

Reframing

Framings of dementia in scientific discourse as well as in media and cultural narratives have material consequences for people's everyday lives. The second section thereby explores how dementia is framed according to existing research agendas as well as in the cultural imaginary, specifically film. The section also points to the potential for critical reframing.

Questions of personhood, self and subjectivity are threaded throughout dementia studies and in Chapter 6 Stephen Katz and Annette Leibing take us on an impressive, critical and reflective journey that traces the diverse and evolving constructions of personhood and related questions in dementia research. They organise these developments according to three thematic stages: 'Disease, Loss and the Medicalisation of Dementia', 'Person-Centred Care and Its Critics' and 'De-Centring Humanism'. Each stage is shown to carry limitations and challenges. For instance, liberal-humanist person-centred approaches have usefully challenged narrow biomedicalised conceptions of dementia as deficit, pre-occupied with cognitive impairment. Nonetheless, as Katz and Leibing observe, person-centred approaches are themselves limited not least in how they overlook the structural conditions of care, where austerity-led cuts to the care system have resulted in a failure to recognise the personhood and rights of both people with dementia and their care partners. At the same time, they argue, even more recent work, which has decentred humanism and disrupted underlying assumptions about time and memory, cannot be regarded as the end of the story. Ultimately, the chapter points to the need for an on-going *critique of the critique* in dementia studies.

Nick Jenkins (Chapter 7) takes further issue with the exceptional position of personhood and the human subject within existing dementia research and offers a radical proposal of 'thinking with animals and other forms of (nonhuman) life' in dementia studies. Jenkins suggests that there is a need for more attention to the links between cognitive ableism and speciesism, and how the othering of those with cognitive disabilities rests on the premise that they are not fully human. Rather than sticking with a human rights discourse, which by definition is exclusionary, a multispecies approach which disrupts notions of humans as indivisible and exceptional could thus offer a path to radical social change, Jenkins argues. Interestingly, what Jenkins' argument suggests is that critical dementia studies do not by default have to pit themselves against the natural sciences or biomedicine. Instead, emerging research within these fields, including studies of the human microbiome and the co-constitution of human and nonhuman cells in our bodies, may lead to other ways of thinking about self/non-self (see also Shildrick, 2021). There may then be alliances to be made to reframe and disrupt existing enactments of dementia.

Overall inattention to questions of power and social inequity in current framings of dementia has been one of the main impulses for this volume. The focus of Maria Zubair's chapter (Chapter 8) is specifically on the silence that surrounds issues of racism within dementia research agendas and the dominance of an unmarked white standpoint. Zubair discusses how minority ethnicities and cultural difference are recursively framed as the problem in research, leaving whiteness unaddressed and invisible. The way dementia is enacted in current research institutions is thus very much a matter of which bodies inhabit and control them. Indeed, critical dementia studies must also be about disrupting the comfortable. The possibilities of upsetting current research agendas require resistant and disobedient researchers who make visible the workings of power. Yet, at the same time, and as Zubair forcefully illustrates, the vulnerable positioning of some scholars due to intersections of race with gender, dis/ability, class and an increasing precarity in academia makes such resistance difficult.

The possibilities for deconstructing cultural framings of dementia are addressed in Sadie Wearing's chapter (Chapter 9), where she explores how recent mainstream films can provide more progressive narratives on dementia. Political and media discourses as well as cultural representations often intermingle with biomedical narratives to frame dementia as a burden. Critical analysis of films and other cultural artefacts are significant for the ways dementia is imagined and can indeed be reimagined as they, in Wearing's words, 'elicit a range of affective responses'. Contemporary films may reproduce longstanding tropes of dementia as catastrophic loss while simultaneously providing ways of rethinking care relations and vulnerability. As Wearing points out, readings of such representations are thereby a crucial aspect of critical engagement with dementia, allowing opportunities for interrogation of popular understandings that circulate about the condition.

Care and control

As we discussed at the beginning of this chapter, the political context of dementia became acutely visible as the COVID-19 pandemic unfolded. It was soon painfully clear how older people in general and older people with illnesses and disabilities in particular were positioned as outside 'frames of grievability' (Butler, 2009), their lives deemed not worth protecting. This betrayal of claims to citizenship is critically explored in the third part *Care and Control*. The chapters in this part in various ways take contemporary crises as a theme, not only the pandemic but also neoliberal austerity politics. Collectively, they highlight the structural violence and precarity imposed on people with dementia, especially those living in long-term care.

Amanda Grenier and Chris Phillipson (Chapter 10) outline a contemporary shift which they refer to as 'precarious ageing'. It is an experience of later life characterised by the withdrawal of institutional supports and universal welfare alongside increasingly privatised care markets. Consequently, they suggest we are witnessing the intersection of intensified biomedicalisation and a wider social and cultural devaluation of ageing subjects. Precarious ageing affects people with dementia in care homes in particular ways. The vulnerability of people with dementia is often understood in medicalised and individualised terms. Yet, thinking with Grenier and Phillipson, the precarity of people with dementia in care homes can be understood as a 'politically induced condition' which leaves people unprotected and exposed.

This exposure is discussed further by Hamish Robertson and Joanne Travaglia (Chapter 11) who draw on Achille Mbembe's concept of 'necropolitics' to explore the political conditions that surround and decide where and how people with dementia may live and die. They take the COVID-19 pandemic as a case in point, examining the structural conditions under which older people with dementia are understood as expendable in the population and thus excluded from treatment and care, or are subjected to harmful and in some cases fatal political interventions. Robertson and Travaglia make a compelling argument for how the position and treatment of people with dementia should not be understood merely as the failure of individual institutions or organisations. Instead, they argue, it is linked to wider questions of population ageing and longstanding ideas of the 'healthy state'. As future crises will inevitably emerge, including new pandemics as well as health crises and climate-change related disasters, these issues will only become of greater relevance and significance to the positioning of people with dementia in society.

The structural violence against people with dementia and care homes as sites for individual and structural harms are also highlighted by Linda Steele, Lyn Phillipson, Kate Swaffer and Richard Fleming (Chapter 12). While care homes are often regarded as therapeutic, benevolent and benign settings, Steele and colleagues introduce a more politicised terminology from critical disability scholarship where care homes are understood as 'carceral'. These institutional settings normalise control, confinement and segregation under the banner of protection. While these kinds of political framings have been rare in dementia studies, they are important not only because they challenge current conditions but also because they provide more radical ways of reimagining care. As Steele and colleagues rightfully point out, ideas of abolition of existing care institutions would require more equitable communities.

However, where there is power and control there is also resistance, which is shown by Andrea Capstick and John Chatwin (Chapter 13). In their argument, what is often perceived in biomedical or psychosocial paradigms as 'challenging behaviour' or 'inappropriate' verbal expressions may instead be understood as forms of cultural resistance in a controlling care environment.

Drawing on Bakhtin's theories, the authors discuss how the people with dementia they observed in their research used humour and 'laugh[ed] in the face of adversity'. While struggling to be heard, in various ways residents tried to resist how they were approached and positioned in everyday inter-actions. Few studies on citizenship and agency in dementia focus on people in care environments and Capstick and Chatwin's chapter thus provides a novel lens for thinking about resistance among those who are often per-ceived as too frail, too impaired or disabled, and lacking a political voice.

Forging alliances

In the final part *'Forging alliances'* of this volume, the authors explore the affinities and coalitions between dementia studies and feminist, queer, crip, critical disability and neurodiversity scholarship. A shared feature across the chapters is how other critical movements and theories contribute to problematising a discourse of consensus and assimilation within demen-tia studies. In contrast to liberal-humanist and citizenship approaches to dementia, which focus on the individual, their rights and responsibilities, the authors in this part underscore the need to turn the gaze towards the normative. This includes for example highlighting the always unstable cate-gories of dementia and 'ablemindedness'.

Hailee Yoshizaki-Gibbons (Chapter 14) explores the potential of conver-gences between critical disability studies and dementia studies. Yoshizaki-Gibbons argues that one of the things to be learnt from critical disability perspectives is how a rights-based discourse does little to challenge state power or neoliberal capitalism and often prioritises the rights of the more privileged within a disabled community. Alongside other chapters in this volume, Yoshizaki-Gibbons calls for a greater focus on intersectionality and argues that dementia should not be regarded as a separate/distinct category but as co-constitutive with race, gender, sexuality, mental health and so on. She points out that marginalised groups are at greater risk of becoming ill with dementias, while the question of who is understood as sane, healthy and rational is also intimately linked to different power asym-metries. Yoshizaki-Gibbons argues that turning to critical disability studies frameworks and concepts such as the 'bodymind', 'debility' and a 'crip of colour-critique' may thus be useful to forge more systemic structural change and social justice.

Overall, difference is a contentious issue in dementia studies, and Linn Sandberg (Chapter 15) focuses on how feminist scholarship can be drawn upon to explore this. Sandberg argues that recent discourses of 'living well with dementia' have sought to underscore the normality/sameness of people with dementia and evaded questions of difference. This kind of approach is still highly invested in narrow and normative Western modernist ideals of active, agentic, autonomous, cognitive subjects. Sandberg suggests that femi-nist scholarship provides ways of thinking of dementia as lived and embodied difference, which does not necessarily equate difference with otherness, and highlights the potential of people with dementia living across different positionalities of forming an epistemic community – a '"demented" standpoint'.

Forging alliances is not only about identifying theoretical and methodological affinities, but very much a matter of coalitions in practice, and of how critical knowledges can inform policy and practice. Wendy Hulko (Chapter 16) explores this challenge through the process of becoming an accomplice and managing to 'walk the talk' through development of critical praxis. This is vital, given longstanding criticism of critical scholarship as effective in dismantling existing frameworks, but often falling short of building a new political apparatus. Hulko offers a case study of the incremental process of shifting from normative assumptions to critical awareness in social care practice. Her chapter provides a valuable insight into how a more critical agenda can be fostered through practice.

Another close companion to critical dementia studies is queer theory, as introduced by Andrew King (Chapter 17). King outlines the potential for queer theory to trouble the commonplace and normative in dementia research, policy and practice. Emerging in the wake of another global health crisis, the AIDS pandemic, queer theory and activism have provided forceful critical tools and resources to deconstruct binaries of healthy/pathological and normal/deviant that are directly applicable to dementia studies. But queer theory also poses pertinent critical questions about normative constructs of time and memory. Indeed, King draws upon queer theoretical work (such as that of Halberstam) to suggest that forgetting may be usefully understood outside the realms of the pathological as a form of disruption to normative chronologies.

Many affinities exist between queer theory and the neurodiversity paradigm, which originally emerged within critical studies of autism, and which is discussed by Linda Örulv (Chapter 18). In her chapter Örulv asks how neurodiversity, a concept that aims to depathologise neurodivergence, can contribute to critical dementia studies. The chapter provides a compelling case study, this time of what a critical methodology might look like for bridging different experiences of 'difference'. Örulv outlines a methodology that draws attention to the unmarked privilege that resides in much mainstream scholarship. Through this, she points to how critical dementia studies might be generative of a new (coalitional) politics that leads to change.

Our concluding chapter, 'Thinking back and looking ahead', is less a conclusion and more an effort to draw together learning from the preceding chapters to map the co-ordinates to guide a critical methodology for dementia studies. With the aim of informing the thinking and approach of researchers and practitioners interested in engaging with a more critical reading of dementia, we bring into dialogue two commentators who have helped inspire this book: Alison Kafer whose book *Feminist, Queer, Crip* (2013) not only integrates different strands of critical thinking and theory but usefully demonstrates how the discourse and dominance of the able-bodied and able-minded intersect in processes of disablement and exclusion. Alongside

Kafer is Patti Lather (2007), a feminist ethnographer, whose own work engages directly with intersections of gender, health and disablement in the experience of HIV and AIDS. Lather draws on this experience to outline a different kind of methodology. Her argument is for uncertainty, unknowing and a lack of confidence as methodological strengths. In this final chapter, we bring these two influences into dialogue and apply the learning to dementia scholarship. We argue for bringing ourselves closer to experiences of dementia while simultaneously moving farther away from dementia as a fixed and stable category of experience.

No big bang

This book grew out of a series of meetings and workshops convened by the Critical Dementia Studies Network.[1] Many ideas and different territories were mapped during these events from diverse perspectives and disciplines that included the participation of campaigners living with dementia. It would be misleading to suggest that what it represents is something new or previously unvoiced. Rather it is the weaving together of many different threads across a variety of disciplines, domains, histories, cultures and practices of dissent. Indeed, Lather (2007) has cautioned against conventional notions of what she describes as a 'successor regime' in narrativising an evolving discipline. She observes this often leads to overblown proclamations of the 'big bang' of a new 'turn' or paradigm. Instead, she argues for a less sequential understanding and a rather different temporality. A more representative portrayal of an emerging critical direction for dementia studies might then involve slow change based upon accretions in practice. This is more about reflecting on what's been missed or left unsaid as it is about the novelty of an alternative framing. It is then as much a matter of thinking back as of looking ahead.

We believe that the time has come for critical dementia studies. Together we are calling for more approaches that problematise, defamiliarise, denaturalise and destabilise common assumptions and orthodoxies in dementia research, policy and practice. This means reflecting upon what we have become attached to, in terms of theories, concepts and methods, and what our habits and attachments enable or impede. We offer this volume as an introduction in a genuine sense – as an invitation or an opening to further dialogue. It is not our intention to fix what critical dementia studies *is*, but to explore what it may *become*. Collectively, we hope the ideas and arguments advanced in this book prove to be a critical moment in the field of dementia studies, one that will inspire future scholarship and ultimately lead to change.

Note

1 Visit our webpages: https://memoryfriendly.org.uk/programmes/critical-dementia-network/.

References

Butler, J. (2009). *Frames of War: When Is Life Grievable?* London: Verso.

Grant, A.J. (2016). Storying the World: A Posthumanist Critique of Phenomeno-logical-Humanist Representational Practices in Mental Health Nurse Qualitative Inquiry. *Nursing Philosophy, 17*(4), pp. 290–297.

Hall, M.C. (2019). 'Critical Disability Theory', in *The Stanford Encyclopedia of Philosophy* (Winter 2019 Edition), E.N. Zalta (ed.). Available at: https://plato.stanford.edu/archives/win2019/entries/disability-critical/.

Jackson, A.Y. (2013). Spaces of Power/Knowledge: A Foucauldian Methodology for Qualitative Inquiry. *Qualitative Inquiry, 19*(10), pp. 839–847.

Kafer, A. (2013). *Feminist, Queer, Crip.* Bloomington: Indiana University Press.

Katz, S. (2003). Critical Gerontological Theory: Intellectual Fieldwork and the Nomadic Life of Ideas. In S. Biggs, A. Lowenstein, J. Hendricks, and J. Hendricks (eds.), *The Need for Theory: Critical Approaches to Social Gerontology* (1st ed., pp. 15–31). Abingdon: Routledge.

Lather P. (2007). *Getting Lost: Feminist Efforts toward a Double(d) Science.* New York: SUNY Press.

Marcus, G.E. and Fischer, M.M.J. (1999). *Anthropology as Cultural Critique: An Experimental Moment in the Human Sciences* (2nd ed.). Chicago and London: University of Chicago Press.

Matsuda, M.J. (1991). Beside My Sister, Facing the Enemy: Legal Theory out of Coalition. *Stanford Law Review, 43*(6), 1183. https://doi.org/10.2307/1229035.

Schraer, R. (2021). 'Dominic Cummings: What Was on His Whiteboard?' *BBC News* (online), 26th May. Available at: https://www.bbc.com/news/health-57254654 (Accessed 1/8/22).

Shildrick, M. (2021). Queering Dementia: Technologies, Visceral Prostheses and Embodiment. *Lambda Nordica, 27*(2–3), pp. 76–101. https://doi.org/10.34041/ln.v27.742.

Part I
Reclaiming and recasting

1   I want to be the orchestrator of my entire fabulous life

Dáithí Clayton

I was born in the United States, although I am Irish. My family came from Ireland, from County Monaghan. I was born and raised in the United States in an Irish Catholic (alcoholic, dysfunctional) family. I was queer from the cradle. I just remember without even having a vocabulary for it, just knowing that I was different, you know – 'a Sissy'. And I survived, so many people did not, but I learned very quickly how to navigate those spaces in-between. Then I came out in the 1970s just five years after the Stonewall Rebellion of 1969, which is what the modern gay rights LGBT+ movement celebrates (there had, of course, been homophile efforts long before that). I have lived my life out of the closet and travelled all around the world: North America, South America, Europe, Africa and Western Asia.

I was a caregiver during the AIDS epidemic. I showed up and lost a whole lot of friends who aren't here any longer (both King, Chapter 17, and Robertson and Travaglia, Chapter 11, further discuss parallels between AIDS and the COVID pandemic). So, I've been at the bedside for the death rattle and all of that. It doesn't have to be awful and horrible; it can actually be a celebration and a joy, depending on how the life is lived, how it's held and what is valued.

Personally, I value my queerness at its core, to the very end, even in this culture that is frequently LGBTQI-phobic, transphobic, ageist and ableist as hell – as I'm finding out! But I will go down fighting to not have my core identity erased by heteronormative care. That's not been my lived experience; I've never been heterosexual in my life, and I don't want my care to be.

Back in the mid-1970s when I came out, we really just had two labels, 'lesbian' and 'gay', and that was it. I was around at that heady time when there were these political debates about how should we proceed? Should we be revolutionary, living outside of an established society? Or, should we assimilate and be just like the good heterosexuals? Well, guess who won? We've got same-sex marriage and gays in the military and all of that, but what a price we paid. So, I was a rebel *with* a cause from the very beginning. I remember early leaders like Audre Lorde in New York City and Barbara Gittings and so many of them were women and women of colour, who advocated for 'smashing the patriarchy' and that's what my life has been about and

DOI: 10.4324/9781003221982-3

continues to be about. So, I first identified as a gay man back in the 1970s and then I evolved in my own life and over time, as more and more letters were added to the big (LGBTQ+) tent. I don't consider myself transgender, but I'm not in the binary any longer (i.e. non-binary). It just seems to fit more and more, and that's who I am.

But I'm still on a journey; wherever I'm at in my life and with my health conditions too, it may change over time – however much time I have available to me. So, this is where I'm at today: non-binary, using pronouns 'he' and 'they'. It was just a little like coming home to myself. Everyone's journey is unique, but I also hear echoes of this in other stories, not only from my own generation but in conversations that I have with younger generations who are inspirational as well. I have, and others of my generation have, so much to teach from our lived experience, but I am also a lifelong learner; it never, ever stops. It has been exhilarating and liberating because I am a liberationist – that's how I've always identified.

I was first diagnosed with prostate cancer at stage two. I had surgery in a tiny little college town in Slovakia and then I went back to the United States for further cancer treatment. In the United States there are several of these LGBTQ-inclusive health care centres, some in San Francisco, LA, Washington, several of them, and well, Chicago had one: the Howard Brown Health Centre. That was very affirming and hugely important for me because they are about the intersectionality of identity and diagnosis and medical support. It was there that they sent me for an MRI brain scan which showed the presence of amyloid plaques and micro-strokes, which were contributing factors to the early onset dementia that I was eventually diagnosed with. It's not easy to adjust to chronic conditions that have no cure – I know where this train is headed! I've been living with both (cancer and dementia) now for nearly ten years and increasingly symptomatic with both. There are surprises on this dementia journey; it's not always a walk in the park, that's for damn sure! However, there are good surprises and gifts along the way, too. What I'm finding is that the journey of discovery never really ends.

Well, since the Trump shitshow started I saw that trainwreck coming and left the United States and went back to Ireland, where I had residency and medical care, and I was hoping to find a rainbow community. I was down in Cork, where there are some wonderful people. Unfortunately, my general practitioner was both homophobic and transphobic. She never, in three years, ever touched my body. She was my doctor, and there was not even a physical examination nor even a touch or anything. I remember when I initially met her about my dementia diagnosis (which had already been determined by MRI and then cognitive function testing in Chicago) and she turned to me and said 'I don't see it'. Oh, really? What does dementia look like to you, doctor? I'll never forget that, and I stopped going to her because I didn't feel safe or respected. It's changing, I know, in both the UK and Ireland and elsewhere, but not nearly enough. No one should be dealing with that in 2022. So, I was down in Cork and I did a lot of volunteer work and advocacy, particularly around older LGBTQI folks and dementia issues, hoping to get a support group up and running but getting nowhere with it. Eventually, I made the decision that nothing's going to change in this country, and I don't have the luxury of time. So, I packed up everything and moved here to Belgium.

When I'm in a safe space I literally let my hair down. I don't always do that even where I live now in very progressive Belgium; this is a new place, a new town right now, where people have been very welcoming, but at least for right now, I wear my hair up and back, but I do still wear my accessories and feminised clothing and all of that. What I really like, and it's happened to me several times here in Flanders and when I was in Turkey and Mexico, is when I am mistaken for a woman or when people aren't sure you know, I love that! Ideally, I would like to be in a genderless society, just let go of all of it and be who we are. In Ireland, they clearly didn't know what to make of me. I did some advocating not only on my own behalf or for my own community, but for all marginalised communities. I am a revolutionary to the very end.

This process of brain atrophy can be slow and it shows up in so many different ways. I try to observe those changes or symptoms as dispassionately as possible, without drama. I've been experiencing a little of what I thought were hallucinations, a bit of wandering; I can't cook on my own safely in the kitchen any longer. I have carers who come into my home now and it's a very intimate thing to have people come into your home. It's absolutely critical to me that they understand who I am at my core, not just tolerate or respect me – I want celebration. Celebrate me! and they do. I have three of them who are just wonderful, I'm so grateful for that.

The first carer who came, and she's still coming, she's coming tomorrow actually. When she learned that I'm a member of the LGBTQ community, well, among other things, she told me about this LGBT club in the nearby town. I haven't been yet, but it sounds fabulous. The second time she came to visit me, she brought a bag full of women's clothes. I didn't ask her to do that, it was simply a gesture that she made that she thought I would enjoy. It turns out she has some remarkably good taste. I was very, very grateful, and it's those kinds of human heart-to-heart interactions that I think are too often missing among the training that modern clinicians receive.

So far so good here in Belgium, but even here there's some work to do. I want to have my advanced directives about who I am and when I can no longer communicate for myself, I want it in writing and not only in English but translated into Dutch and I want it made very clear, I don't want prayers. I don't want artificial resuscitation either, or breathing machines or anything like that. I would like a disco ball, thank you very much. That's when I was coming of age and celebrating the end of my yellow brick road, that's hugely important. I'm having that which I didn't get in my home country of Ireland, and I don't think it's unique only to Ireland; I know it's true in the UK and probably even here in Belgium. I mean it's easy to recognise the rabid hateful homophobes and transphobes. What's much, much more insidious is 'Oh, we treat everyone the same' – Oh yeah? Well, in treating everyone the same, what happens for older people of the LGBT community? You're erasing their identity because that sameness is almost always heteronormative care in the context of your nuclear family – your mother, father, kids – but don't impose that on me, particularly when I am at my most vulnerable.

Some organisations are doing remarkably good, inclusive work, not just with the LGBT community but with BME communities, and so many different marginalised communities and all around intersectionality with ageing brain issues. There are now at least seven LGBTQI safe spaces for people living with dementia. I've been Zooming (teleconferencing) with one in London for over a year and a half now, there's one in Manchester. Later today I'm going to be Zooming with the fabulous folks in Brighton, at Switchboard. That's my Rainbow family of support. I've been campaigning for something similar in Ireland for over two years but still nothing. 'We treat everyone the same' – it's so clueless. And that's the thing, too, about this brave new post-COVID world we inhabit—all this Zooming—it's still a connection, virtual or otherwise, and absolutely a lifeline. Later today, I'm going to dial into the Brighton Group. It's mostly these older lesbians from all over the UK who have just welcomed me and we're going to get together, eventually. My mobility is rapidly declining, but I can get on a Eurostar train to be able to have a weekend with my rainbow family of support and I want them with me to the very end.

Doctor M. is my primary care physician here in Belgium. She's a wonderful young woman 50 years my junior. I was referred to her by the transgender information point at the local university. First thing she asked me was which pronouns I preferred using – that was great, that's all I'm looking for. That would never happen in Ireland. Here in Belgium and in other EU states, they have euthanasia and assisted suicide. I want that choice available whether I avail myself of it or not. I want to be the orchestrator, not only of the end of my life, but my entire fabulous life. It's a conversation that I've already begun having, it's a quite a rigorous process. I don't want the medical community deciding 'put them on artificial breathing machines, let them have 20–30 more years of whatever they call life'. No, I want to be able to make that decision for myself, not the state, not the church, not the justice system – me. It's my life, you don't get to decide, you don't know better than I do.

So, all I have is my pension, that's all I have right now, and it's stretched as far as I can. I know that there are thousands and thousands of older folks in deep shit right now, but I'm still here. I'm still doing the best I can for as long as I can and I will continue looking for, and not just looking for, but demanding support. I won't settle for less – I'm not built that way. I've heard these horror stories about not just people with dementia but older folks tethered to their beds in care homes. Well, part of that appeals to my bondage fetish but seriously, I don't want to be drugged into submission, and I know that's what they do in Medicare settings (in the United States). It might sound clichéd, but I am who I am and I want to remain that way for as long as I'm able. It's not all bad in here but I've had conversations with my doctor particularly around pain management because it can be painful, osteoarthritis and all of these things. When I need it, I want more than paracetamol or a fucking cup of tea. I want morphine for that shit! And she assured me that I'll have that available to me, so I'm OK with this journey. I really am. I just want to be affirmed by the people who take care of me – that I am who I am to the very end.

Here in Europe, I think more than ten years ago in Stockholm, they opened the first LGBTQI-inclusive care home specifically for older folks – the Rainbow House. It has a very long waiting list and I've been on it for many years because I want to die among queer folks. I think I may be a teeny-weeny little bit heterophobic, and I own that. But wouldn't it be fabulous? Gay bingo, Drag Queen bingo, just be who you are to the very end. Celebrate that and don't just allow it on Rainbow Pride week, I want Pride every fucking day of the year.

2 Small quantities at a time

On music, poetry and social media

Ronald Amanze

This is the first-hand narrative of Ronald Amanze who had a stroke and sustained a brain injury before being diagnosed with dementia a couple of years later. The chapter interweaves Ronald's story with poems about his everyday life that he publishes regularly on his Twitter account.

My mum and dad were both born in Jamaica. They came to the UK as part of the Windrush generation with my elder sister Shirley, with whom I am very close. Reggae and ska music from the Caribbean underpinned my upbringing. It was always played at family gatherings. As a young man, I had a wide circle of friends, and we were in and out of each other's homes with no consideration of race, colour or creed.

As time passed, we went to youth clubs, where the main music was reggae. I remember Marcia Griffiths and Bob Andy singing 'Young Gifted and Black', and 'Liquidator' by Harry J. Allstars, Toots and the Maytals. But not just reggae – The Jacksons, Carol King, The Beatles, The Rolling Stones. Great music. As kids, we were always into the latest fashion. In the skinhead era, we wore Ben Sherman shirts, DM boots, Harringtons and a Crombie coat. I always find it interesting that skinheads are sometimes associated with racism. In my community and the world I grew up in, I never saw or experienced any of that. I was conscious of my colour, and the mixing with other colours was part of the beauty of my youth.

> June 19th 2022
> In the Dementia world.
> I'm often reading about research programs.
> And wonder. When SOME (Only some)
> Professionals and academics talk about seldom heard communities.
> What do they mean by that.
> Are they also talking about
> The romantic voices in our communities
> Like Ronalds <3

DOI: 10.4324/9781003221982-4

When I was in my late teens, I began to read. I read amazing books. By Angela Davis or Malcolm X. I became aware. Occasionally, people would joke, 'What's a Black man like you doing with a Scottish name like Ferguson?' I didn't take issue with it, but I did become curious about my name and my heritage. When I was reading about Africa, there was a name – Amanze – which means 'the quality of a king'. And so I adopted that because it identified me as who I was, culturally. When I went into the music industry, Ronald Amanze became my pseudonym.

June 22, 2022
When they see me coming
With my sparklers and my twigs.
I guess they says.
Look there comes Ronald again.
Trying to stand up to the machine.

There is blatant racism in our society. Often, I think what leads to racism is cultural misunderstanding. People seem to misunderstand me. I am energetic and passionate. But that behaviour is not the norm for certain parts of England. And I wonder when they see I am Black, do they interpret that more negatively than they would normally?

April 25th 2021
As I could not find any Black books written on the subject of dementia
By people of my heritage from the perspective of someone with a lived experience.
I had to learn from my experiences.
Which is one reason why I aspire to write a book.
So others may learn from my journey.

History has become much more important to me over the last few years. I had a stroke, and sustained a brain injury. Two years later I was diagnosed with dementia. With dementia, people began to talk a lot about memories. I realised I didn't have a lot of memories – not of growing up. So now I call my auntie in Jamaica and ask her about Jamaica and about my mum and dad. I even wrote a song about it called 'Black History'.[1] When I consider my heritage, it saddens me to think about what Black people had to go through. I know the exclusion that Black people have felt.

Over the last few months, during coronavirus lockdown, I feel very strongly that I have been culturally misunderstood by the council, and discriminated against. They are a big bureaucracy, and they have power. And I don't. And it leaves me feeling threatened and feeling constantly anxious.

March 28th 2020
Need time to think about things.

When phoned up out of thin air expected to discuss things
Without fore Notification. It confuses and frightens me,
Yesterday I had an interesting call from
Someone who said they were my new social worker.
WOW. That is my 8th social worker.

March 31st 2020
True story. When asked how I am. I just say I'm ok.
But today I am bored and exhausted with social isolation and fatigue
Sometimes It feels my freedom has been relentlessly revoked. Nonetheless, no matter how socially inclined I am.
I am sticking to the rules.

August 6th 2020
Due to the COVID 19 Lock down
I've certainly experienced a change of circumstances
Nonetheless despite the anxiety and stress
In some respects I have started to grow like a tree.
With branches evolving out of me.
As my poor unruly happy Brain has started to lean towards the Sun.

November 14th 2021
As I'm exhausted with always being told to wait.
For another meeting, Or for another futile debate
Under no illusions and not complaining.
As I do understand how heritage and stigma influences perception.
So Happy and Ok I've decided to just smile and move on.

August 2nd 2022
Interesting 3.05 am.
Been awake thinking.
When things seem to matter to me.
I'm not taken seriously.

There is a real need to educate people about dementia. Alzheimer's Society has been amazingly helpful during that time.

April 15 2022
Honestly I'm not being critical nor complaining.
Its just my nonessential opinion.
But speaking from experience. And observations.
I believe most support services are designed to encourage their clients
To be dependent on medication and reliant on their services.

Getting my diagnosis was sad. But it has galvanised me to make the best of my life and live a meaningful life. I want to live every moment, and address incorrect notions. I am not frail. I do not need support all the time. Some-times, I might need support, but I am more likely to need empathy and encouragement and understanding.

> January 24th 2021
> Though they know I struggle to explain myself.
> Stumble over words and lose my way in what I aim to say
> Yet nonetheless so many people have been inviting and including me
> in conversations.
> How beautiful and nice.
> On a separate note real conversations always make me smile
> February 24th 2021
> I've been invited to many talks where I try not to share an opinion.
> Simply as I struggle to explain myself in words???
> Plus my thinking needs time to consider what I feel and wish to say.
> As all too often what I think and what I feel,
> Seems to come out in an alternative way

Some things make people uncomfortable and dementia is one of those things. If you have dementia, it is beautiful to have real conversations. But it feels awkward. So in a way, we need to be inspired to talk about dementia. I came up with this idea about encouraging people to talk about dementia, but through music and arts and poetry. Sabrina Jantuah and Cheryl Elliott from Alzheimer's Society motivated and encouraged me to progress it, and I am so grateful to them.

> January 30th 2021
> Perhaps one reason why I think I am turning in to a tweeting machine.
> (so to speak)
> Is simply because I lose focus early in conversation.
> I stray in my conversation. And I find it more reliable and comfortable.
> To explain myself in small quantities at a time.

People began to send in their submissions by email. Just a few at first, and then dozens. Something remarkable happened. It became called 'Talk Dementia' and was moved to Twitter (@arts_dementia). Now there are hun-dreds of entries. It is growing like a tree. It has sprung all of these branches.

I am conscious of my language. I stumble over words. But with poetry and music, I feel comfortable in the way I communicate and express myself. In art, I cannot make a mistake – I am making a new language. There is no restriction to my conversation. I can be expressively real and free. I can mix words with African drumming and reggae and ska. When I am at my lowest, it is the very definition of social prescribing.

> July 26th 2022
> Beyond the storm-lashed corridors of my brain,

Through social prescribing and nurturing alternative ways,
To talk about and share the many burning issues and conversations
in my brain,
Especially the happy beautiful debates,
I now write poetry, dementia diaries and song

I see Talk Dementia as like a tour bus. There is a mainstream bus that visits lots of areas. But there is also our bus, and it goes to the areas that the mainstream bus doesn't stop at – especially poor or marginalised communities. It makes people feel better through social prescribing. Talk Dementia gives me freedom of expression where I don't have to tiptoe around the conversation. I feel grateful and excited that I can build on something. This will keep me active and in line with a world that I want to be in.

May 26th 2022
I am unsure how it got in there.
But I have just found a lush
Beautiful garden inside of me.

Acknowledgements

A previous version of this chapter has been published by the Alzheimer's Society UK in October 2020. See https://www.alzheimers.org.uk/blog/ronald-amanze-talk-dementia-music-culture.

Note

1 https://www.youtube.com/watch?v=xdbOU9MUrv8.

3 Who knew a pothole could bring it all back?

Patrick Ettenes

This is a small chapter from my own life journey about what it means to be a Dementia Activist or an Ambassador, and the expectations that come with it. In 2019, I won the National Diversity Award, for LGBT Positive Role Model of the Year. Funnily enough I had literally been about to give up. Looking back, I think I was trying to hold myself accountable for a lot of people *and* speak on their behalf but when I won the award, it gave me a bit of a spark. I had messages come in from all around the world; people wrote in from Barbados, Trinidad, Panama, Canada, and the Netherlands. It was really touching. Some of the messages were so thoughtful and caring that I still have them to this day. When I got the award and I saw those messages, I realised I had a responsibility. I came to realise – that's my job now.

Trying to change things

After being diagnosed with dementia (due to frontal lobe atrophy), I realised there were services missing. Being me, I went out and started to develop them. Back in 2017, I made a video with the Alzheimer's Society for a project called 'Bring Dementia Out'.[1] It was only a ten-minute video and took about a month to make. The video entailed travelling to different parts of the country and interviewing people who identified as members of the LGBTQ+ community. I was basically investigating what it was like living with dementia or caring for someone with dementia from within the LGBTQ+ community, asking about the challenges people faced and their fears. It is one thing to speculate but another to hear it from the horse's mouth.

At the end of two years, the project finished. The video did well, we achieved a great deal and so I assumed it would all continue. I honestly believed that someone would take it on and allow us to continue the work. Well boy was I wrong: 'Money Patrick, it takes money'. I was told there was no available budget. You could imagine my disappointment so I asked: 'How much money would it take?' 'About £80,000'. I smiled and said, 'Sure ok give me a month, I'll get you your money'. Everyone in the office burst into laughter... A slight mockery maybe and a slight kindness towards my

DOI: 10.4324/9781003221982-5

delusional state. Well, it took about two months until I had secured the funding (and more). We even got linked in with *Supernova*, the movie (discussed further in Chapter 9). Who knew that our little project could get linked with a worldwide movie! For one year I received the funding for a project that did much in a short space of time and hopefully helped to change things.

The project is now linking with Dementia United, a co-ordinated programme of services and support across Greater Manchester.[2] The city has the second largest LGBT community in the UK, and I now have a support group for people from across the Northwest. Some people are understandably terrified of dementia. Think about a trans person having to go into a care home, the risks they face. Many care providers don't have the patience and they don't have the knowledge of how to support someone who is trans, so I realised there's a lot of fear. More recently, I'm helping to set up the first LGBTQ+ Dementia support group for Malta.

Struggles and loneliness

So far, all's well and good, but behind the scenes is where the true battle lies – like a monster under the bed. I was struggling on a personal level. Yes, I'm helping other people, but what's happening for me by the time I closed the front door or when that laptop shuts, the phone calls end, or I reach home from a meeting away? The emptiness to my personal life was becoming more visible to me. I was feeling as if my relationships were falling apart because people just didn't want to accept my dementia, and all that came with it. I don't just have dementia; I also live with PTSD, am recovering from a break down, and am still learning to normalise my nerves, adapting to a whole new body, and recovering. Yet, people have tried to take advantage of me when they knew I had dementia. 'Oh, don't worry, I'll be the next of kin' and all this sort of stuff. They would be pushing for it and I'm like 'And maybe after next of kin you want to have power of attorney over me?' Even friends: 'Oh yeah, we never had that conversation Patrick, that's your dementia kicking in'. I mean like 'How fucking dare you?!' 'Everyone else remembers the conversation, but you use my condition to get away with it'. In our (LGBT) community we have always supported each other, and our chosen family has educated us. But my experience of dementia has made me see my community in a different light.

Here in Manchester where I live now, I know a lot of people, and I do a lot of good work, but on a personal social level Manchester hasn't always been the most accepting place with me. I don't feel as if I fit in. Even within my own relationships and with friends here, I don't have a 'best friend'. Back in Wales, there's a friend of mine who's known me for about 21 years; we met on the stairs of a club called Trade in London. He's my memory bank; he tells me all the stories of our youth about the adventures we used to have and the things we used to do, and I cry sometimes. He says, 'Don't cry, don't get upset that you don't remember these things, I'll remember them for you' – and that's wonderful. But I don't have anyone here who does that.

The charity 'LGBT Foundation' that I work for is the one that saved my life, the people there support me like no other. So, there are aspects of the community that saved me. I owe them everything but they're not in my personal life. In fact, my personal life with dementia is really screwed up. When COVID happened and the LGBT Foundation closed and everyone went home, I saw nobody. I couldn't see my doctor, psychological help stopped, help with substance abuse stopped, the Alzheimer's support worker no longer came over, and I couldn't see my family for about three years. That had been my support line – that was my safe zone.

Home, love, and memory

So, I went home, back to Barbados, and I spent three months there. It was the best time of my life. Of course, we still had lockdown over there, but I was with my best friend, I was with people that cared for me. My best friend there (who I think of as my Gay mother) has known me since I was 15 years old. When he gave me a hug I felt love for the first time. Like I actually *felt* love coming from him. Love is meant to be a mental thing, but I felt a physical thing and I went, 'Oh my God, this is amazing'. I realised how many people are sitting in those care homes and they don't feel any of that. People ask, 'why do you need to hold someone's hand with dementia?' Well, because human touch is so important.

Back in Barbados and I was driving around on my own, I had the memories and confidence to do so. I had friends asking 'Are you OK? Are you on your own? Do you want me to stay with you?' My best friend said, 'This is your home, this is where you were brought up. This is where your core memories are' and it was true. My family brought me things when I was ill, and it was just wonderful. I felt supported, like no one could penetrate and get to me because I had family and love around me. My memories came back when I was in Barbados because I hit a pothole while I was driving and I remember hitting that pothole with every car I had. Who knew a pothole could bring it all back? I remembered sitting in the back seat as a kid with my parents hitting that same pothole, then being able to drive the first time and hitting that same hole. That pothole reminded me of the kind of memories my friend was trying to explain to me. Core memories, something so trivial as a hole in the ground could bring back memories I thought I'd lost. Thank you pothole!

You see, in Barbados, my LGBT friends are like family, something I describe in my talks as 'Chosen family'. Within the LGBTQ+ community a lot of us don't have actual blood family, but we decide for ourselves who is our family. And these individuals are as close or closer to us than those who are relatives. A lot of LGBTQ+ people were ostracised from their family and communities for being gay. Studies show that this can leave emotional scars, even trigger events much later in life, and when situations happen where we need to speak to health officials, we might not have the 'traditional' family member, but a Chosen family.

I guess I'm telling you this because, whenever I went to appointments, they would wonder why I was alone. For instance, one time when I felt like I was falling apart, I was asked why my mother couldn't call on my behalf! I called and asked for help, but only got help after my mother intervened. She rang in and the same week I was given an appointment. That's when the receptionist said, 'Why didn't you get your mother to call?' I said, 'She lives 5000 miles away'. This is where I find the work I do important. I'm a bit of a fighter, and I realised that not everyone in a similar situation would say something. How many other LGBTQ+ people would have experienced such attitude, and just walked off, never accessing support? This is where I have to be strong for everyone around me and I think that's why I sometimes feel as if I could fall apart, I just want to go off the rails, just to be vulnerable sometimes because I'm exhausted.

Navigating a dementia diagnosis

In the last couple of years, I've noticed a decline in my ability to cope with stress. The stress and pressure alone could lead to a blackout, which means that I don't remember anything for five to ten minutes. I don't even remember who I am. When it first happened, I was absolutely mortified, because I was sitting there with a suitcase, at Euston station (London). I blinked, and then I went, 'Oh my God, where am I?' I had no memory of getting there, how long I was there, or what city I was in. All I knew was that I was at a train station, and I needed to get to Manchester. I tried to remember who I was, but nothing came to mind – no family memory; no past, present, or future thoughts. It was as though I awoke after 100 years and was planted right there. I wanted to scream, but I knew that wasn't right. I stood so still, terrified. Eventually the memories came back, and I walked to the train.

It's horrible to know you cannot travel like you used to. People see me on holiday, but they have no idea of the fears that run through my mind, and precautions I take to make sure certain events don't befall me. Because what would happen if I was away, and I blacked out for an hour? How do I communicate to others what's going on? They would laugh at a young man who says he cannot remember. When I tell people I don't remember them, and I have dementia, they laugh in my face. Some men, although I explain everything, still can't understand why their mug (face) and the two hours I spent fucking with them weren't the highlight of my life and why they aren't engraved on my memory. I don't have time to remember all of them… priorities my dear, priorities.

Dementia has taken some things from me – all those barriers are slowly being depleted. It takes away those small fundamental bricks that build up those walls over the years. That's how dementia affects your brain. It doesn't just take away things, like when you forget what a key is, but it also takes away parts of your personality that you worked so hard to get hold of. I was given my diagnosis three times, twice retracted, and the third time I had the Alzheimer's Society worker sat next to me and the psychologist said, 'You have dementia'. The Alzheimer's worker said, 'We were there when you were given your diagnosis and we stand by you'. The uncertainty over my diagnosis left me with real difficulties in trusting any medical practitioner; nothing seemed certain, and at times it felt like disbelief at my condition. I've seen this many times before; many people within the health-care service believe that if you are mentally unwell, you should LOOK IT. And if you're able to speak for yourself, then clearly to them, nothing is wrong. But what do mental health issues look like? What does a person with dementia look like? Over the years I've noticed that once I say I have demen-tia to some, that to them, I am instantly considered stupid, and clearly nothing I say matters; my views, thoughts, or perceptions aren't valid just because I have dementia. So, being an activist started to become more and more important to me.

Gender and sexuality

I came to England originally to have a sex change, and I never went ahead with it because the operations were very invasive back then. I'm 39 now, but back then, the surgery wasn't the best. I would never have been able to have an orgasm if I were a woman, so I didn't go ahead with it. The older I get, the harder it is to contain that feminine side of me. I am wiser now, not to give a fuck. People will say 'Oh my God, you're a bit feminine'. I say, 'Go hug a landmine, I just can't deal with you and your internalized homophobia'. I have always been able to switch between masculine and feminine, and I look amazing. At my first conference, I dressed in a suit and gave my pres-entation. As soon as I was done, I went back to the hotel, and three hours later, I was a beautiful heiress from the 1920s and they were all amazed. People were like, 'Oh my God, you look fantastic'. But that's the art, that's the beauty of it, and I love it. But while that part of me is important, I came to the decision that I'm not going to transition.

This isn't why I came back to the UK; it wasn't to transition, but to find the balance within me. I still identify as trans; I am trans and I am non-binary and I am he/she and that's what I say my pronouns are. I sometimes perform drag, as a way to look and embrace that which is ultimately beau-tiful about being a woman. The only time I think like a 'man' is when I do substances and for some reason my masculinity comes out. When I'm in the bedroom, I have learned to enjoy my dominant side, a side of myself I never previously liked because a certain kind of masculinity was beaten into me as a kid and forced upon me. Not all was bad – being the son of a police officer, I trained in the martial arts, I was shooting guns before I played with dolls, and some days I felt like a mixed-race Lara Croft. I noticed that side of myself is more alive now than ever, and it's a good thing. I wonder how many other trans women are going through the same thing, or trans men? What is it about dementia that unlocks the sides of ourselves we have hidden? No partner, no one is going to say 'Oh you can't. I don't like you dressing up'. I'm sorry, but she needs to come out. It's a fucking dress and I want to wear it and sit and paint my nails. Often you don't know what version of yourself is going to come through.

Bridging work

I fit into a lot of categories, and a lot of dimensions. I also have HIV, and I used my platform for HIV to develop a platform for dementia. My work is becoming international and continues to grow. Some of the people have come up to me face-to-face saying that my articles and other work I've done has saved their lives. I work for an organisation called Black Beetle Health that supports people from the LGBTQ+ BPOC (Black, and People of Colour) community, and they do a lot of support work around mental health, HIV, and substance abuse that is tailored for people of colour, and I've helped develop their toolkits. I did a lot of work for eight to ten years around HIV, and now I'm helping develop guides around HIV and substance abuse.

So, here I am discussing what dementia is and that's predominantly white (as Zubair discusses in Chapter 8). There was not one person of colour that I interviewed when I was talking to people from the LGBT community. Now I'm realising this gap exists and I need to start representing people of colour and I do, I know racism. I am a person of colour and I realise that there's a lot of microaggressions received over the years from racism, from people, over a long period of time. I have lived with that and realise that when it comes to dementia and race, that's a huge thing. So, I'm the glue that binds people together. If it weren't for me, the Alzheimer's Society would not have met the LGBT Foundation, the LGBT Foundation would never have hosted Bring Dementia Out, and the Guinness Housing Trust would have never run their training. And now I'm bringing Black Beetle Health to join them. I'm the common denominator, I'm bringing a lot of organisations together. Being an advocate isn't about 'showcasing' yourself for organisations, it's about stepping out of them to where you could be needed for those who don't have such organisations.

I have my mental health issues, I still have to manage life with HIV, I still have to deal with loneliness, and I still have to deal with my personal life and do all the admin. One of my other jobs finally got me an accessibility assistant but I need a personal assistant for my personal life; there's so much I have to do, and I have to manage that. I believe God gave me this condition so I could help others. I once said my HIV was the best thing that ever happened to me, and now I'm starting to feel like dementia might also be.

I always said as a teenager I would change the world. I want to help others; no one needs to be left alone like I was: misunderstood and frightened. So maybe I will change the world.

Notes

1 Here's a link to the video we made: https://www.youtube.com/watch?v= Tskv2GFG5L8.
2 Here's a link to details of Dementia United, including an interview with me: https://dementia-united.org.uk/about-us/.

4   Nobody is allowed to offend us – Not by language, nor by attitude

Helga Rohra

My name is Helga Rohra, and I live in München (Munich), Germany. I was diagnosed with Lewy Body Dementia at 54 years old, and Alzheimer's disease was added three years ago.

I started as a dementia activist because I saw that we needed a change in society. The outlook on people with dementia was: we are old, we are not speaking up for ourselves, we have no self-determination. We are in a way guided by our relatives and different organisations. I felt it was important to listen to us and to get our experience and that's how I started. I volunteered myself.

I started as a dementia activist noticing that there was no post-diagnostic support at all for people diagnosed at younger ages. Alzheimer's societies as well as other stakeholders were well prepared to counsel the relatives of people with dementia, who were in a very advanced stage of dementia. The main aspects that were considered were: care, nursing homes, legal affairs and case management for the care partner. I needed a completely different counselling: how can I be enabled to continue with my new life on this dementia journey? I still have many abilities! See me as a person, not only from a pathological point of view. Being diagnosed doesn't mean the end of life! On the contrary, I felt that as a part of society I wanted to contribute and be included in working life and social life too. But nothing existed to support that.

Alzheimer Europe has yearly conferences, and there was a general meeting where they decided various things referring to people with dementia, including what kind of research should be conducted. Obviously, different representatives of all countries were there, but I was the only one touched by dementia. I was sitting quietly in the front in order to understand, and I took notes and then I said: 'Why don't we have a group of people with dementia who work with you and who tell their opinions about what *we* need? We can speak up for ourselves'. And they said: 'Do you think this is possible?' And I said: 'I volunteer myself'.

I had the courage to speak up that time because if you look at my biography, I always wanted change. I started by being very politically active in my local area (that is Bavaria, Germany), then in Munich. And I was always

DOI: 10.4324/9781003221982-6

active because my son is a special child. He has a form of autism and I started at a very young age to fight, let's call it 'fight', for these children who have special needs, so I was already involved in political activities, asking how I can change something. Today, my son is working at the airport. He has studied and still has special needs, but I am convinced that many people with dementia can be similarly supported if you see the person, not only the diagnosis, to better include them in society (see Chapter 18 for further discussion of parallels between dementia and neurodiversity). And so I had this motivation, and yes, I wanted to speak up.

My first international conference about dementia – this time attending as a person with dementia – was in Thessaloniki. It must have been about ten years ago. I met my mentor Richard Taylor (USA) and the activist Kate Swaffer (Australia); it was such an incredible turn in my life! I learned that campaigning is the only way to raise a voice for people living with dementia in my own country. Dementia knows no borders; we stayed in close contact to learn from each other and to develop ways to motivate thousands of other people with dementia to speak for themselves!

I started to work on the Board of the Alzheimer's Society in Munich. That was a completely new perspective for all those employed at the Society. After five years, without constructive projects supporting the inclusion of people with dementia at young ages, I decided to leave that Board. Instead, my whole energy and passion was dedicated to the 'European Working Group of People with Dementia' at Alzheimer Europe. I was the Chair for four years and later two years as part of the Steering Group. That European group of people with dementia made me strong; I was included in projects, working in a team with professionals, being valued. I started with the first homepage of a person with dementia, offering lectures and workshops together with professionals.

Today, after more than 12 years, my life is almost a 'career' in dementia: appearing on stage over 1,000 times in front of very different audiences. My four books in German have been translated into English, Romanian and Bulgarian. I never stop raising my voice together with other people living with dementia all over Germany and our border countries: Austria and Switzerland.

My experience so far? Many more people with dementia need to be on stage, to be actively involved in working groups, to participate as co-researchers and to be portrayed in a positive way in the media. We are all heroes who started pioneering for the cause at a young age! We need to be empowered and have a voice in political decisions referring to our lives. You should never forget: we are the real experts by experience! My campaigning keeps me mentally and physically strong and I myself will continue raising awareness.

I am confident and I have a dream: if you have been diagnosed with dementia, tell your boss at work and your colleagues. Do not feel ashamed; go on working in a team. Tell your family and friends and no one will feel scared to death or distance themselves! Raise your voice in local parliaments for our rights – for dementia being treated as a disability – and feel empowered despite having dementia! (German: trotzDEM = despite having dementia)

To be a dementia activist means to be qualified! Each of us is the result of a former life, before getting diagnosed. Each of us is the result of a very specific biography! In addition, my personality will not change, at least in the early stages of dementia. Having always been interested in trying new things, with a high level of communication, being open-minded, hardworking, being trained and especially being passionate for what I do and being able to light that fire in my friends – all of these are touched by dementia. These are features needed by a dementia activist.

However, having experience from a professional point of view in the field of dementia is also vital to campaigning. No voice can be strong enough without solidarity at the very basic level: with all care partners, with professionals in different dementia fields and with people living with dementia combined. This requires a unique combination of different skills and attributes. Firstly, a positive attitude towards all the losses involved with dementia is needed. Also, the ability to be a motivator for others diagnosed to rise up and speak up in public. It helps to be eloquent in media contacts and to be up-to-date with news from dementia research. It's also important to participate actively in projects and to be a speaker at Alzheimer conferences and other events. Being well-connected via social media is also useful but most of all, having a commitment to dementia advocacy as a mission. ALL of these features really keep a brain active – and a person happy.

To speak as a person with dementia, as a strong campaigner, you need daily contact with your friends touched by dementia as well as with their care partners, friends and families. Only in such a strong relationship can I know about all the obstacles encountered by my friends. Obstacles either in legal matters – inclusion in the workplace – or in social matters. We exchange ideas if somebody is attacked. Let me give you an example. Some weeks ago a doctor on Twitter attacked one of my friends, a dementia activist. He saw her at a conference and commented on how she talks. He is a neurologist and dementia specialist, and he said on Twitter, 'if all my patients were like this person, I think I wouldn't have any patients at all'. He asked, 'How is it possible [for someone with dementia] to talk in such a structured way?' Yeah, it was an attack, you know, and the women (dementia activists), no matter whether they were in Singapore, Japan, Germany or Bulgaria, all wrote to this man and responded to his attack and said, 'You have no experience, you don't know that people with dementia can speak up for themselves'.

I remember this one time. I presented my first book. I've since written further books, but it was the first one, and it was entitled *Stepping Out of the Shadows*, and I was invited to the Frankfurt book fair by the organiser to speak in front of the audience. I started to speak and to read, and almost at once somebody raised a hand – I couldn't even say, 'let me finish my sentence'. This person stood up and said, 'I can't believe that you have dementia. You are sent by a theatre company. Shame on you'. I was very upset, with tears in my eyes. But I held the microphone and I have a very good technique of breathing from meditation. So I was breathing and I said:

> I don't know who you are. You didn't even present yourself, Sir, but it is disrespectful to question. Do you think somebody with cancer would stand on stage and say 'I have cancer and will talk about my experience' and someone would say, 'No, you don't have cancer?'. I'm not prepared to talk to you anymore.

I started breathing again and I took a sip of water. So, from the very beginning, I adopted a very clear attitude; they are not allowed, nobody is allowed, to offend us by language, nor by attitude. The man who questioned me was actually from the hospital, from the neurology department, the chief for neurological diseases, mainly dementia. But he had never seen somebody who was like me; I was 54 at that time, I talked for myself and I was able to answer questions (similarly both Clayton and Ettenes discuss their experience, as people with young onset dementia, of scepticism and the policing of diagnostic categories by health professionals).

There are people who question the diagnosis of women diagnosed with dementia. Men are not questioned about their diagnosis. When it's the woman who speaks up, 'She doesn't have dementia. She can't have dementia'. It always happens and you know what I say? I'm very strong.

> Would you like me to send you all my PET scans and so on, but I'm not here to talk about my diagnosis, I'm here to change the view in society. I'm here to speak up for all those who are not able to speak because we have millions who are not able, really not able, and some others are too shy and they need support.

I feel the sadness and wishes of my fellows – and of course I can represent them.

I inform them via Zoom (teleconference) or by telephone, or even in live meetings or in social media groups, about the outcome of a conference or workshop. We evaluate, we plan and we even guide the newly diagnosed to be able and motivated to speak publicly about their needs after being diagnosed at a younger age with dementia.

My friends empower me in my 'job' as a strong campaigner! I feel though that I cannot represent marginalised groups of people with dementia. Referring here either to their geographical situation (maybe German or English isn't their first language) being immigrants' or simply a lack of know-how with digital technology to join Zoom meetings. This aspect is of course a future challenge for stakeholders, for politicians and for each society: how do we include marginalised groups? Together with Alzheimer Europe, we worked carefully and thoroughly on a paper regarding inclusion of LGBT and queer people who are diagnosed with dementia![1] A big first step in the history of raising awareness. We need more 'dementia leaders' trained, working together with dementia professionals!

I am confident the future will exist in working together, empowering each other, and realising the benefits and ethical challenges in all fields. 'Heterogeneity' and 'authenticity' are the keywords! Research needs campaigners – policy needs them as well – over 11 million people with dementia in Europe need us too! Our message is definitely: together WE CAN!

Note

1 https://www.alzheimer-europe.org/resources/publications/2021-alzheimer-europe-report-sex-gender-and-sexuality-context-dementia

5 Recognising Birkby

Living and caring with dementia

Wendy Hulko, Marsha Griffith and
Birkby Griffith

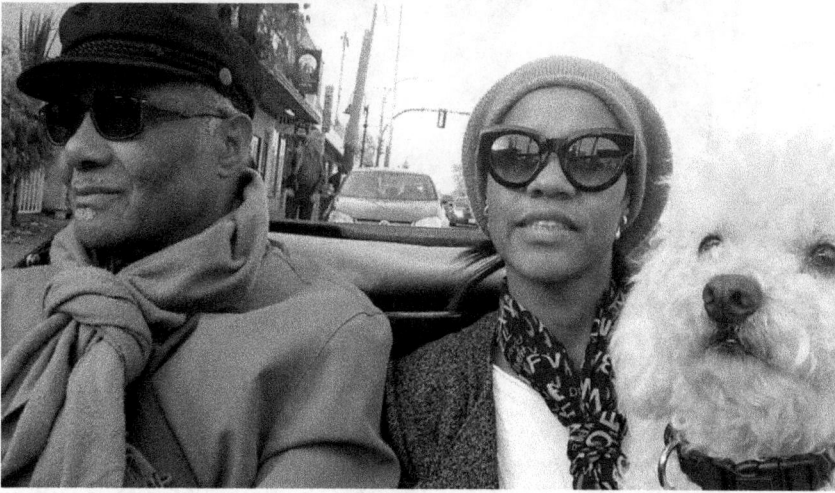

Figure 5.1 Chillin' in the Triumph with Yummy [dog].

The purpose of this photo-essay is to share glimpses into the daily lives of Marsha and Birkby, a family carer and a person living with dementia, and offer insights into the different ways in which Marsha supports her 'papa' and ensures that he is treated with respect and kindness by others (Figure 5.1).

In January 2014, Marsha Griffith returned to British Columbia (BC), Canada, from Asia, where she'd been teaching English for over eight years, first in Japan and then in Korea; she planned to stay with her parents for a few months before starting a new teaching position in Saudi Arabia. Instead, Marsha became a care partner for her papa Birkby who had recently been diagnosed with Alzheimer Disease (AD); while this was an unexpected deviation from her life plans, Marsha took on this role willingly to ensure her papa could be cared for at home – with love and respect. Marsha and Wendy (co-authors of this chapter) have been close friends for over 35 years and know each other's parents well; both sets of parents live near Sidney, BC, in the same agricultural area (Figure 5.2).

DOI: 10.4324/9781003221982-7

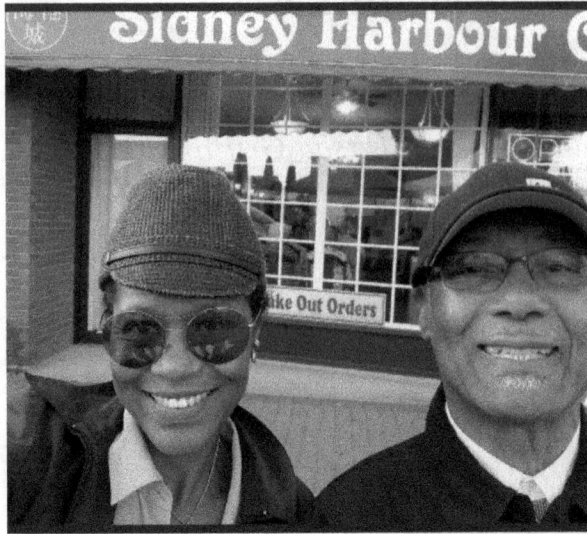

Figure 5.2 Marsha and Birkby in Sidney by the Sea in 2015.

From the age of four, when Marsha first remembers visiting her father at his work at Glendale Lodge (a facility for people with developmental disabilities in Victoria, BC), Birkby instilled in her the lesson that everyone deserves a quality of life and respect. Marsha's approach is based on her family's teachings and her experience working intermittently at her mother's group home for adults with developmental disabilities. Her own approach to caring for her father includes a lot of smiles and laughter – whether Marsha is putting on a charcoal mask at home or she and her papa are going on an outing in the Triumph, as seen below (Figure 5.3) and in the photo that began this chapter.

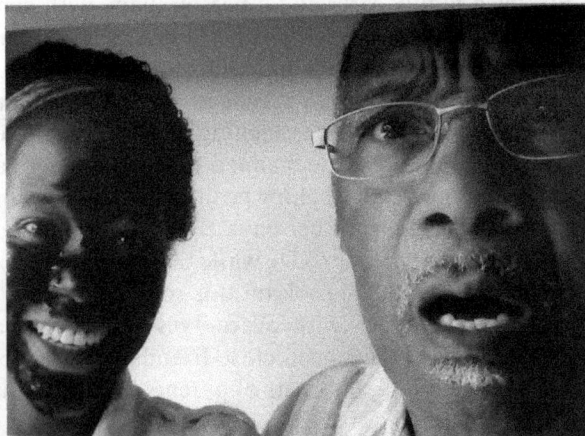

Figure 5.3 Selfie of Marsha (with charcoal mask) and Birkby in 2015.

Over the following years, Marsha shared photos and videos of her father and updated Wendy on their daily lives and activities and events in which they took part. This included the British Columbia Seniors Games in both 2015 and 2016. Birkby had been a competitive distance runner and he and Marsha had trained and competed together occasionally. Wendy and her nephew are runners as well and accompanied Birkby on a run during these early years of dementia, gently encouraging and guiding him, while Marsha followed along in the car. Below is an e-mail Marsha sent to Wendy on August 31, 2015, detailing their experiences at the 2015 BC Seniors Games, and to which we have added emphasis.

> *thanks for ur interest in the senior games. t'was a learning experience for me: **i was totally oblivious to papa not knowing the significance of the starting words and when to go....lanes, when to move in to the 1st**..... he also began to have little patience for waiting his turn. he was never one to warm up before racing, so getting him to do it now was a challenge. i think he strained a hamstring on the 1st day. So, he warmed a little the following days. **bronze in the 100m, 5th in 200m, 5th in 400m, 6th in 800m** (he was assigned the 7th lane and didn't move in until the 2nd lap), we missed the 5000m walk 'cause they started 45 min early. i failed to hear the announcement the day before. that would have been his "for sure" gold... no relays since they didn't have enough men for a team.*
>
> *i was disappointed that they turned him away from the banquet friday night because i left his registration badge in the hotel. burnaby to north vancouver on a friday takes a long time. i wrote a letter to the society to express that disappointment.*
>
> *most of the athletes are serious, hard-core competitors. **i think birkby and i were noticed by most since we were always together and being visible minorities.** as i was getting my dad to stretch blah blaah, a few came up and asked if i was a physio therapist or what happened to my dad; had he been like this all his life.....weird. **i guess only healthy cognitively alert people had taken part before.***
>
> *one of the starting marshals and the starter tried helping us out a bit by allowing me to stand next to him to tell him to go, when the gun went off for his last race.*

In these early years of Marsha's care partnering, Birkby's wife/Marsha's mother maintained her normal routine, which included meals out, social events with friends and travel. The latter caused Marsha some concern, as seen below in the October 3, 2015 e-mail Marsha sent to Wendy after her parents had left for a vacation in Cuba with two other couples.

> *...gong show at the griffith house... i saw my parents off last night. talk about the blind leading the blind, amateur travelers... i forgot to thank u for ur offer of the dementia card; my mom probably wouldn't use it. worrying does me no good. **restless sleep last night wondering how papa handled the stress of traveling + the cold he suddenly got...** [emphasis added]*

*i hope all those people who promised to help, get rid of their excitement and follow thru. **from what i saw at yyj [Victoria airport], my papa was left standing alone in the middle of nothing.** (i spied, with my little eye, after they went thru security). [emphasis added]*

Marsha had observed changes in the ways her parents' friends interacted with her papa – or rather, failed to interact with him – and thus was aware of the fact that "dementia seems to act as a very powerful solvent on many kinds of social ties" (Taylor, 2008, p. 319). Like her parents, Marsha embraced collectivist approaches to caring. For Marsha, this ethos came mainly from being the daughter of two Caribbean migrants who, despite both having trained at St Margaret's Hospital in England, held the cultural belief that family members care for one another. Marsha had internalized the cultural message that "*you do not stick them [parents] in homes.*" She accompanied her parents on trips to their countries of origin – Barbados for her father and Jamaica for her mother – in their early years of living and caring for dementia (Figures 5.4 and 5.5).

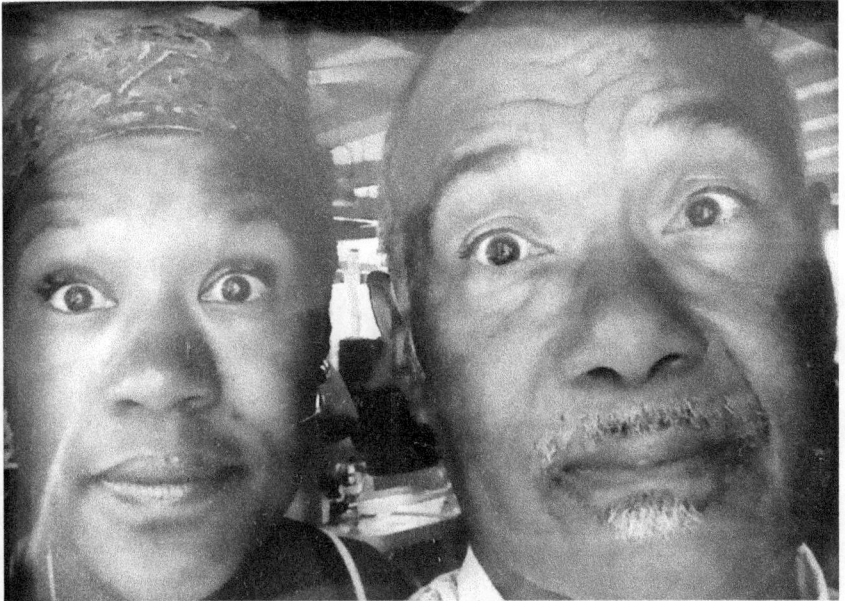

Figure 5.4 Selfie of Marsha and Birkby in Barbados in 2015.

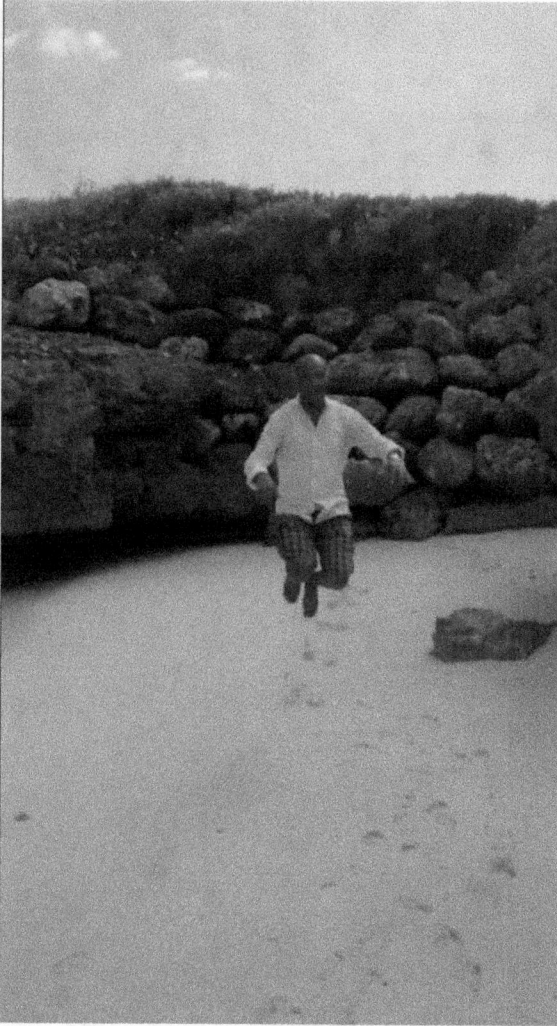

Figure 5.5 Birkby jumping in Barbados in 2015.

2016 BC Seniors Games

Based on their experiences the previous summer, Marsha was better able to prepare herself and Birkby for their second BC Seniors Games. Thus, it was a far better experience and resulted in a medal, as seen in the photo of Birkby on the podium (Figures 5.6 and 5.7).

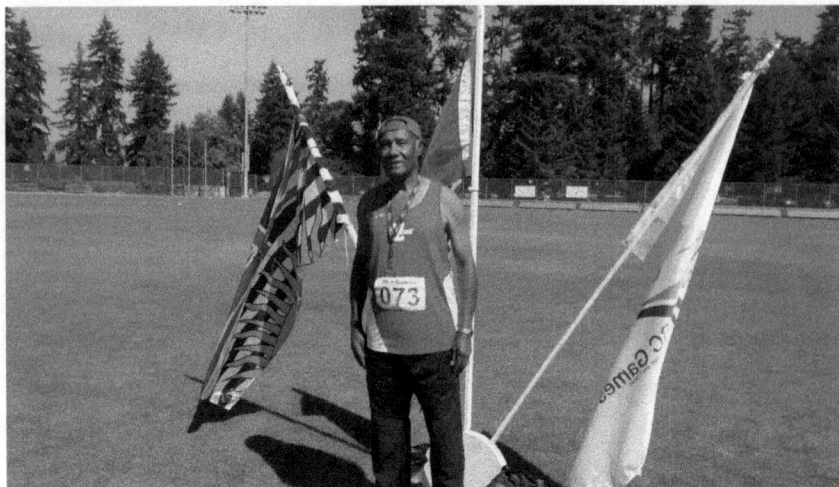

Figure 5.6 Birkby on the podium, having won bronze in the 55-metre dash (men 70+).

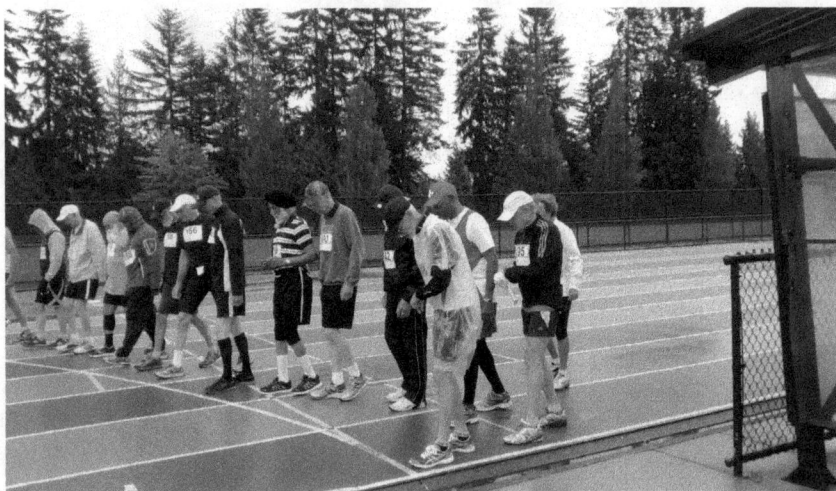

Figure 5.7 Birkby at the starting line for the 5,000 Metre Run/Power Walk.

At the same Games, Birkby did not complete the 5,000 Metre Run/Power Walk. Marsha explained why in an August 2016 e-mail to Wendy:

He got disqualified after lap 8 of 12.5 'cause he started to run when he saw my big camera… Such a show off… He felt like a celebrity anyway (Figure 5.8).

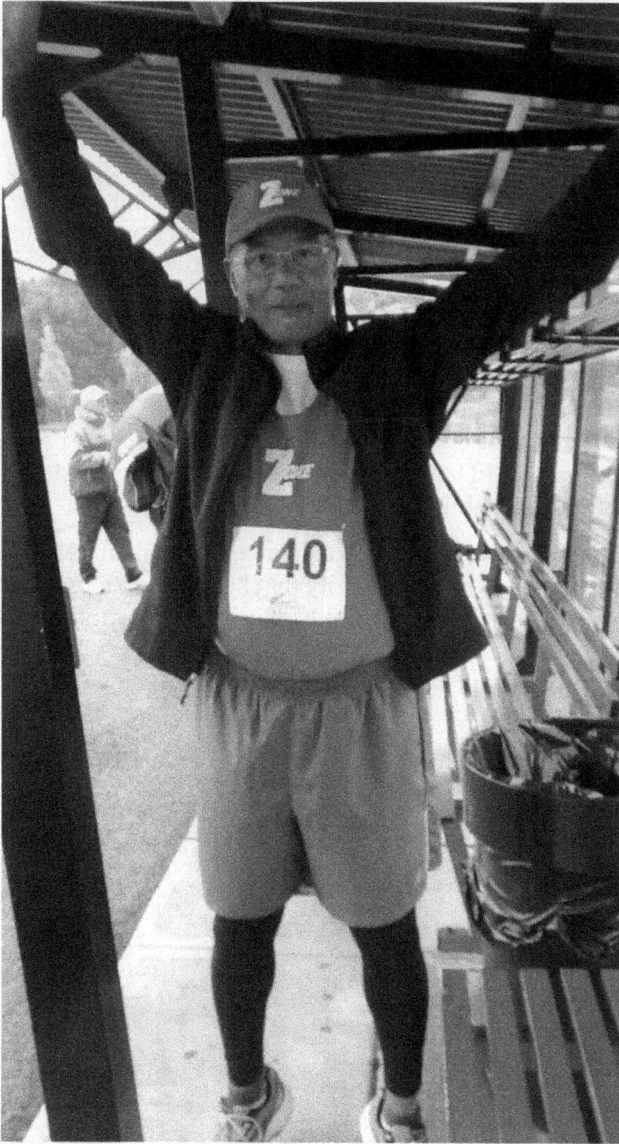

Figure 5.8 Birkby, the celebrity.

In addition to maintaining her father's identity as a competitive athlete, Marsha ensures her papa is well dressed, as he was always a sharply dressed man before he was diagnosed with Alzheimer's. Marsha and her father engaged in a series of activities recommended by critical dementia scholars who view memory as relational and embodied: "people who are no longer able to speak coherently may often still take part in, and enjoy, activities such as walking, dancing, or singing that rely on embodied procedural memory" (Taylor, 2008, p. 328; see also Basting, 2009; Kontos et al., 2021).

Dancing and singing

Four years into caring for her papa, Marsha remained concerned about the impact of travelling and social events on Birkby, though she now accompanied her parents on trips, as detailed in a February 5, 2018 e-mail she sent to Wendy (1). The next day she reflected in a follow-up e-mail on changes to her parents' social life and their routine at home (2).

1   We went to Vegas and Palm Springs in December. [It was] exhausting for me.
2   He is a bit more confused, especially in the evening. If he isn't in his PJs by 8, it is almost a calamity. That can be a prob[lem] when they are out 'til late. It still happens, but not as much. Ma mére [my mother] is slowing down a bit.

While Birkby was no longer able to run or compete in athletic events, dancing continued to be a favourite activity that he and Marsha enjoyed at home. In the early years, the Griffiths continued to go out dancing and Marsha and I both accompanied her parents to a club before their trip to Cuba in 2015, and we all danced for several hours. Music and dancing have always been intergenerational activities associated with Caribbean culture and family for the Griffiths (Figures 5.9 and 5.10).

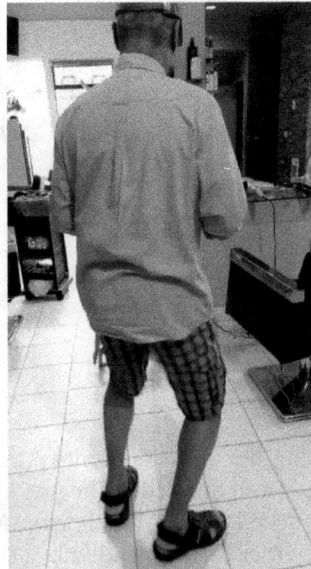

Figure 5.9 Birkby dancing at the hair salon.

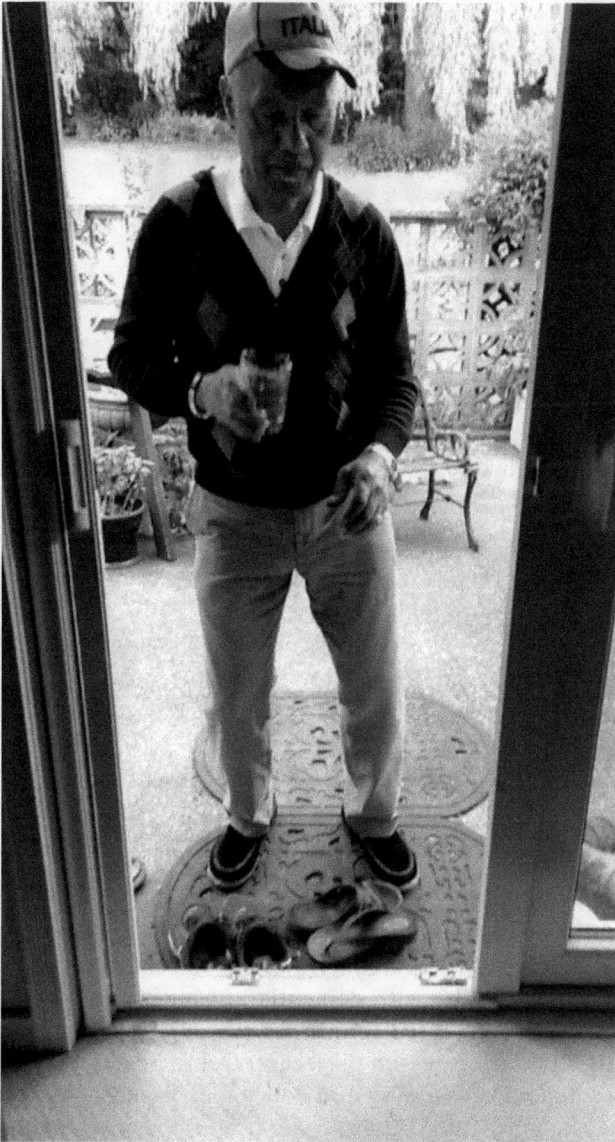

Figure 5.10 Birkby dancing at home.

Dance and movement therapy with persons living with dementia has a long history in the UK (Coaten, 2001; Whiteside, 2020) and arises from the belief that dance is another means of communicating. It can also promote playfulness and sociability (Kontos et al., 2021). The positive effects of dance can be seen in the numerous short videos Marsha has taken of her father dancing since she became his primary care partner (Figure 5.11).

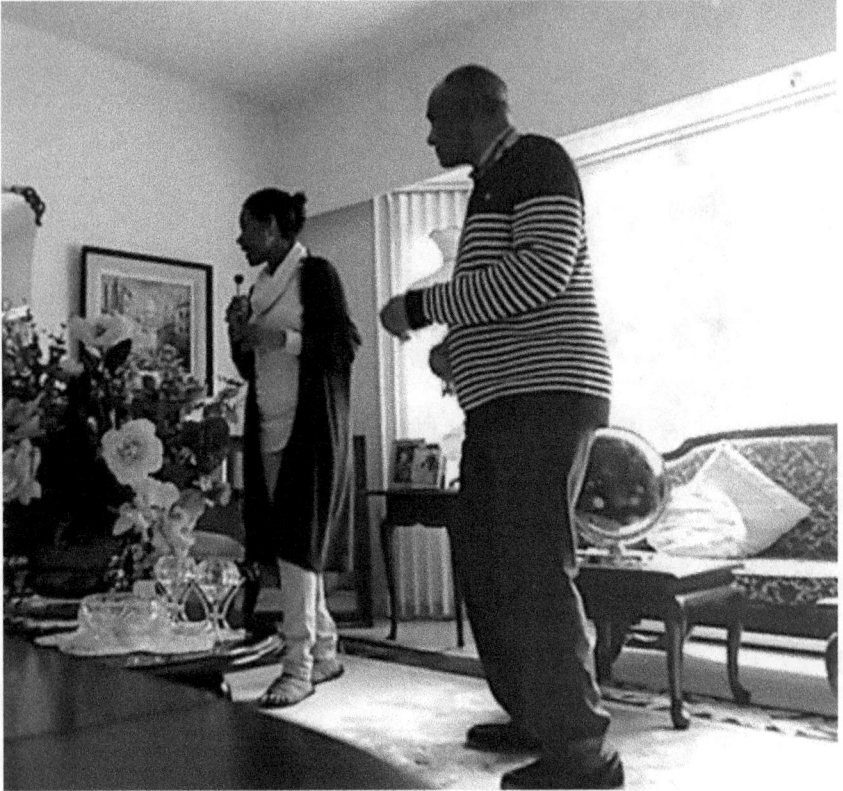

Figure 5.11 Marsha and Birkby singing and dancing at home.

In 2019 dancing and singing together at home became a public shared activity for Birkby and Marsha when they became involved with Voices in Motion (2022). This is an intergenerational choir made up of high school students and older adults with dementia and their care partners and at the end of each season, they perform for the public. What began in 2018 as an interdisciplinary research project by Debra Sheets of the University of Victoria's School of Nursing and colleagues from Sociology, Psychology, and Music grew into a non-profit society and was able to continue throughout the pandemic via Zoom (Craigie, 2020; Sheets et al., 2020) (Figure 5.12).

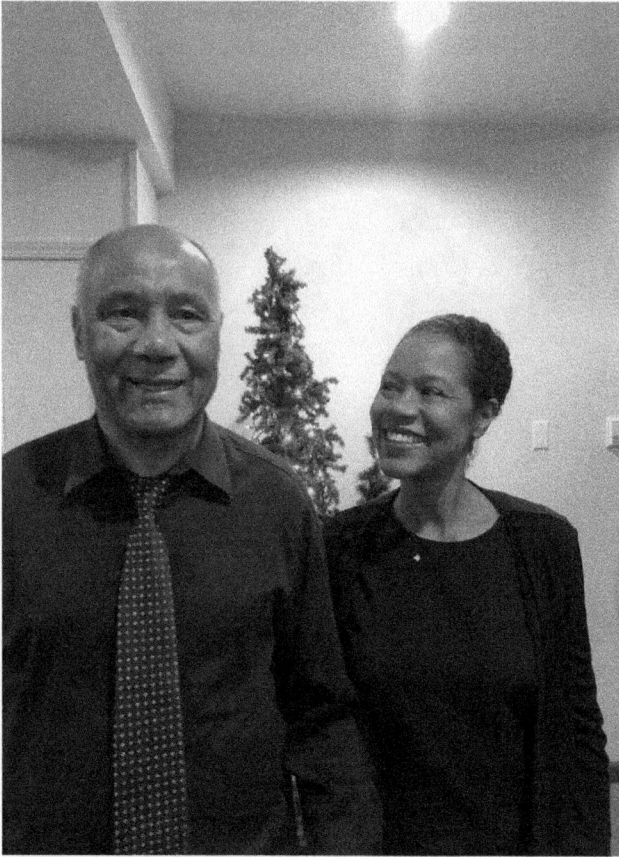

Figure 5.12 Ready for the Choir.

The COVID-19 pandemic

Once the COVID-19 pandemic began in March 2020, Birkby's world became much smaller as programmes were suspended and his verbal communication skills and mobility decreased. He also had to adjust to people coming to the house, as this was new for him. As Marsha said, "He's not stupid, he just doesn't want to do things" (June 6, 2022). Given this, Marsha advises greeting her papa with "Good morning Birkby, how are you?" and advises those coming to the house to tell him who they are and why they are there, as she believes this would go a long way towards making him receptive to care from strangers. Marsha knows to go at the same pace as Birkby – to walk or climb *with* him – as can be seen in the photos below, and wants others to do the same (Figures 5.13 and 5.14).

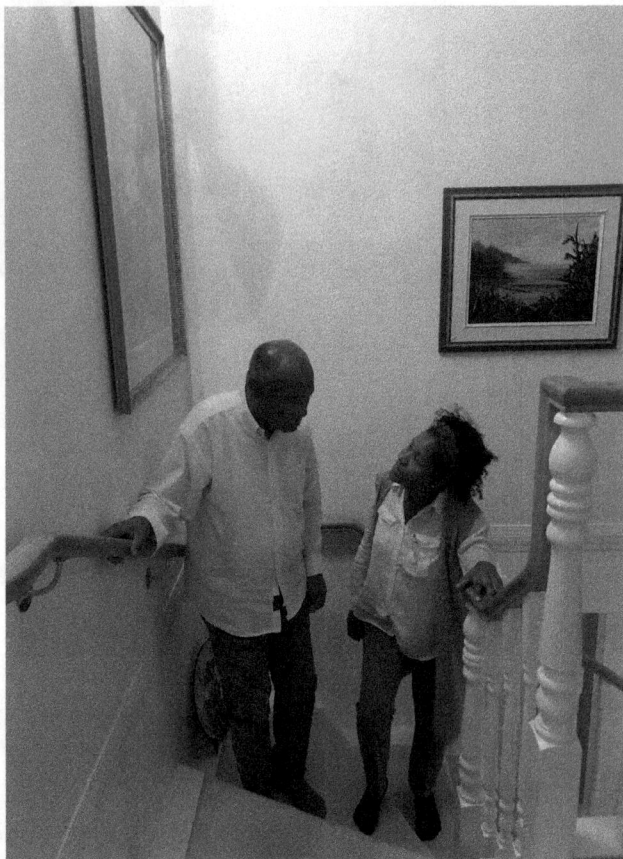

Figure 5.13 Climbing stairs together.

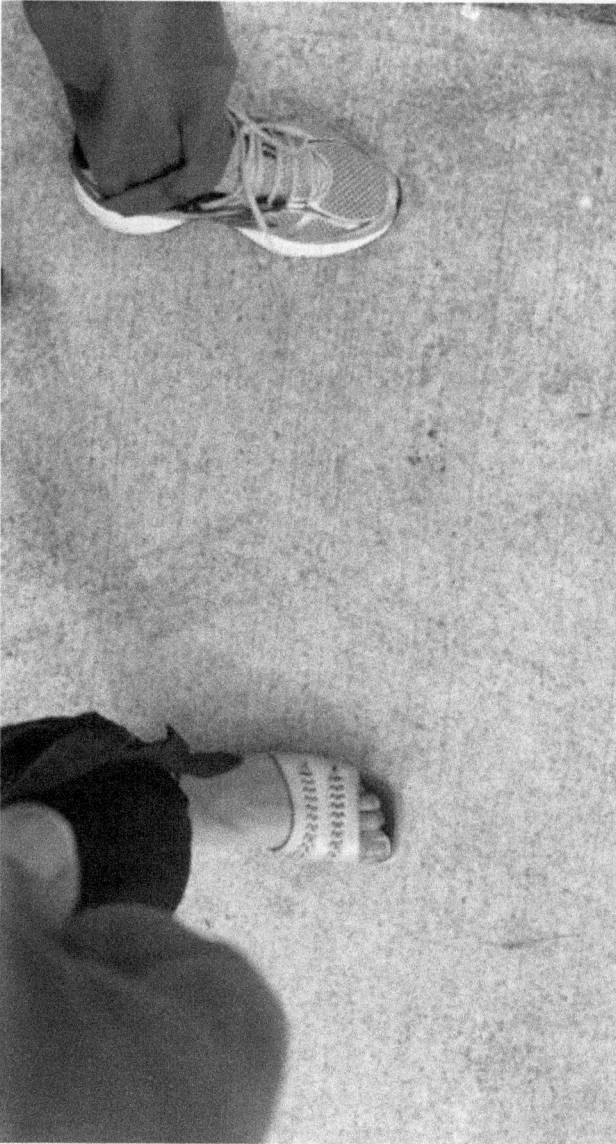

Figure 5.14 Walking at the same pace.

Reflecting on two years of caring for her papa during the pandemic, Marsha identified various changes and the impact of lockdown upon her father. Overall, there was less interaction with people as programmes were cancelled and consequently more time spent at home with Marsha. Everyday

tasks and activities like getting in and out of the car started to be a challenge, which eventually meant no return to his day programmes. "I don't
like this rush, rush anymore," Birkby suddenly and surprisingly said after
sitting in silence with Marsha. She noticed that his speech decreased a lot –
five words at a time at most and that he went from using a fork to using
a spoon (he liked to scoop). Sometimes Birkby would eat on his own but
would then stop, despite still being hungry. He also stopped going out on
drives with Marsha or accompanying her on errands.

Eventually, Marsha noticed that Birkby had stopped getting out of the
chair on his own. A transfer belt was a lot of help, as was the power lift chair.
Overall, mornings became slower. Marsha would swing Birkby's legs around
to help him get up after giving him breakfast in bed most days; bendable
straws became very helpful. It was also becoming increasingly hard to keep
appointments (e.g. X-rays, lab work) as it was difficult to get Birkby up and
moving and into and out of the car (Figure 5.15).

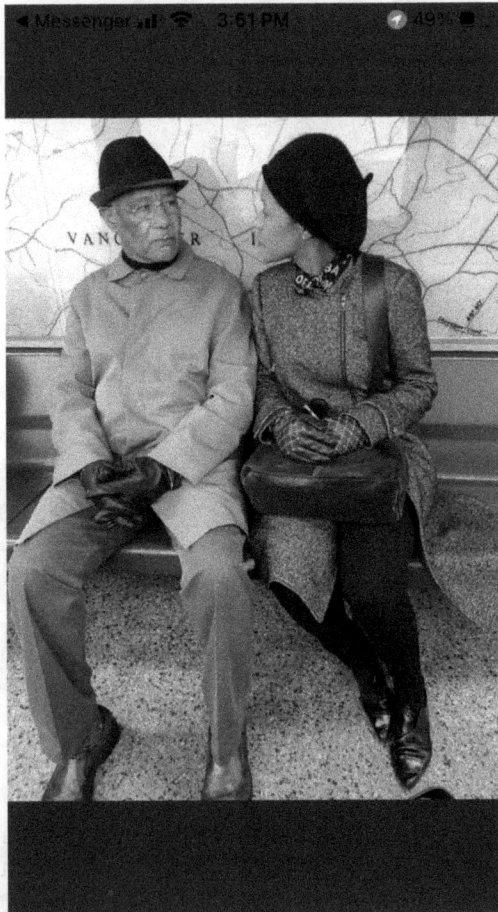

Figure 5.15 Birkby and Marsha Mill Bay ferry.

Marsha summarized her approach to caring for her father and what makes Birkby's daily life 'pretty perfect' in an e-mail to Wendy on August 26, 2022:

> all i know is that my dad is much more aware than we know. and i am his daughter (stay-at- home daughter) who isn't so trusting of having hired help care for my daddy.
>
> he doesn't need to talk. he likes being with his family. simply being in the same room is enough. but when you add eye contact, smiles and laughter, [that] makes it pretty close to perfect (Figures 5.16 and 5.17).

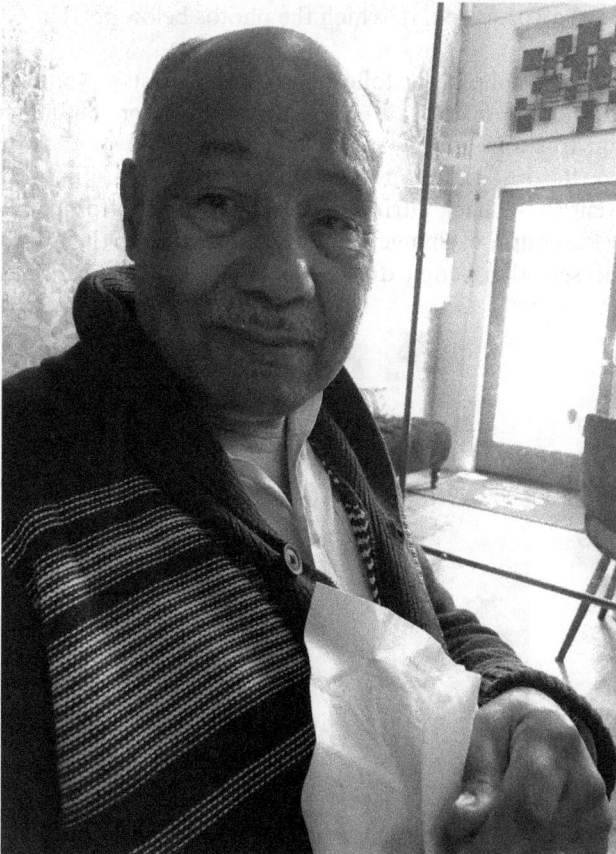

Figure 5.16 Birkby at Saveur restaurant.

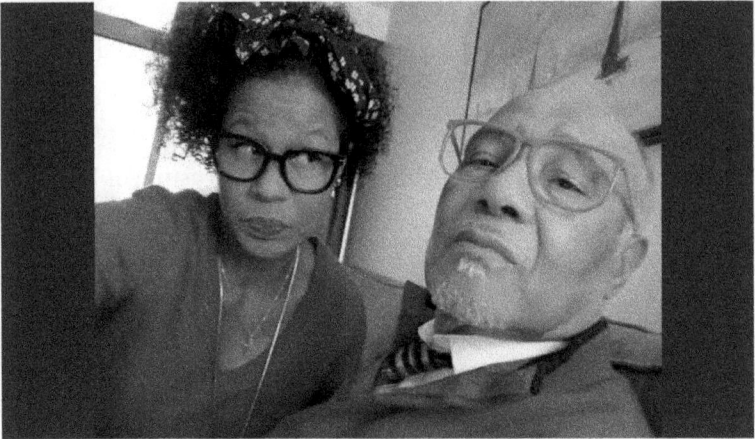

Figure 5.17 Birkby and Marsha's Christmas staycation.

In July 18, 2022 e-mail, Marsha wrote to Wendy about a recent outdoor wedding they had attended, to which the photos below pertain.

> My dad surprised us as he followed wedding guests to stand as the bride entered and began to walk down the aisle. Prior to that, he seemed reluctant to stand on his own or to even want to stand from a seated position. But he would not sit again. We were seated in 2nd row so he and i went to the back during the ceremony in an effort to allow others to view the couple exchange vows. He chose to go to the DJ. He was also happy to see other people dressed up (Figures 5.18 and 5.19).

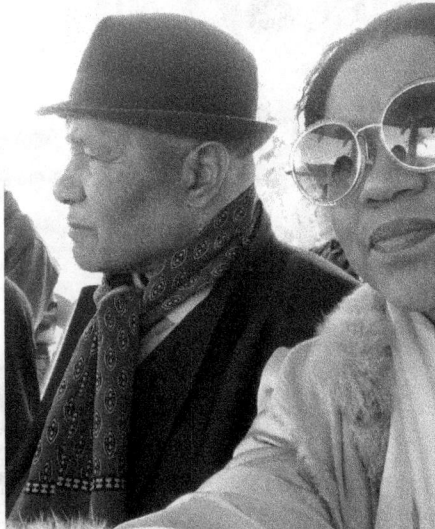

Figure 5.18 Marsha and Birkby at an outdoor wedding.

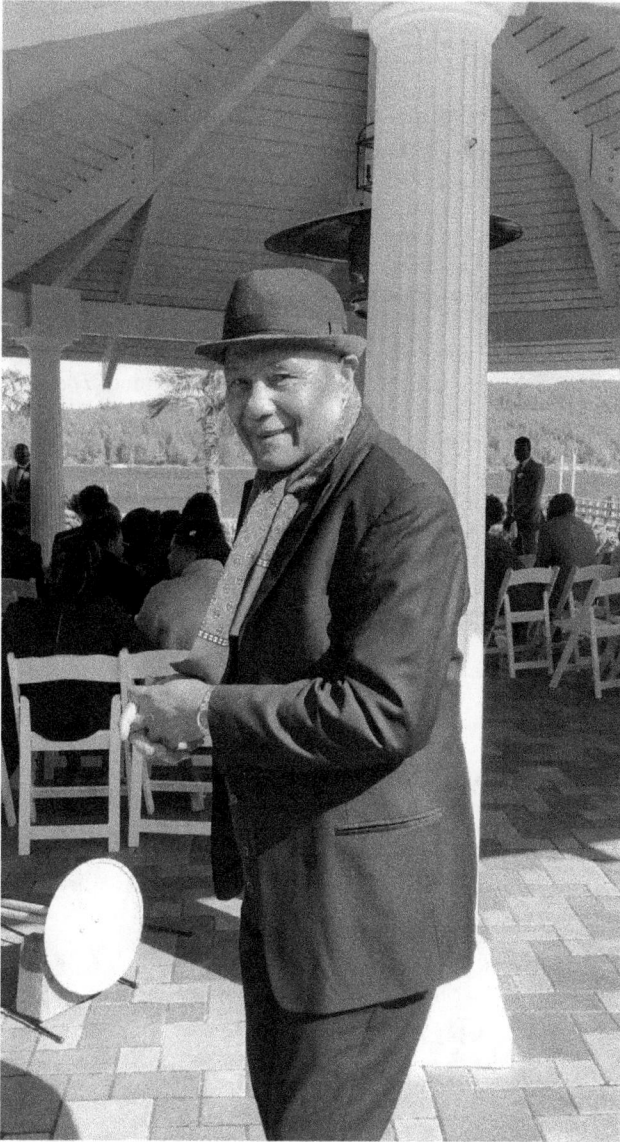

Figure 5.19 Birkby at the wedding in April 2022.

The purpose of this photo-essay has been to highlight ways in which persons with dementia can be assisted to continue living and enjoying life through engaging in activities that have personal and cultural significance. As the photos and e-mails indicate, Marsha draws on her familial and cultural teachings and makes use of her knowledge of her papa Birkby and his Caribbean culture to ensure Birkby is provided with quality of life and respect.

References

Basting, A. (2009). *Forget memory: Creating better lives for persons with dementia.* Baltimore, MD: Johns Hopkins University Press.

Coaten, R. (2001). Exploring reminiscence through dance and movement. *Journal of Dementia Care, 9*(5), 19–22.

Craigie, G. (2020, May 8). Debra sheets. *CBC Radio on the Island.* Available at: https://soundcloud.com/universityofvictoria/debra-sheets-may-8-2020-cbc-radio-on-the-island (Accessed 4/9/2022).

Kontos, P., Grigorovich, A., Kosurko, A., Bar, R.J., Herron, R.A., Menec, V.H., & Skinner, M.W. (2021). Dancing with dementia: Exploring the embodied dimensions of creativity and social engagement. *Gerontologist, 61*(5), 714–723. DOI: 10.1093/geront/gnaa129.

Sheets, D., Smith, A., MacDonald, S., Phare-Bergh, E., & Bergh, R. (2020, May 7). In our choir, people with dementia sing. Now it's Zooming. *The Tyee.* Available at: https://thetyee.ca/Culture/2020/05/07/Choir-Dementia-Zooming/.

Taylor, J. (2008). On recognition, caring and dementia. *Medical Anthropology Quarterly, 22*(4), 313–335. DOI: 10.1111/j.1548-1387.2008.00036.x.

Voices in Motion. (2022). *Social singing counters stigma and discrimination.* Available at: https://voicesinmotionchoirs.org/research/ (Accessed 6/9/2022).

Whiteside, B. (2020). *Time to dance: Exploring the experiences of a dementia-friendly program.* Scottish Ballet. Available at: https://www.scottishballet.co.uk/join-in/sb-health/time-to-dance (Accessed 8/9/2022).

Part II
Re/framing

Part II

Reframing

6 'Lost in time like tears in rain'

Critical perspectives on personhood and dementia

Stephen Katz and Annette Leibing

Near the end of the film *Blade Runner* (1982), Roy Batty, the dying human-machine 'replicant' played by actor Rutger Hauer, reflects upon his short life in a touching well-known monologue, lamenting that 'All those moments are lost in time, like tears in rain'. Batty's words not only express the fleeting value of a life's accumulated experience and knowledge in the face of death, but also evoke or at least perform his human-like emotions, despite the short duration of his mercenary existence. Thus, Batty's status is confusingly liminal, as evident by the surprised reaction of character Rick Deckard (Harrison Ford), the detective sent to hunt him down. Here, liminality exists not between types of life transitions nor biographical trajectories, but between different types of selves encountering each other: Batty is both 'us' and 'not us', and while we are intrigued by the appearance of his humanity, we also distrust the dangerous unpredictability of his not-really-human brain, even as he clings to his losses in a very human way.

This cinematic scene is evocative of the self-other liminal status familiar to us because it frames encounters with individuals diagnosed with dementia,[1] where interior, personal life is assumed to be continually fragmenting, unreliable and uncontrollable. In large part, this assumption is due to the historical construction of Euro-Western concepts of personhood itself, characterised by certainty, rationality, agency, memory and individuality (Laceulle, 2018). These are also enduring culture-bound ideals with their own moral prescriptions (Leibing, 2019). In the dementia field, throughout the 20th century, these assemblages of personhood merged at first with a disease-based model of dementia and the medicalisation of those diagnosed with it. Thus, they have also become the target of critical scholars who seek more tolerant and less restrictive understandings of the person with dementia. It is this juxtaposition between dementia and concepts of self and personhood, terms used interchangeably here, that this chapter examines. We are taking a closer look at how such concepts became embedded within the development of dementia research itself and, as a consequence, practices of care, along with the critical ideas they inspired. Our position follows Barbara Prainsack's assertion that '[t]he key to ... medicine that fosters solidarity and is sensitive to people's needs lies in being cautious about what

DOI: 10.4324/9781003221982-9

idea of personhood we use and promote' (2014, p. 652). While the history of dementia is a complex story of science and culture, one interwoven with the biopolitics of ageing itself, this chapter outlines three overlapping stages of dementia research and the lineages of personhood concepts that inhabit them for our purposes. Conclusions ponder ideas for future research that looks more to community models of care and collective traditions of support and is less burdened with resolving problems of individual personhood and liminality.

Stage 1: Disease, loss and the medicalisation of dementia

Neuropathologist Alois Alzheimer's documentation of his first and famous patient Auguste Deter, at the dawn of the official discovery of Alzheimer's Disease (AD) in 1906,[2] is an account of the gradual dissolution of the woman's personal life from her early 50s until her death. 'I have kind of lost myself', he quotes Frau Deter as saying (Maurer and Maurer, 1998, p. 145). In fact, Dr Alzheimer not only diagnosed a brain pathology (post-mortem), but one that had apparently fragmented the memory, coherence and emotional stability of his patient – the very attributes of conventional personhood. Frau Deter and later other patients were seen as too young to be suffering from the dementia symptoms of old-age senility; hence, their puzzling presentation of 'senile dementia' became the starting point for what became the modern Alzheimer's disease movement (Ballenger, 2006a; Fox, 1989). The movement, especially since the 1960s and with the acceleration of neurological research, promoted AD as a powerful articulation of concerns about ageing itself. Leading gerontological figures such as Robert N. Butler, the first director of the American Institute on Aging in 1974, urged the replacement of the ageist image of 'senility' with that of AD as deserving of public funding, since he advocated that AD was a disease separable from the normal ageing process itself.[3]

At the same time, the image of AD as an age-related problem *in* but not *of* old age continued to galvanise the AD movement as it has quickly become a global phenomenon, with World Health Organization (WHO) and other reports citing increasing numbers of older persons diagnosed with AD, along with dire predictions for the future sustainability of systems and resources of care (e.g., WHO, 2017). Following Butler, as medical experts and dementia policy advocates believed that the disease model relieved older people from being labelled as naturally 'senile' or even earlier as 'being dangerously mad' (Leibing, 2005), the medicalisation of dementia created other issues of exclusion, stigmatisation and neglect. As Ballenger claims, the gerontologic disassociation of senility with ageing created a division between positive 'successful' agers and those afflicted with disease, such as AD, that became a separate entity that 'seems to create at least as much public fear and loathing about old age as did the expansive concept of senility out of which it was carved' (2000, p. 98).

The AD movement's aim of supplanting the historical ageism of 'senile dementia' was also premature because the lines connecting memory loss as a disease of the mind, a pathology of the brain and a detriment to self-hood were actually further strengthened as the cases of AD diagnoses grew (Ballenger, 2006b). Meanwhile, historical notions of self and personhood were left largely unquestioned as the default definitions of civilised humanity (Ballenger, 2006a; George and Whitehouse, 2021; Lock, 2013). Adding to these dilemmas was the obvious problem that, as ageing populations became increasingly associated with the risks of dementia, the search for cures, development of drugs, expansion of diagnostic technologies and neurological explanations of cognitive impairment favoured by the scientific community were not necessarily advancing nor improving care for persons diagnosed with dementia. For this group, personhood remained characterised by loss, isolation and dissolution, accompanied by public images of Zombie-like terror and suffering (Behuniak, 2011; Zeilig, 2014).

These developments form the crux of this first stage of contemporary dementia research. As the sciences of ageing optimistically rendered previous ideas about senile dementia as obsolete, they transformed AD into an isolated and singular disease whose mysteries became the property of medical research, clinical technologies, pharmaceutical funding and hopes for an eventual cure. In turn, they also re-stigmatised and alienated the very people such developments were designed to help by relegating their humanity to the pathologies of their tangled brains (Beard, 2016; Whitehouse, 2008).

Stage 2: Person-centred care and its critics

In Stage 2 of dementia research and culture, the focus shifted more sharply to issues of care, especially after it became evident that the once-hopeful pharmacological interventions had no major impact on the course of the dementia syndrome, although these medications continue to be widely prescribed (Leibing, 2014). The limitations of the medical modelling of AD and its harmful effects of institutional isolation for people diagnosed with it became especially problematical. Instead, non-medical approaches were sought that proposed more humane care practices identified with alternative concepts of personhood that rejected the bleak helplessness of subjective loss and emptiness. Stage 2 researchers and practitioners, whose great variety in backgrounds cannot be captured within the scope of this chapter, commonly proposed that the perceived liminality of being both human and non-human for persons with dementia could be ameliorated if ideas about human rights, compassionate healthcare ethics and, above all, *person-centred care* (PCC) were integrated into dementia therapeutic practices and care environments.

PCC was inspired by the work of Tom Kitwood (1937–1998), a social psychologist and 'personhood pioneer' who in the latter part of his career laid out the ethical principles to moor the care of a person with dementia to practises of empathy, respect, dignity, communication and reciprocity (Kitwood, 1997). For Kitwood, 'person-first' practices took into account the immediate living conditions of a person with dementia and their inter-dependence with others, as well as training caregivers to utilise different and more appropriate sensory skills, such as focused listening, observing and touching. The PCC framework asserted that if the needs of the care recip-ient and respect for their moral status were properly met, apart from the demands of institutional schedules and efficiencies, then problems of agi-tation, depression, sleeplessness, poor appetite, inactivity and even accel-erated cognitive decline might be remedied, while lessening the need for behaviour-modifying medications.

PCC became a rallying cry for the dissident voices in the latter decades of the 20th century, who criticised the mistreatment of persons diagnosed with dementia and attacked mainstream assertions that subjective life in demen-tia is bound for irrecoverable collapse (although final stages of dementia remain a challenge). Such mistreatment included over-medication, isolation in closed wards, physical abuse and regular neglect (especially in countries with pro-profit health economies). On a grander scale, PCC appealed as a revolution in dementia care, bringing together non-science experts with philosophical, artistic, literary and spiritual backgrounds, with the aim to re-imagine dementia as a shared human condition rather than an isolated and isolating disease. Above all, for Kitwood and his associates, such as Steven Sabat (2002) and Stephen Post (2006), it is the facilitation of expres-sion of selfhood, as the deep and continual human quality that under-lies individuality even for persons with dementia, that is the most crucial care-giving task. Thus, in the PCC perspective, for people with dementia who are treated well, self and personhood are not simply lost because they continue to animate biographical connectivity. They are always, at least partially, 'preserved' (Palmer, 2013), as recuperative interventions through inventive exercises in music, dance, theatre, elder clowning and storying that target 'the enduring self' seek to demonstrate (Berenbaum et al., 2017).

Since Kitwood's time, the popularity of PCC has grown to influence pro-fessional strategies and practices, sometimes for budgetary and managerial reasons. Texts such as *The Dementia Manifesto* (Hughes and Williamson, 2019), government long-term policy reports such as Ontario's 'Patients First' (2015), housing organisations such as the Eden Alternative (https://www.edenalt.org/) and a robust literature on training guidelines, such as those provided by the Alzheimer's Society of Canada (2011), attest to the adaptation of PCC into programmes of care. As the Alzheimer Society of Canada framework recommends: 'Person-centred care should be incorpo-rated into all aspects of care regardless of the resident's condition or stage of the disease' (2011, p. 19). Thus, PCC advanced from a critical movement recognising the value of the expression of selfhood in dementia to become a promising administrative programme in dementia care, even where original

PCC mandates became distorted or simplified in the process. As Fazio and colleagues state, 'Recognizing that selfhood persists, learning about the complete self, and finding ways to maintaining selfhood though interactions and conversations are fundamental components of person-centred care for people with dementia' (2018, p. S11). And because people with dementia are dependent on others, their interpersonal relationships are crucial, such that 'The other person, the caregiver, is needed to offset degeneration and fragmentation and sustain personhood. The further the dementia advances, the greater the need for "person-work"' (p. S12).

However, this hyphenated term 'person-work' opens onto one of the more contentious issues in PCC, which is the status of the caregiver and respect for their personhood. In Canada, for example (the authors' home country), this issue is particularly salient because labour conditions in long-term care residences suffer from severe understaffing, poor salaries and demanding schedules. As well, research reports illustrate how care workers have little decision-making authority and inadequate training time for new initiatives and technologies. In one study, researchers found that care workers experience a 'near impossibility of providing relational care, that is addressing residents' emotional, social, existential and spiritual needs' (Banerjee et al., 2015, p. 32). These workers sometimes used their own unpaid labour and free time to fill in the gaps. A recent special issue of the *Journal of Clinical Nursing* reviewed research on the barriers of PCC for people living with dementia from the perspective of nursing staff (Kong et al., 2021), finding conditions of insufficient resources and poor and unsupportive relationships within the residence itself. While Kitwood claimed that poor care was a form of 'a malignant social psychology' to be countered by his 12 interactions of 'positive person care' (Kitwood, 1997, pp. 119–120), neither he nor his followers adequately considered the training, labour and emotional implications of these tasks for caregivers (Davis, 2004), nor the basic structural changes required to allow care workers and family caregivers to enact the recognition of persons with dementia according to PCC principles (Leibing, 2019, 2021).

A related problem in PCC raised by critics and central to this chapter is the question of the meaning of 'person-centredness' as an ethic of care practice (Dewing, 2008, p. 3). Care-giving for persons with dementia is already an asymmetrical relationship where the status of personhood, however vague, is conferred by others (without dementia). As Higgs and Gilleard remark,

> The problem with adopting a personhood-centred approach to helping people with dementia is that it fails to recognise the distinction between these two aspects of personhood, namely, the standing of persons and the capabilities of personhood. By failing to recognise the distinction, this approach risks placing the burden of responsibility on other persons, other selves, to sustain the personhood of individuals with

dementia (in the sense of preserving people with dementia's capacities for personhood), as well as sustaining the due moral concern for them.

(2016, p. 25)

Indeed, we may question whether better care or empathetic nursing necessarily requires a PCC managerial programme at all, including its extensive agendas and tasks for sustaining agency, well-being, self-expression and identity. And in cases of advanced dementia, if the only agent is the care provider, for the care recipient this can mean that 'there may be an end to needing to express oneself, and an end, even, to wanting to be someone' (Higgs and Gilleard, 2016, p. 134).

Critics of these and other problems with PCC, while recognising its benefits and bold radicalisation of Stage 1 medical models, have looked to different ideas about self and personhood in order to further critical dementia studies. These mark a departure from Stage 2 and its development of PCC and give rise to Stage 3 of dementia research based on broad concepts of relationality, embodiment, discontinuity and materiality.

Phase 3: De-centring humanism

The universalising notions of person and selfhood implicit in PCC and its one-way models of care became targets of critical dementia researchers who share a general project of de-centring or revising traditional notions of self and personhood and their associations with dominant formations of power. These include contributions adapted from feminist and theoretical work in phenomenological embodiment, post-humanism, post-structuralism, decolonialism and materiality studies. For example, embodiment in dementia is one of the central discoveries of the work of Pia Kontos. While she maintains the importance of selfhood for persons with dementia, she explores how it is expressed in bodily, rather than strictly cognitive, ways (Kontos, 2015; Kontos et al., 2017). Kontos uses a 'pre-reflexive' phenomenological notion of embodied selfhood, whereby the capacities, senses, routines and repertoires accumulated in a person's life via their bodies remain important meaning-making resources for being in the world, even if individual status has been fragmented. Thus, for Kontos and her colleagues, dementia-related behaviours often treated as disturbing such as wandering, incoherence or non-compliance should be seen more empathetically and closer to other typical activities that suggest life-long bodily dispositions, representing a person's distinctly persistent self from a non-neurocentric perspective. In this approach, arts-based and story-telling programmes are encouraged because they 'draw significantly on the body's potentiality for innovation and creative action, and significantly support non-verbal communication and affect' (Kontos, 2015, p. 176).

Nicholas Jenkins (2014, see also Chapter 7), in his interpretation of bodily relationality, adds that care interventions should not aim to 'repair' the broken self nor recover the former self as much as enliven the relationality of the 'inter-embodied self'.

> Contrary to person-centred approaches, the inter-embodied self does not require a unified or coherent narrative in order to thrive. On the contrary, our inter-embodied selves may be more fruitfully conceptualised as montages; polyphonic repertoires of voices and experiences that co-exist in dialogical relationship to one another; constantly updating, constantly changing.
>
> (Jenkins, 2014, p. 133)

For this kind of relational and bodily framework to influence care, the idea of individual linear narrative time itself is also questionable, since inter-bodied knowledge is an exchange among individuals within conjoint world-making activities unbounded from the individual her-/himself. Here world-making is also a collaboration of the material agents, both human and non-human, and their ever-changing contexts. These might include things, smells, sounds, atmospheres, machines, colours and textures. As Nicky Hatton explains, dementia care and living environments are a 'moving materiality' that is felt, not just inhabited, and may involve components that cannot be seen or touched (Hatton, 2021, p. 74). Even sleep in these environments, assumed to be an individual's disengagement from the material world, may be a form of negotiation about personal time and boundaries or a defence against being overwhelmed, and as such enable residents to move into a strategic and deliberate 'slow time' in order to create distance from structured managerial temporality (Hatton, 2021, p. 165). Lee and Bartlett (2020) also develop a 'material lens' to detail the overlooked but vital relational world of objects, possessions and living spaces for people with dementia living in a care residence, advocating for a 'material citizenship' to counter the loss of material control.

Some of these propositions accord with a wider post-humanist movement in ageing studies that attempts to de-centre the continuities of self, biographical coherence and autonomous agency that define the status of the human subject in conventional humanism. Post-humanism is both a recognition of those who have been violently marginalised as less-than-human and polarised into being 'other' (Braidotti, 2020), and a critique of universalising notions of individuality that gave rise to a 'regime of the human' (Tsing, 2015, p. 19). In the case of dementia, post-humanist critiques recognise that care is more than a relationship between two people, but involves a 'constant flux of tools and technologies, behaviours, embodiments, economies and ecologies' (DeFalco, 2020, p. 51). Further research linking post-humanist thinking to dementia draws upon studies of decolonising and Indigenous knowledges and their expansive collaborative visions and 'two-eyed approaches' (Webkamigad et al., 2020) of collective identities, healing landscapes and community resources (see Asker and Andrews, 2020;

Povinelli, 2016). For example, the value of 'place-ing' dementia care among the Southern Inuit of Labrador (Pace, 2020) or the Chocktaw interpretation of memory loss as the mind being spiritually 'elsewhere' (Grande, 2018; Henderson and Henderson, 2002), along with other Indigenous ways of understanding dementia (Hulko et al., 2019), contest the colonial legacy embedded within settler gerontologies about individual loss and alienation (see also Chapter 16).

Another dimension of Stage 3 dementia research is poststructuralist studies that challenge the re-traditionalisation of sexual identities within the personhood movement (Sandberg, 2021; Sandberg and Marshall, 2017; Silverman and Baril, 2021). For these writers, the pressure to express a selfhood linked to a continuity with a hegemonically gendered past contributes to the crisis of loss of self for persons with dementia. However, according to these critics, dementia is more an experience of a changing self rather than one in need of recovery framed by PCC concepts of personhood (see also Chapter 15 and 17 in this volume). Indeed, one of the key themes of Stage 3 dementia research is its deconstruction of normative forms of selfhood and identity associated with taken-for-granted expectations of continuity in time in dementia care. For example, Anne Basting's work has demonstrated how creative imagination and its benefits for persons with dementia are best recognised in the co-created co-presence apart from assumed continuities of the past (Basting, 2009, 2020). As Basting says,

> Creative care is an agreement between people to imagine themselves, each other, and their worlds a little differently. It is an invitation to shape the world together. For people denied the tools for world-shaping, this invitation can be a profound and life-changing act of healing.
>
> (2020, p. 57)

In his work on dementia and memory, Katz also questions how memory itself is a historical conceptualisation (2012, 2013), and is exploring how living with dementia may be a window onto the experience of non-continuous temporalities (Katz, 2021), akin to Henri Bergson's idea about the fluid co-existence of past and present memories (Bergson, 1939; Deleuze, 1988). For Bergson, memories include dreams, fantasies, possibilities and mirages that exceed location in linear time, such that memory

> is not a possession – although it may be recollected and uttered in the possessive and thus attributed to an individual as a content of consciousness or the brain. Pure memory is in excess of recollection, actuality or consciousness. It is we who belong to memory, to different planes of the past.
>
> (Al-Saji, 2004, p. 228)

This idea of an intermingling, rather than a continuity, of points in time undermines the essentialist sense of individual identity and resonates with a different kind of duration as the term is defined by Elizabeth Grosz:

> Duration is that which undoes as well as what makes: to the extent that duration entails an open future, it involves the fracturing and opening up of the past and the present to what is virtual in them; to what in them differs from the actual, to what in them can bring forth the new. This unbecoming is the very motor of becoming, making the past and present not given but fundamentally ever-altering, virtual.
>
> (Grosz, 2005, pp. 4–5)

This exciting idea of duration of temporalities – to undo and to make, to un-become and to become, to create and to alter memory, to live in a multitude of temporal flows – is a way of de-centring the limits of purely humanist personhood and rethinking how memory loss can be part of the duration of temporality.

Returning then to our introduction, Batty's self-reflection of being 'like tears in rain' when applied to dementia could mean the 'soul-searching' in persons often described as having lost their selves. But it can also be read as a wish to enlarge the scope of personhood itself, as belonging to a wider community of diverse citizens of the kind that relational, materialist and post-humanist writers promote. Such an approach moves the focus away from the individual self, which ultimately remains the 'other' (Leibing, 2018) even within personhood approaches, and instead prioritises the environmental contexts, conditions of existence and landscapes of ageing around the needs of the individual living with dementia. It is this approach that frames our questions for further research in the Conclusions.

Conclusions: Both rain and tears

The three stages of dementia research summarised above represent important reflections about our humanity, encapsulated by debates about self and personhood, memory and time, authenticity and vulnerability, agency and dependency, and individualism and relationality. They further show that Prainsack's warning – that the kind of personhood we propagate is not without consequences – needs to be considered in our discussions around dementia care and more generally about all kinds of care, including self-care. Following the medically dominated Alzheimer's Movement in Stage 1, Stage 2 was framed by the need to recognise the previously unacknowledged individual and her ('lost') self – the separation of the single tear from the rain, to return to our cinematic metaphor. Dementia research in Stage 3 proposes an altered direction: zooming away from the single tear as a specific agent (at risk of disappearing in the rain) to perspectives that reconnect the tear to the rain by transcending anthropocentric ideas and conceiving the person with dementia as entangled in embodied, relational or more-than-human relations and environments. And while both Dementia stages 2 and 3 are important advances over Dementia stage 1 and overlap in their compassion for the lives of persons living with dementia,[4] both suggest areas for further research that encompass context, policy, cultural and structural factors that shape all dementia care.[5] At the same time, we cannot ignore the reality that people living with dementia are still individuals who suffer and need support and who must be recognised as such. However powerful are the critiques that transcend gendered, disabled and colonised elements of personhood, these may not be sufficient to ensure a vision of best practices of care (see Leibing, 2019).

For example, Leibing's ongoing anthropological work in Brazil illustrates how personhood (a term not used in Brazil) is situated in contexts of family and professional care that provide an interactive series of relationships that both include and relieve the individual with dementia of the pressures of self-care. Brazil is a culture based on reciprocity and strong communal interdependency in, at the same time, a deeply divided and hierarchical society (DaMatta, 2020). The absence of a dependable social net manifests in the necessity of creating one's own connections, both within and outside family relationships, along with negotiating the ways in which gendered family care labour is organised. The person with dementia, often infantilised as being in a completely dependent state that excludes the search for personhood, is still part of a greater constellation made up of predominantly family relations. This set of circumstances explains why, for example, it is unacceptable for older people to arrive unaccompanied at geriatric clinics. As anthropologist Cintia Engel (2020) shows, for the less privileged in Brazil, the complicated and extremely stressful ways of embedding a family member with dementia in the multiple networks of care resources require a mobilisation of family members, community and related institutions in a constant patchwork of care-related activities. This patchwork also intersects with the communal overtones of the pharmaceutical market in Brazil.[6]

Brazil is but one example of the cultural inseparability between a person with dementia, caregivers, family, community and the relations, resources, medications and pathways of access that mobilise around them, even in the poorest of circumstances. In their recent book, *American Dementia: Brain Health in an Unhealthy Society* (2021), George and Whitehouse argue that real change in dementia care and brain health depends on reversing the deepening social inequalities, accelerating environmental destruction, and growing precarity and instability of living communities (for both human and non-human inhabitants). The evidence of dropping incidence rates of dementia in several countries due to better access to educational and health resources signals to these authors that 'winning the struggle for a fairer political-economic order where prosperity is more inclusively shared and the public's health and well-being is once again aggressively protected will provide the conditions for *everyone* to build greater resilience to brain aging' (p. x). Carol Brayne, one of the first researchers to alight on falling dementia rates in the UK, when asked in an interview about what would lower dementia risks further in the future, responds:

> I'd think about maternal health, about the environment in which children grow up and their education. I'd think about health interests and the way we educate children to understand their own risks and the good that they can do themselves. I would want to look at the whole system; not only the health aspects across the life course, but how we can encourage localities and governments to implement strategies, whether it be laws, transport systems, or ways to address local communities that are sensitive to the risks.
>
> (New Medical Life Sciences, December 7, 2015)

In these scenarios in Brazil, America, the UK and across the world, where politics, society, history and collective action are the resources now and into the future that shape and change dementia care, personhood is much bigger than the individual. Personhood is polymorphic and entwined with 'socio-material modes of togetherness' (Duclos and Criado, 2019, p. 161), as they are made and un-made in multiple sites, diverse temporalities and heterogeneous distributions. Together, as our chapter has outlined, the relationship between personhood and dementia as a relative modern problem of ageing has tapped into a deep and reflecting well of historical meaning about the dilemmas of human sociality. Roy Batty may have been right that liminal life is lost like tears in the rain, but both are made of the water that constitutes all existence and connects all things.

Notes

1 Dementia is an umbrella term for a number of conditions with changing nosologies and aetiologies over time, of which Alzheimer's disease is the most well-known form.

2 In reality the condition had been described before, but Emil Kraepelin's influential textbook on psychiatry (1910) attributed the 'discovery' to his friend and colleague Alois Alzheimer (Berrios, 1996).

3 After Serrano-Pozo et al. (2017), funding of dementia research started in 1975 and budgets steadily increased, reaching an amount of around $8 billion (US) worldwide in 2010, and started then to decline slowly.

4 An exceptional example is the project Carpe Diem in Québec, where there is not only person-centred care as a central philosophy but also the provision of a home-like house and care where providing autonomy and, as much as possible, an experience of 'normal' life for residents is central, even if considerable risks are taken, such as letting residents walk alone in the streets of Trois-Rivière where Carpe Diem is located. Less is known about how such models deal with the needs of persons with an advanced dementia. https://alzheimercarpediem.com/lapproche-carpe-diem/lapproche-carpe-diem/.

5 Some of these issues have been approached by critiques of personhood in dementia as a problem of citizenship and disability (Baldwin and Greason, 2016; Bartlett and O'Connor, 2007).
6 The empirical data have been previously published in Leibing et al. (2019). Also see Leibing (2021) on the vascularization of Alzheimer's disease and its impact on geriatric care.

References

Al-Saji, A. (2004) 'The Memory of Another Past: Bergson, Deleuze and a New Theory of Time', *Continental Philosophy Review*, 37, pp. 203–239.

Alzheimer Society of Canada. (2011) *Guidelines for Care: Person-Centred Care of People with Dementia Living in Care Homes*. Toronto: Alzheimer Society of Canada.

Asker, C., and Andrews, G. (2020) 'The Understated Turn: Emerging Interests and Themes in Canadian Posthuman Geography', *The Canadian Geographer*, 64(4), pp. 551–563.

Baldwin, C., and Greason, M. (2016) 'Micro-Citizenship, Dementia and Long-Term Care', *Dementia*, 15(3), pp. 289–303.

Ballenger, J.F. (2000) Beyond the Characteristic Plaques and Tangles: Mid-Twentieth-Century US Psychiatry and the Fight against Senility. In P.J. Whitehouse, K. Maurer and J.F. Ballenger (eds.), *Concepts of Alzheimer Disease: Biological, Clinical and Cultural Perspectives*. Baltimore, MD: Johns Hopkins University Press, pp. 83–103.

Ballenger, J.F. (2006a) *Self, Senility, and Alzheimer's Disease in Modern America: A History*. Baltimore: Johns Hopkins University Press.

Ballenger, J.F. (2006b) 'The Biomedical Deconstruction of Senility and the Persistent Stigmatization of Old Age in the United States'. In A. Leibing and L. Cohen (eds.), *Thinking about Dementia: Culture, Loss, and the Anthropology of Senility*. New Brunswick: Rutgers University Press, pp. 106–120.

Banerjee, A., Armstrong, P., Daly, T., Armstrong, H., and Braedley, S. (2015) '"Careworkers Don't Have a Voice:" Epistemological Violence in Residential Care for Older People', *Journal of Aging Studies*, 33, pp. 28–36.

Bartlett, R.L., and O'Connor, D.L. (2007) 'From Personhood to Citizenship: Broadening the Lens for Dementia Practice and Research', *Journal of Aging Studies*, 21(2), pp. 107–118.

Basting, A. (2009) *Forget Memory: Creating Better Lives for People with Dementia*. Baltimore: Johns Hopkins University Press.

Basting, A. (2020) *Creative Care: A Revolutionary Approach to Dementia and Elder Care*. New York: Harper Collins.

Beard, R.L. (2016) *Living with Alzheimer's: Managing Memory Loss, Identity and Illness*. New York: New York University Press.

Behuniak, S.M. (2011) 'The Living Dead? The Construction of People with Alzheimer's Disease as Zombies', *Ageing & Society*, 31, pp. 70–92.

Berenbaum, R., Tziraki, C., and Mazuz, K. (2017) 'The Enduring Self: Personhood, Autonomy and Compassion in the Context of Community-based Dementia Daycare Centers', *Journal of Compassionate Health Care*, 4(1). DOI: 10.1186/s40639-017-0037-z.

Bergson, H. (1939[1896]) *Matter and Memory* (trans. N. Paul and W. Palmer). New York: Zone Books.

Berrios, G.E. (1996) 'Cognitive Impairment'. In G.E. Berrios (ed.), *The History of Mental Symptoms, Descriptive Psychopathology Since the Nineteenth Century.* Cambridge: Cambridge University Press, pp. 173–207.

Blade Runner (1982), Ridley Scott (director), H. Fancher and D. Peoples (screenplay), Warner Bros (distribution).

Braidotti, R. (2020) '"We" Are in This Together, But We Are Not One and the Same', *Journal of Bioethical Inquiry*, 17, pp. 465–469.

Brayne, C. (2015) Interview with Dr. Carol Brayne, *New Medical Life Sciences*, December 7.

DaMatta, R. (2020[1998]) *Você Sabe Com Quem Está Falando? Estudos Sobre o Autoritarismo Brasileiro.* São Paulo: Rocco.

Davis, D.H.J. (2004) 'Dementia; Sociological and Philosophical Constructions', *Social Sciences and Medicine*, 58, pp. 369–378.

DeFalco, A. (2020) 'Towards a Theory of Posthuman Care', *Body & Society*, 26(3), pp. 31–60.

Deleuze, G. (1988[1966]) *Bergsonism* (trans. H. Tomlinson and B. Habberjam). New York: Zone Books.

Dewing, J. (2008) 'Personhood and Dementia; Revisiting Tom Kitwood's Ideas', *International Journal of Older People Nursing*, 3(1), pp. 3–13.

Duclos, V., and Criado, T.S. (2019) 'Care in Trouble – Ecologies of Support from Below and Beyond', *Medical Anthropology Quarterly*, 34(2), pp. 153–173.

Engel, C.L. (2020) *Partilha e cuidado das deme ncias: entre interações medicamentosas e rotinas.* PhD thesis, University of Brasilia, Department of Anthropology.

Fazio, S., Pace, D., Flinner, J., and Kallmyer, B. (2018) 'The Fundamentals of Person-Centered Care for Individuals with Dementia', *The Gerontologist*, 58(S1), pp. S10–S19.

Fox, P. (1989) 'From Senility to Alzheimer Disease: The Rise of the Alzheimer Disease Movement', *Milibank Quarterly*, 67, pp. 58–102.

George, D.R., and Whitehouse, P.J. (2021) *American Dementia: Brain Health in an Unhealthy Society.* Baltimore, MD: Johns Hopkins University Press.

Grande, S. (2018) 'Aging, Precarity, and the Struggle for Indigenous Elsewheres', *International Journal of Qualitative Studies in Education*, 31(3), pp. 168–176.

Grosz, E. (2005) 'Bergson, Deleuze and the Becoming of Unbecoming', *Parallax*, 11(2), pp. 4–13.

Hatton, N. (2021) *Performance and Dementia: A Cultural Response to Care.* Cham, Switzerland: Palgrave MacMillan.

Henderson, J.N., and Henderson, L.C. (2002) 'Cultural Construction of Disease: A "Supernormal" Construct of Dementia in an American Indian Tribe', *Journal of Cross-Cultural Gerontology*, 17(3), pp. 197–212.

Higgs, P., and Gilleard, C. (2016) *Personhood, Identity and Care in Advanced Old Age.* Bristol: Policy Press.

Hughes, J.C., and Williamson, T. (2019) *The Dementia Manifesto: Putting Values-Based Practice to Work.* Cambridge: Cambridge University Press.

Hulko, W., Wilson, D., and Balestrery, J.E. (eds.) (2019) *Indigenous Peoples and Dementia: New Understandings of Memory Loss and Memory Care.* Vancouver: University of British Columbia Press.

Jenkins, N. (2014) 'Dementia and the Inter-embodied Self', *Social Theory & Health*, 12(2), pp. 125–137.

Katz, S. (2012) 'Embodied Memory: Aging, Neuroculture, and the Genealogy of Mind', *Occasion: Interdisciplinary Studies in the Humanities*, 4, https://arcade.stanford.edu/occasion/embodied-memory-ageing-neuroculture-and-genealogy-mind.

Katz, S. (2013) 'Dementia, Personhood and Embodiment: What Can We Learn from the Medieval History of Memory?', *Dementia*, 12(3), pp. 303–314.

Katz, S. (2021) 'Time, Memory and Dementia: A Becoming/Un-becoming Approach', Critical Dementia Network Symposium *Temporalities of Dementia*, December 3.

Kitwood, T. (1997) *Dementia Reconsidered: The Person Comes First.* Buckingham: Open University Press.

Kong, E.-H., Faan, H.K., and Hyejin, K. (2021) 'Nursing Home Staff's Perceptions of Barriers and Needs in Implementing Person-Centred Care for People Living with Dementia: A Qualitative Study', *Journal of Clinical Nursing.* DOI: 10.1111/jocn.15729. Online ahead of print.

Kontos, P. (2015) 'Dementia and Embodiment'. In J. Twigg and W. Martin (eds.), *Routledge Handbook of Cultural Gerontology.* London: Routledge, pp. 173–180.

Kontos, P., Miller, K.-L., and Kontos, A.P. (2017) 'Relational Citizenship: Supporting Embodied Selfhood and Relationality in Dementia Care', *Sociology of Health and Illness (Special Issue: Ageing, Dementia and the Social Mind)*, 39(2), pp. 182–198.

Kraepelin, E. (1910) *Psychiatrie* (8th ed.). Leipzig: Barth.

Laceulle, H. (2018) *Becoming Who You Are: Aging, Self-Realization and Cultural Narratives about Later Life.* Bielefeld: Transcript Verlag,

Lee, K., and Bartlett, R. (2021) 'Material Citizenship: An Ethnographic Study Exploring Object–Person Relations in the Context of People with Dementia in Care Homes,' *Sociology of Health and Illness*, 43(6), pp. 1471–1485.

Leibing, A. (2005) 'The Old Lady from Ipanema: Changing Notions of Old Age in Brazil', *Journal of Aging Studies*, 19(1), pp. 15–31.

Leibing, A. (2014) 'The Earlier the Better: Alzheimer's Prevention, Early Detection, and the Quest for Pharmacological Interventions', *Culture, Medicine & Psychiatry*, 38(2), pp. 217–236.

Leibing, A. (2018) 'Situated Prevention: Framing the 'New Dementia', *Journal of Law, Medicine & Ethics*, 46, pp. 704–716.

Leibing, A. (2019) 'Geriatrics and Humanism: Dementia and Fallacies of Care', *Journal Aging Studies*, 51(2), pp. 1–7.

Leibing, A. (2021) 'The Vascularization of Alzheimer's Disease: Prevention in "Global" Geriatric Care'. In A. Leibing and S. Schicktanz (eds.), *Preventing Dementia? Critical Perspectives on a New Paradigm of Preparing for Old Age.* New York and Oxford, UK: Berghahn Books, pp. 40–64.

Leibing, A., Engel, C., and Carrijo, E. (2019) 'Life through Medications: Dementia Care in Brazil', *ReVista Harvard Review of Latin America*, Winter (part II). https://archive.revista.drclas.harvard.edu/book/leibing-change-title.

Lock, M. (2013) *The Alzheimer Conundrum, Entanglements of Dementia and Aging.* Princeton, NJ: Princeton University Press.

Maurer, K., and Maurer, U. (1998) *Alzheimer, Das Leben eines Arztes und die Karriere einer Krankheit.* Munich: Piper.

Ministry of Health and Long-Term Care (Ontario). (2015) *Patients First: Action Plan for Health Care*. Toronto: Government of Ontario.

Pace, J. (2020) '"Place-ing" Dementia Prevention and Care in NunatuKavut, Labrador', *Canadian Journal on Aging*, 39(2), pp. 247–262.

Palmer, J.L. (2013) 'Preserving Personhood of Individuals with Advanced Dementia: Lessons from Family Caregivers', *Geriatric Nursing (New York, N.Y.)*, 34(3), pp. 224–229.

Post, S.G. (2006) '*Respectare*: Moral Respect for the Lives of the Deeply Forgetful'. In J.C. Hughes, S.J. Louw and S. Sabat (eds.), *Dementia: Mind, Meaning, and the Person*. Oxford: Oxford University Press, pp. 223–34.

Povinelli, E.A. (2016) *Geontologies: A Requiem to Late Liberalism*. Durham: Duke University Press.

Prainsack, B. (2014) 'Personhood and Solidarity: What Kind of Personalized Medicine Do We Want?', *Personalized Medicine*, 11(7), pp. 651–657.

Sabat, S.R. (2002) 'Surviving Manifestations of Selfhood in Alzheimer's Disease: A Case Study', *Dementia*, 1, pp. 25–36.

Sandberg, L.J. (2021) '"I Was the Woman, He Was the Man": Dementia, Recognition, Recognisability and Gendered Subjectivity', *Humanities and Social Sciences Communications*, 8, p. 85. DOI: 10.1057/s41599-021-00758-1.

Sandberg, L.J., and Marshall, B.L. (2017) 'Queering Aging Futures', *Societies*, 7(3), p. 21. DOI: 10.3390/soc7030021.

Serrano-Pozo, A., Aldridge, G.M., and Zhang, Q. (2017) 'Four Decades of Research in Alzheimer's Disease (1975–2014): A Bibliometric and Scientometric Analysis,' *Journal of Alzheimers Disease*, 59(2): pp. 763–783. DOI:10.3233/JAD-170184.

Silverman, M., and Baril, A. (2021) 'Transing Dementia: Rethinking Compulsory Biographical Continuity through the Theorization of Cisism and Cisnormativity', *Journal of Aging Studies*, 58, p. 9. DOI:10.1016/j.jaging.2021.100956.

Tsing, A.L. (2015) *The Mushroom at the End of the World, On the Possibility of Life in Capitalist Ruins*. Princeton, NJ: Princeton University Press.

Webkamigad, S., Warry, W., Blind, M., and Jacklin, K. (2020) 'An Approach to Improve Dementia Health Literacy in Indigenous Communities,' *Journal of Cross-Cultural Gerontology*, 35, pp. 69–83.

Whitehouse, P.J. with George, D. (2008) *The Myth of Alzheimer's*. New York: St. Martin's Press.

World Health Organization (WHO). (2017) *Global Action Plan on the Public Health Response to Dementia*, 2017–2025.

Zeilig, H. (2014) 'Dementia As a Cultural Metaphor', *The Gerontologist*, 54(2), pp. 258–267.

7 Multi-species dementia studies

How moving beyond human exceptionalism can advance dementia's more critical turn

Nick Jenkins

Introduction: 'Hic sunt dracones'

Ever since Levi-Strauss (1964) noted that animals are good to think with, scholars have been arguing for greater consideration of nonhumans within social theory. With the rise of 'the animal turn' (Ritvo, 2007), attending to humanity's relations with the more-than-human world (Abram, 1996) has expanded considerably, finding expression in academic disciplines as diverse as sociology, psychology, history and geography, and within interdisciplinary fields, including Science and Technology Studies, Gender Studies and, more recently, Ageing Studies. Several new *'isms'* have emerged in an attempt to define this growing area of theorising, most notably *inter-speciesism* (e.g. Alexis, 2020), *trans-speciesism* (e.g. Matsuoka and Sorenson, 2018) and *multi-speciesism* (e.g. Kirksey and Helmreich, 2010). It is beyond the scope of this chapter to give a detailed account of what each *'ism'* entails. However, following Kirksey and Helmreich (2010), the term 'multi-speciesism' is used throughout this chapter as a useful hypernym when referring to ways of thinking with (and of thinking about) dementia studies' relations with the more-than-human world.

As argued elsewhere (Jenkins et al., 2021), the field of dementia studies has been slow and arguably somewhat resistant to embrace attempts to think with animals and other forms of (nonhuman) life. Such hesitancy is understandable, given how people with dementia have, for centuries, been excluded from what Tom Kitwood (1937–1998) referred to as the 'Personhood Club' (Kitwood, 1997). Given that we are *still* struggling to ensure people with dementia are recognised as persons – with the full corollary of rights that such standing entails – do we *really* want to start bringing animals and other nonhuman life forms within the 'lens of the dementia debate' (Bartlett and O'Connor, 2007, 2010)? Surely, this way, *hic sunt dracones* ('Here be dragons')!

In advocating for (a more) critical dementia studies, Ward and Sandberg (2019, see also Chapter 19) argue for new collective affinities and flexible coalitions between researchers, activists and critical scholars. Dementia's critical turn, they argue, has potential to advance less homogenising forms of discourse and to de-territorialise dementia from being an exclusive domain

DOI: 10.4324/9781003221982-10

of the applied health and social care disciplines, and more firmly draw it into critical gerontology and critical disability studies. This chapter makes a case for including multi-speciesism as a sympathetic 'messmate' (Haraway, 2008) to this cause. Whilst multi-speciesism takes much from critical theory it is not, exclusively, a field of critical inquiry. Studies in human-animal interaction (HAI), for example, draw as much on mainstream social theory (e.g. symbolic interactionism) as from critical perspectives. However, what (a more) critical multi-speciesism offers dementia studies, this chapter argues, is the ability to move *beyond* reliance upon re-packaged and re-constituted forms of liberal humanism, in pursuit of a more radical ontological-epistemological-ethical project. In the sections that follow, this chapter provides a brief introduction to multi-species dementia studies, as an emerging sub-field of inquiry, before offering some tentative thoughts on how critical multi-species dementia studies can enable radical alterity in dementia.

Why (a more) critical multi-species dementia studies?

Human societies, cultures and civilisations are inherently multi-species. As such, and as Bryant (1979, p. 417) observes, we 'can no more appropriately ignore the zoological dimension, than an analysis of drama can ignore the seminal actors in a play'. To think with *Zoë*[1] in dementia is not, therefore, a niche area of inquiry, neither is it exclusively for those who 'like' animals (Wolfe, 2010). Rather, multi-species dementia studies can be understood as an attempt to 'adjust our conceptual apparatus in ways that redirect attention, bring heightened acknowledgement [of the more-than-human world], and enable new ways of seeing' (Jenkins et al., 2021, p. 2). As Jenkins and colleagues argue, multi-species dementia studies has clear potential to advance research, policy and practice – from advancing our understandings of interspecies caring in later life, to exploring the role animals play in shaping our understandings of, and responses to, dementia's disease pathology.

Advancing a more *critical* multi-species dementia studies, however, involves disrupting and destabilising the ideology of human exceptionalism that has, for the last two centuries, pervaded this field of enquiry. Since the late-18th century, human exceptionalism has been at the centre of our attempts to define dementia and to understand that which dementia affects. Humans, according to exceptionalist logic, are distinct from all other sentient forms of life. Their unique attributes and endowments (principally the capacity for reason, self-awareness and episodic memory) serve to make humans worthy of superior moral consideration. Human exceptionalism is foundational to modern capitalism and the modern episteme (Foucault, 1966), as well as the dehumanisation of people with disabilities (Goodley, Lawthorn and Runswick-Cole, 2014).

As Scull (1979) highlights, prior to the European Enlightenment, 'insanity' was widely associated with descent into the animal realm and a fall from the status of *Man*. This ontological position underpinned most early 'treatments' for psychiatric illness, including beatings, blistering and purging, which were deployed by the physicians of the age in their attempts to tame the animal spirits of 'the insane'. Whilst the *Moral Treatment* movement of the early 19th century sought to challenge this worldview and bring Enlightenment science into psychiatric nosology, the dehumanising of people living with progressive neurocognitive conditions has continued well into the 21st century. Dehumanisation continues, not *despite* our attempts to recognise the exceptional and indivisible humanity of people with dementia but, at least in part, *because* of them. By emphasising the exceptional and indivisible humanity of people with dementia, normative understandings of the human (as a category of being that is superior to and set apart from all other forms of life) remain the hegemonic model for thinking subjectivity. Following Wolfe (2003, 2010), this presents critical dementia studies with a difficult choice. On the one hand, appealing to the essential and indivisible humanity of people with dementia leads to pragmatic gains, such as greater freedoms to life, social participation and health, as well as greater freedoms from torture and the arbitrary deprivation of personal liberty. On the other hand, by drawing upon normative understandings of human beings as indivisible and exceptional subjects, dementia studies risks essentialising the very oppressive ideology that it is seeking to challenge. As will be argued in the following sections, a more critical multi-species dementia studies offers alternative approaches for thinking about subjectivity, which are less unconsciously anthropocentric and more response-able (Haraway, 2016) for the radical alterity that we, as an epistemic community, are seeking to create. In the sections that follow, this chapter explores three key areas where multi-species thinking can lead to radical innovations in dementia. These key areas are connecting cognitive ableism with the ideology of speciesism, exploring the embodied experience of dementia across species and moving beyond (human) rights-based approaches to dementia.

Connecting cognitive ableism with speciesism

To move beyond human exceptionalism involves recognising the ways in which cognitive ableism *intra*-acts (Barad, 2007) with the ideology of speciesism, so as to create mutually re-enforcing systems of oppression.

Carlson defines cognitive ableism as 'a prejudice or attitude of bias in favor of the interests of individuals who possess certain cognitive abilities (or the potential for them) against those who are believed not to actually or potentially possess them' (Carlson, 2001, p. 140). Since the 1980s, dementia studies has well recognised the pernicious effects of cognitive ableism upon the lives of people living with progressive neurocognitive conditions. Eurocentric understandings of humans as rational, independent agents capable of exercising choice and practising self-regulation have been criticised for disabling people with dementia and facilitating their exclusion from the Personhood Club (see, for example, Lyman, 1989). Where dementia studies has been less effective, however, is positioning cognitive ableism within its wider set of institutional, political, social and economic structures. As Hulko (2004) argues, exploring how oppression in dementia intersects with other sites of discrimination, such as gender, race and class, has been largely neglected within dementia research. As Bartlett et al. (2018) similarly argue, common forms of address used in dementia studies, including 'the person with dementia', carry implicit assumptions that socio-material factors such as gender do not matter when, clearly, they do. Whilst awareness of how neurocognitive disorder, age, gender and race intersect is growing within dementia studies, an equally important ideological system has received virtually no attention: namely, speciesism.

Popularised by Charles Darwin (1809–1882), the origins of species – as a concept – can be traced back to the centuries preceding the European Enlightenment, to the naturalist John Ray (1627–1705) who, in *Historia Plantarum*, introduced the concept to refer to the fixed and unchangeable classifications of organisms within which only limited variations may occur (Aldhebiani, 2018). In the 19th century, species and speciation[2] became central within early scientific attempts to define dementia as the *Fourth Species of Mental Derangement* (Pinel, 1806). It was not, however, until the middle of the 20th century that modern understandings of species, as a population that can only reproduce amongst itself to the exclusion of all others, were first established by the evolutionary biologist Ernst Mayr (1904–2005). Species-*ism*, then, may be understood as 'prejudice… in favour of the interests of members of one's own species and against those of other species' (Singer, 1975). Such systemic prejudice, according to Singer, is the only plausible explanation for humanity's treatment of nonhuman animals who, like humans, possess the capacity to experience pain, suffering and happiness.

As Wolfe (2003, 2010) argues, critical scholarship has largely failed to recognise the role that speciesism plays in the oppression of human and nonhuman populations alike. Wolfe (2003, p. 1), for example, states that:

> … debates in the humanities and social sciences between well-intentioned critics of racism, (hetero)sexism, classism, and all other -isms that are the stock-in-trade of cultural studies almost always remain locked within an unexamined framework of speciesism. This framework, like its cognates, involves systematic discrimination against an other based solely on a generic characteristic—in this case, species.

With the rise of posthumanist and new materialist ontologies, during the early decades of the 20th century, critical scholars have started to explore connections between speciesism and other forms of institutionalised oppression, including cognitive ableism. Braidotti (2013, p. 15) argues, for example, that equating subjectivity with 'consciousness, universal rationality, and self-regulating ethical behaviour' carries 'essentialist and lethal connotations' for bodies that are branded as Other (including nonhuman animals) who, through such discourse, become relegated to the 'less than human status of disposable bodies'. In order to move beyond speciesism, Braidotti argues, we need thinking tools for understanding subjectivity that are not predicated upon a hierarchical and essentialised division between the human and the nonhuman. In other words, we (humans) 'need to become the sorts of subjects who actively desire to reinvent subjectivity as a set of mutant values and to draw our pleasure from that ...' (Braidotti, 2013, p. 93). With its emphasis on de-centring rationality and promoting more inclusive understandings of embodied personhood, dementia studies offer an ideal site through which to develop our more mutant subjectivity (see also Chapter 15 and 17 in this volume).

Embodied subjectivity in dementia (across species)

Destabilising human exceptionalism compels us towards more 'mutant' understandings of embodied subjectivity (Braidotti, 2013), yet this goes against the grain of over two centuries of thinking within dementia studies. Since the late 18th century, attempts to understand the psychosocial seque-lae of dementia have been framed within an epistemological framework rooted in liberal humanist ontological assumptions about what it means to Be a person. This has served to make investigating the embodied experi-ence of dementia an exclusively human affair. If, for example, nonhuman animals do not possess either a sense of self, a family, a theory of mind, the capacity for reason or episodic memory, then they are, *ipso facto*, incapable of losing them. Over-reliance upon humanist phenomenology and symbolic interactionism within qualitative dementia research has served mainly to re-enforce this epistemic position. According to the 'founding father' of symbolic interactionism, G.H. Mead (1863–1931), humans alone are capable of generating and communicating meaning. If so, then attempts to generate thick, empathetic understandings of the embodied experience of dementia (*verstehen*), which are so central to qualitative dementia research, are only possible when both the observer and the observed are human.

There are several reasons, however, for challenging such an anthropo-centric worldview. As Arluke and Sanders (1996) and Sanders (2009) high-light, studies in ethology and ethnozoology suggest that some nonhumans are indeed capable of some forms of symbolic interaction, albeit in qualita-tively different forms to that of humans. Mammals capable of rules-based play, for example, appear to attach symbolic properties to physical objects (e.g. stick = toy/play), display an ability to take turns and create a 'shared definition' of the game (Arluke and Sanders, 1996; Sanders, 2009). As such, Arluke and Sanders argue that assertions that only humans are capable of generating and communicating meaning appear to be based more on *specie-sism* than on robust empirical evidence.

Animal bodies are also cable of experiencing age-related neuro-cogni-tive conditions. Studies in veterinary medicine, for example, suggest that the generation of senile plaque and neurofibrillary tangles that are char-acteristic of Alzheimer's Disease (AD) in older adults is also present in the brains of older nonhuman mammals diagnosed with Cognitive Dysfunction Syndrome (CDS). Such similarities in pathology between AD in humans and CDS in nonhumans have led some, such as Prpar Mihevc and Majdic (2019), to argue that AD and CDS are but two facets of the same disease. If nonhuman mammals are capable of experiencing age-related cognitive disorder, and are capable of being affected by the advent and progression of such conditions, then one can only summise that *speciesism* lies at the heart of why their embodied experiences have been systematically 'forgot-ten' (Davies, 2012) within qualitative dementia research.

Even within the human body, the embodied experience of dementia is not an exclusively human affair. Research from across the fields of biology, ecol-ogy, cybernetics and systems theory has highlighted how relations between the human and the nonhuman, at the microscopic level, are central to the accomplishment of human selves. Contemporary understandings of hori-zontal gene transfer, for example, suggest that in excess of 100 genes within the human genome originated from nonhuman species (Sheldrake, 2020), whereas endosymbiosis – the process in which one cell exists inside another cell, typically with mutual benefit – has long been theorised as providing the basis for the evolution of mitochondrial DNA (Gray, 2017; Margulis, 1970). In addition to cells within cells, the human microbiome is thought to con-stitute a universe of over 39 trillion microbial (nonhuman) cells, accounting for up to 3% of human body mass. These microbiota perform vital functions including, amongst other things, storing fat, activating genes, replacing damaged cells and preventing illness. As such, microbial relations within, for example, the gut and large intestine, are thought to play a pivotal role in brain functioning, influencing how affective states such as anxiety, agi-tation and depression are experienced (see, for example, Foster and Mcvey-Neufield, 2013; Lach et al., 2018).

Whole systems understandings of human subjectivity radically destabilise Enlightenment-based myths that persons are both indivisible and autopo-etic (i.e. self-producing and self-maintaining). As Gilbert, Sapp and Tauber (2012) poignantly argue, taking a relational view of life leads to the conclu-sion that humans have never been 'individuals', in the conventional sense of the term. Rather, whole systems understandings of human subjectivity appear better aligned with non-Western knowledge systems that have, for centuries, highlighted the *dividual* nature of personhood (Strathern, 1990) and humanity's inter-being (Nhat Hanh, 2017) within the more-than-human world.

Exploring the embodied experience of dementia across species offers dementia studies an opportunity to break free from its reliance upon 'com-pensatory' models of human subjectivity (Braidotti, 2013), within which human exceptionalist logic is simply inverted (rather than rejected) in the pursuit of more 'dementia friendly' understandings of embodied experience.

Kitwood (1997), for example, argues that people with dementia often display elevated levels of emotional engagement, whereas the rest of 'us' in our 'customary patterns of over-busyness, hypercognitivism and extreme talkativity' do not (Kitwood, 1997, p. 5). Aside from chronically lacking in empirical evidence, such assertions do little to challenge exceptionalist thinking. In contrast, by understanding the ways in which being affected by dementia is shaped by relations within the more-than-human world (at both the inter-corporeal and intra-corporeal level), we may begin to develop a clearer sense of the 'mutant subjectivities' which Braidotti (2013) alludes to.

Beyond (human) rights-based approaches

Rejecting human exceptionalism compels us to move beyond the language of (human) rights, in the pursuit of radical social change.

Parallel to the rise of the *Social Citizenship* movement (Bartlett and O'Connor, 2007, 2010), (human) rights have become the central framework through which activists, researchers, policy makers and practitioners have sought to challenge discrimination and pursue greater social justice in dementia. During the 21st century, legal frameworks such as the *Universal Declaration of Human Rights* (1948), the *International Covenant on Economic, Social and Cultural Rights* (1966) and the *Convention on the Rights of Persons with Disabilities* (2006) have so far provided the basis upon which global dementia policy is formulated (see, for example, World Health Organization, 2017 and as discussed in Chapter 12).

Whilst human rights-based approaches (HRBA) have led to tangible advances for many people with dementia, (human) rights are not the panacea that they are often held up as being. As D'Souza (2018) argues, (human) rights have a problematic history as their origins are intricately entangled with campaigns of colonialism and the forced displacement of indigenous populations that stem from the European Enlightenment project. Whilst, D'Souza argues, the language of (human) rights is much less radical now compared with when it was first introduced, during the period of the French Revolution, the demand for more rights has become ubiquitous within many contemporary social movements. Correspondingly, the number of (human) rights recognised within international law has increased from 30 (in 1948) to over 300. What is more difficult to observe, D'Souza argues, is any positive correlation between the proliferation of rights and changes in the socio-material conditions within which oppressed populations live and struggle. Thus, D'Souza argues, we need to shift critical focus away from asking, 'What do *we* want rights to achieve?' and towards asking, 'What do rights actually *do?*' Why, for example, are those in positions of power often so eager to adopt the language of (human) rights?

D'Souza (2018) is not the first critical scholar to question the emancipatory potential of rights. O'Neil (2005), for example, argues that the 'normative approach' to rights requires that institutions and individuals (rather than the State) are responsibilised for ensuring that the right to life, liberty, food, healthcare and other basic rights are met. This, O'Neil argues, leads to the creation of complex legal and bureaucratic landscapes within which those responsibilised for upholding rights become subjected to increased levels of surveillance, control and (ultimately) blame. As Rose (1985) argues, we need to consider the politics that underpin the language of rights and recognise that 'posing demands in terms of rights and entitlements as means of directing social resources' (p. 199) does little to disrupt our reliance upon human exceptionalist forms of moral reasoning.

By developing approaches that are not based upon speciesist notions of moral worth, multi-species theorising may help connect the pursuit of social justice in dementia with broader agendas for social change, including changes to the ways humans treat nonhuman life. In seeking to develop a trans-species framework for social justice, Matsuoka and Sorenson (2018) highlight how Iris Marion Young's five faces of institutionalised oppression (*exploitation, marginalisation, powerlessness, cultural imperialism, violence*) can identify points of connection in the oppression of human and nonhuman beings, thus providing a theoretical foundation for practising multi-species, anti-oppressive social work. In a similar vein, critical approaches to power and personhood within the field of dementia studies may help us to develop and deepen our affinities with the more-than-human world (see also discussion in Chapter 6). Behuniak (2010), for example, argues that Western understandings of Personhood expose people with dementia to *exploitative, manipulative*, and *competitive* forms of power. In contrast, rooting personhood in the embodied capacity to experience vulnerability enables people with dementia to access *nutrient* and *integrative* forms of power. Following Behuniak, both the human and the nonhuman 'have the potential of becoming vulnerable' and thus both 'should be the focus of our ethical responsibility of responding' (Behuniak, 2010, p. 237). Our shared capacity to be made vulnerable in dementia compels us to cultivate ways of 'collective knowing and doing' (Haraway, 2016, p. 36) that, following Behuniak, harness the power to Be. Following McShane (2018), attending to the ways in which we are made vulnerable through dementia can lead to new ways of responding to our increasingly precarious ecological situation. In this context, our shared vulnerability to, and in, dementia may be instrumental in cultivating what Tsing (2015) and Tsing et al. (2017) refer to as the 'Arts of Living' – new strategies for thriving ecologically, politically, economically and socially within the ruins of contemporary capitalism.

Concluding thoughts

This chapter has sought to offer some insights into how multi-species thinking can aid the critical turn in dementia studies. As should hopefully be clear, to explore dementia from the position of multi-speciesism is not to 'animalise' people with dementia nor anthropomorphise the experiences of nonhuman subjects. Yet, cultivating a more critical multi-species dementia studies is likely to face challenges on two primary fronts: first, there are those who will resist the rise of critical perspectives in dementia *per se*, as refocusing attention on oppression and liberation in dementia does not tend to align well with the 'strategic plans' of universities and public funding bodies. In this hostile climate, multi-species approaches will need to demonstrate their relevance, not just to advancing critical scholarship but to addressing a much wider set of social, economic and political questions that we now face, as we strive to find ways of living and dying well, together, on an increasingly damaged planet (Haraway, 2016; Tsing et al., 2017). Second, there are those working within critical traditions who may resist consideration of nonhumans as subjects within transformative scholarship. This is understandable, as to fully consider animals as embodied subjects within modern-day assemblages of dementia raises difficult and emotive issues, especially surrounding the use (or abuse) of animals in biomedical dementia research. If not handled carefully, a more critical multi-species dementia studies has the potential to surface some highly divisive fault lines. And yet, to not move beyond our reliance upon human exceptionalism in the search for a more radical ontological, epistemological and ethical project risks something equally problematic; namely, re-enforcing the centuries-old, well-intentioned belief that reliance upon the liberal humanist project will somehow lead to a more 'enlightened' approach to dementia across the world.

Notes

1 From the Greek, meaning 'life'.
2 The process through which species evolve.

Bibliography

Abram, D. (1996). *The Spell of the Sensuous: Perception and Language in a More-Than-Human World*. New York: Vintage Books.

Aldhebiani, A. (2018). Species Concept and Speciation. *Saudi Journal of Biological Sciences* 25(3), pp. 437–440.

Alexis, N. (2020). Beyond Compare: Intersectionality and Interspeciesism for Co-liberation with Animals. In: Fischer, B. (Ed.). *The Routledge Handbook of Animal Ethics*. New York: Routledge, pp. 502–515.

Arluke, A. and Sanders, C. (1996) Regarding animals, Philadelphia: Temple University Press.

Arluke, A. and Sanders, C. (2009). *Between the Species: Readings in Human-Animal Relations*. Boston, MA: Pearson Education, Inc.

Barad, K. (2007). *Meeting the Universe Halfway: Quantum Physics and the Entanglement of Matter and Meaning*. Durham: Duke University Press.

Bartlett, R., Gjernes, T., Lotherington, A.-T. and Obstefelder, A. (2018). Gender, Citizenship and Dementia Care: A Scoping Review of Studies to Inform Policy and Future Research. *Health & Social Care in the Community* 26(1), pp. 14–26.

Bartlett, R. and O'Connor, D. (2007). From Personhood to Citizenship: Broadening the Lens of the Dementia Debate. *Journal of Aging Studies* 21(2), pp. 107–118.

Bartlett, R. and O'Connor, D. (2010). *Broadening the Dementia Debate: Towards Social Citizenship*. Bristol: Policy Press.

Behuniak, S. (2010). Toward a Political Model of Dementia: Power as Compassionate Care. *Journal of Aging Studies* 24(4), pp. 231–240.

Braidotti, R. (2013). *The Posthuman*. Cambridge: Polity Press.

Bryant, C. (1979). The Zoological Connection: Animal-Related Human Behavior. *Social Forces* 58(2), pp. 399–421.

Carlson, L. (2001). Cognitive Ableism and Disability Studies: Feminist Reflections on the History of Mental Retardation. *Hypatia* 16(4), pp. 124–146.

Coole, D. and Frost, S. (2010). *New Materialisms: Ontology, Agency and Politics*. Durham: Duke University Press.

Davies, G. (2012). Caring for the Multiple and the Multitude: Assembling Animal Welfare and Enabling Ethical Critique. *Environment and Planning D: Society and Space* 30(4), pp. 623–638.

D'Souza, R. (2018). *What's Wrong with Rights? Social Movements, Law and Liberal Imaginations*. London: Pluto Press.

Foster, J. and Mcvey-Neufield, K. (2013). Gut–Brain Axis: How the Microbiome Influences Anxiety and Depression. *Trends in Neuroscience* 36(5), pp. 305–312.

Foucault, M. (1966). *The Order of Things: An Archeology of the Human Sciences*. London: Routledge Classics.

Gilbert, S., Sapp, J. and Tauber, A. (2012). A Symbiotic View of Life: We Have Never Been Individuals. *Quarterly Review of Biology* 87(4), pp. 325–341.

Goodley, D., Lawthorn, R. and Runswick-Cole, K. (2014). Posthuman Disability Studies. *Subjectivity* 7(4), pp. 342–361.

Gray, M. (2017). Lynn Margulis and the Endosymbiont Hypothesis: 50 Years Later. *Molecular Biology of the Cell* 28(10), pp. 1285–1287.

Haraway, D. (2008). *When Species Meet*. Minneapolis: University of Minnesota Press.

Haraway, D. (2016). *Staying with the Trouble: Making Kin in the Chthulucene*. Durham: Duke University Press.

Hulko, W. (2004) *Dementia and Intersectionality: Exploring the Experiences of Older People with Dementia and Their Significant Others*. Stirling: University of Stirling (Unpublished PhD thesis).

Jenkins, N. et al. (2021). Multi-Species Dementia Studies: Contours, Contributions and Controversies. *Journal of Aging Studies* 59, p. 100975.

Kirksey, S. and Helmreich, S. (2010). The Emergence of Multi-Species Ethnography. *Cultural Anthropology* 25(4), pp. 545–576.

Kitwood, T. (1997). *Dementia Reconsidered: The Person Comes First*. Buckingham: Open University Press.

Lach, G., Schellekens, H., Dinan, T. and Cryan, J. (2018). Anxiety, Depression, and the Microbiome: A Role for Gut Peptides. *Neurotherapeutics* 15, pp. 36–59.

Levi-Strauss, C. (1964). *Totemism*. Boston, MA: Beacon Press.

Lyman, K. (1989). Bringing the Social Back in: A Critique of the Biomedicalization of Dementia. *The Gerontologist* 29(5), pp. 597–605.

Margulis, L. (1970). *Origin of Eukaryotic Cells: Evidence and Research Implications for a Theory of the Origin and Evolution of Microbial, Plant, and Animal Cells on the Precambrian Earth*. New Haven: Yale University Press.

Matsuoka, A. and Sorenson, J. (2018). *Critical Animal Studies: Towards Trans-species Social Justice.* London: Rowan & Littlefield.

McShane, K. (2018). Loving an Unfamiliar World: Dementia, Mental Illness and Climate Change. *Ethics and the Environment* 23(1), pp. 1–16.Nhat Hanh, T. (2017). *The Art of Living: Peace and Freedom in the Here and Now.* New York: HarperCollins.

O'Neil, O. (2005). The Dark Side of Human Rights. *International Affairs* 81(2), pp. 427–439.

Pinel, P. (1806). *A Treatise on Insanity.* Strand: Messers Cadell & Davies.

Prpar Mihevc, S. and Majdič, G. (2019). Canine Cognitive Dysfunction and Alzheimer's Disease–Two Facets of the Same Disease? *Frontiers in Neuroscience,* 13, p. 604.

Ritvo, H. (2007). On the Animal Turn. *Daedalus,* 136(4), pp. 118–122.

Rose, N. (1985). Unreasonable Rights: Mental Illness and the Limits of the Law. *Law & Society* 12(2), pp. 199–218.

Said, E. (1978). *Orientalism.* New York: Pantheon Books.

Sanders, C. (2009). Close Relations between Humans and Nonhuman Animals. In: Arluke, A. and Sanders, C. (Eds.). *Between the Species: Readings in Human-Animal Relations.* Boston: Pearson Education Inc., pp. 45–52.

Scourfield, P. (2005). Social Care and the Modern Citizen: Client, Consumer, Service User, Manager and Entrepreneur. *British Journal of Social Work* 37(1), pp. 107–122.

Scull, A. (1979). Moral Treatment Reconsidered: Some Sociological Comments on an Episode in the History of British Psychiatry. *Psychological Medicine* 9(3), pp. 421–428.

Sheldrake, M. (2020). *Entangled Life: How Fungi Make Our Worlds, Change Our Minds, and Shape Our Futures.* London: Vintage Books.

Singer, P. (1975). *Animal Liberation: A New Ethics for Our Treatment of Animals.* London: Bodley Head.

Strathern, M. (1990). *The Gender of the Gift: Problems with Women and Problems with Society in Melanesia.* Berkeley: University of California Press.

Tsing, A. (2015). *The Mushroom at the End of the World: On the Possibility of Life in Capitalist Ruins.* Princeton: Princeton University Press.

Tsing, A., et al. (2017). *Arts of Living on a Damaged Planet: Ghosts and Monsters of the Anthropocene.* Minneapolis: University of Minnesota.

Ward, R. and Sandberg, L. (2019). Calling for (a more) Critical Dementia Studies. https://memoryfriendly.org.uk/programmes/critical-dementia-network/blog/calling-for-a-more-critical-dementia-studies/ (Accessed: February 11, 2022).

Wolfe, C. (2003). *Animal Rites: American Culture, the Discourse of Species, and Post-humanist Theory.* Chicago: University of Chicago Press.

Wolfe, C. (2010). *What Is Posthumanism?* Minneapolis: University of Minnesota Press.

World Health Organization. (2017). *Global Action Plan on the Public Health Response to Dementia 2017–2025.* Florence: World Health Organization.

8 Reframing 'ethnicity' in dementia research

Reflections on current whiteness of research and the need for an anti-racist approach

Maria Zubair

Introduction

Dementia research is characterised by a noticeable focus away from issues of 'race', racism and racialised social inequalities, not least when accounting for experiences of dementia within minority ethnic communities. In this chapter, I take into account the specific silence (even implicit denial and/or concealment) relating to 'race', racism and racialised social inequalities within dementia research relating to minority ethnicities. Conceptualising this silence and/or denial as a form of whiteness[1] (Ahmed, 2007a, 2007b; Bhambra, 2017), I present a number of critical reflections around how this whiteness of public health discourses and research agendas relating to dementia has important implications for knowledge production, social justice and social change. This discussion takes issue specifically with the particular conceptualisations of 'ethnicity' (Torres, 2015, 2019; Zubair and Norris, 2015) within the wider public health discourses around dementia and presents a critique regarding how these white discourses work as a mechanism to shift responsibility and blame collectively to members of the disadvantaged minority ethnic communities who are persistently constructed and represented as a 'problem' (Brotman, 2003; Torres, 2006; Zubair and Norris, 2015; Zubair and Victor, 2015). I argue, in particular, that the essentialist white dominant framings of (minority) 'ethnicity' within current dementia policy and research – that focus predominantly on a discourse of minority ethnic 'cultural difference' – neglect the lived realities of racialisation and marginalisation as experienced by minority ethnic people. These framings thus de-politicise the issue of (in)equitable minority ethnic access to dementia diagnosis, care and support.

Placing a strong emphasis on the need for a decolonisation of research agendas and frameworks with respect to dementia research, I argue here for the need for dementia researchers undertaking research with minority ethnic populations to also adopt anti-racist approaches to knowledge production. The adoption of such approaches would help highlight, challenge and counter (rather than silence, conceal or ignore) the racialised character of current knowledge production within this academic field. I highlight and

DOI: 10.4324/9781003221982-11

reflect upon, in detail, what I identify as the currently dominant Western (and white) framings of the dementia 'problem' with respect to minority ethnicities and the likely harms of such framings for minority ethnic populations. I contend that countering such dominant white framings of the minority ethnic dementia experience and dementia care inequalities needs to be a key priority for a critical dementia research agenda concerned with positive social change.

Minority ethnic dementia research as a white project

For an understanding of how current dementia research relating to minority ethnicities may be conceived of as being predominantly a white project (or, in other words, a white social and political endeavour – whether this happens consciously or habitually as routine, taken-for-granted, ways of understanding the issues), we can begin by considering this research sub-field's current relation to whiteness. Some of the pertinent questions we may want to reflect upon and consider include: in what ways is this sub-field of research informed by a white worldview? How is whiteness located and positioned, or positions itself (in its embodied, ideological and/or political forms) within this sub-field of research and its practice – including within its structures and research-related organisational hierarchies, spaces, methods and processes? How does this whiteness, in turn, also get reinforced and reproduced not merely within the research but through the research itself?

I will return to the questions outlined above during the course of my discussion in this chapter, but first I would like to start by noting a key observation that has been made by Ahmed (2007a) and, time after time, also by other scholars of 'race' and cultural studies (see, for example, Bell and Hartmann, 2007; Dyer, 1997; Fanon, 1963; Frankenberg, 1993; Hall, 1992; Headley, 2004) regarding the invisibility and unmarked character of whiteness which exists:

> ... as the absent centre against which others appear only as deviants, or points of deviation ... Whiteness is only invisible for those who inhabit it, or those who get so used to its inhabitance that they learn not to see it, even when they are not it ... Spaces are orientated 'around' whiteness, insofar as whiteness is not seen. We do not face whiteness; it 'trails behind' bodies, as what is assumed to be given.
>
> (Ahmed, 2007a: 157)

Ahmed (2007a) elaborates further on the normativity and privilege of whiteness whereby invisible marks of privilege – for example, even just possessing a white name or a body that is perceived to be white – bestow a certain power to white bodies to extend their reach in the spaces that they inhabit. This, Ahmed (2007a) notes, is unlike the experience of other bodies that are *not* white. As Fanon (1986: 109–111) has also previously observed in relation to bodies racialised as black, the latter bodies that are not white are likely to be constrained by the 'third-person consciousness' of their own body when these come into contact with those that are white – experiencing their being in such contexts through others, as 'the movements, the attitudes, the glances of the [white] other' fix them there. Building on and reinforcing Fanon's analysis, Ahmed (2007a: 161) observes that the bodies that are visible and marked by being *not* white remain restricted in what they can do, stopped in their movements or actions, and even 'diminished as an effect of the bodily extensions of [white] others'. White bodies, however, she argues, 'do not have to face their whiteness; they are not orientated "towards" it', and since their whiteness 'goes unnoticed', 'they do not get "stressed" in their encounters with objects or others', instead their bodies 'trail behind' in the performing of action and 'do not get in the way of an action' (2007a: 156).

Ahmed's (2007a) and Fanon's (1986) observations relating to how whiteness operates as a normative, invisible mark of racialised privilege – that while remaining unnoticed and invisible in its workings, affects unequal power relations with those marked and racialised as others – are critical to my own argument here regarding dementia research involving minority ethnicities as being a white project. As highlighted previously by various critical 'race' and cultural studies scholars with regard to the relationship between privileged and marginalised social positions (see, for example, Ahmed, 2007a; Fanon, 1963, 1986; Spivak, 1988, 1993), white privilege includes the white power from a privileged normative position to objectify, define, label, characterise, silence, stop and diminish the marked racialised others who are not white.

Of particular significance to my argument here is also Ahmed's (2007a: 157) observation that spaces acquire the shape and 'skin' of the bodies that inhabit them and are more orientated around some bodies than others. She specifically notes how '... institutional spaces are shaped by the proximity of some bodies and not others: white bodies gather and cohere to form the edges of such spaces'. I use Ahmed's (2007a) observations relating to the whiteness of spaces and their different orientations and proximity to different racialised bodies to extend an argument that academic and scholarly spaces (in this case, the academic and scholarly space of dementia research) are also oriented around whiteness, insofar as whiteness is not seen and remains unnoticed as an assumed given. Here, I refer to the whiteness of the academic, scholarly and research space as not something reducible to the presence of bodies with white skin that inhabit that space in larger numbers. Instead, I understand whiteness, following Ahmed (2007a: 158–159), as 'a way of inhabiting space' also beyond (or even despite) the more obvious materiality of one's body (as it appears to other bodies within that space). Whiteness inhabits, for example, through specific (white) orientations, ideologies, perspectives, sensibilities and sensitivities which allow claiming the space 'by the accumulation of gestures of "sinking" into that space', such that one is at ease with one's (embodied, social and ideological) environment, fits in, and by fitting into the space disappears from view (Ahmed, 2007a: 158–159).

Above, I have outlined some of the observations from critical 'race' and cultural studies that I view as pertinent to the sub-field of dementia research focusing on minority ethnicities. Now, I shall discuss the particular relevance of these observations to how we may understand the whiteness of this academic sub-field. These observations provide a useful framework for developing an understanding, particularly around how a largely unmarked academic research whiteness coheres to foster and promote a specific dominant white worldview with respect to its racialised others. Such a worldview is steeped in an essentialising discourse on the *other* (Fanon, 1963, 1986; Hall, 1992; Said, 1978). Moreover, this academic research whiteness, with its hegemonic perspectives relating to the experience of dementia within minority ethnic communities, may never become apparent, visible or noticed without a critical reading of the academic research. The latter would entail examining its processes along with some critical reflection around the role that it plays in essentialising, determining and silencing the peoples that are the focus of its interest – minority ethnic persons and communities.

My argument regarding current dementia research focusing on minority ethnicities as being predominantly a white project of knowledge production relates to two key aspects of this body of research. First, the specific structures of academic research development and organisation (as with research in most other academic fields beyond dementia research) mean that different racialised bodies (and institutions) are placed differentially. This is in terms of the power dynamics concerning both the conduct and control of the research (Burman, 2012; Nimako, 2012; Smith, 1999; Tamdgidi, 2012; Zubair and Victor, 2015). This power differential, based on the type of proximity to the research (and its control), works as a resource for whiteness. Whiteness thus takes the lead in not merely identifying the research agendas and what is worthy of research attention but also determining the framing of the issue(s) under consideration (Nimako, 2012; Smith, 1999). The result is a body of academic research led by whiteness, using white framings of the identified issue(s), and casting a white gaze on racialised others. Second, following on from the above, the implicit white conceptual, ideological and political underpinnings of this research reinforce and legitimise the racial status quo and its associated inequalities at the expense of the racialised others. This is the case even where these underpinnings of research may reflect the habitual or routine, taken-for-granted, knowledge and understanding of researchers shaped through a context of academic whiteness and coloniality of knowledge (Burman, 2012; Tamdgidi, 2012).

For further elaboration of my argument regarding this whiteness of dementia research, I now turn my attention towards a more specific analysis of the particular white worldview this research encompasses and facilitates in terms of its specific discourses, representations and positioning of minority ethnicities. As I do so, it is important to also highlight here that both the essentialism and tendency for silencing and negating alternative perspectives and voices within this sub-field of research are supported by a wider context of academic whiteness and coloniality (Burman, 2012; Nimako, 2012; Smith, 1999; Tamdgidi, 2012). The spaces of academic research, scholarship and knowledge production are orientated around white bodies and whiteness more generally to the extent that this normative whiteness (and its ideological hegemony) remains unnoticed by those that habitually inhabit these white spaces (Ahmed, 2007a). The experience of this whiteness and its normative discourses is, however, different for bodies and persons who are not at home in these spaces given their different relationship to whiteness, and for whom whiteness is not so invisible. I return here to Fanon's (1986: 116) description of the white gaze in terms of the experience of black bodies 'being dissected under white eyes, the only real eyes'.

Using such ideas as a starting point, there is a whole host of important interlinked questions to consider, with reference to dementia research focused upon minority ethnicities. These include:

- How exactly does whiteness and the white gaze position itself within this sub-field of dementia research?
- What (and who) is its focal point of attention, interest and observation?
- What does it take for granted, fail to see, or even turn a blind eye to?
- How does it look upon and perceive those that it sees as the 'others'?
- What does it do with respect to essentialising the latter's difference?
- How does it silence the perspectives and voices of these 'others'?

Let me share a personal anecdote here which usefully illustrates some of the ways in which academic whiteness operates in a research context. Specifically, I outline what this means for understanding the issue of minority ethnic positioning and representation under the white gaze of dementia research:

> I accompany a white senior academic colleague from my university to a meeting with a local South Asian community group organised around dementia. The purpose of this meeting is to undertake some initial work around building research contacts within the community in preparation for putting together a programme of research activities involving a focus on dementia within the local South Asian communities. The meeting starts and, after brief introductions, I am assigned the task of taking notes of the discussion by my senior colleague. My senior colleague is given the floor to open up the meeting with a brief introduction of the meeting's purpose. The senior colleague starts to explain the importance of the proposed programme of research activities by first

contextualising and framing 'the problem' that needs to be addressed
through undertaking the research – the identified issues of concern are a
lack of timely diagnosis of dementia among minority ethnic communities, and a lack of use of dementia services which is identified as putting
those living with dementia within these communities at a disadvantage.
As the senior colleague describes the issue, they also frame it contempo-
raneously in a specific way by adding, "It's not because there is racism.
The issues are more complex – there are language and cultural barriers
[to service access and provision for minority ethnic groups] ... There is
a clear need to raise awareness among BAME communities ...".

The senior academic in the anecdote above pre-defines the barriers to minority ethnic people's access to dementia diagnosis and services as not being
related to racism, even before they have embarked on their identified programme of research. This is the case even when there is a noticeable absence
of any significant piece of existing dementia research that has specifically
explored and/or systematically discredited the role of racialisation and/or
racism in minority ethnic people's experiences of dementia and/or their lack
of access to, and/or engagement with, dementia-related services. While I felt
an urge in that moment of time to point out this knowledge gap in the field
of dementia research, which continues to be organised largely around whiteness, my own status as an unestablished early career researcher working in a
subordinate role held me back from speaking.

In making sense of this anecdote, I return here to the observations made
earlier in this discussion relating to the privileged normative position of
whiteness, white bodies and white standpoints, which allows them to extend
their reach in the spaces that they inhabit without being noticed or having
to face their whiteness. My senior colleague's framing of the issues in this
regard was neither surprising nor stood out as unusual enough to warrant any
comment or dialogue among those present at the meeting. This is because,
within a broader context of the normative academic whiteness of dementia
research, the senior colleague's perspective, which silenced the role of 'race',
racism and racialised inequalities through the problematisation of minority
ethnic cultures instead, was already well-supported – even endorsed – by the
whiteness of the existing body of dementia research involving minority ethnicities (see, for example, Adamson, 2001; Berwald et al., 2016; Blakemore
et al., 2018; Bowes and Wilkinson, 2003; Mackenzie, 2006; Mukadam et al.,
2015). This perspective is further supported by wider white public and policy discourses such as those encapsulated within the UK's Prime Minister's
Challenge on Dementia (see, for example, Department of Health, 2015).

I looked around at the group of people attending the meeting, to see if
anyone would challenge the potential whiteness of such a perspective, but
everyone appeared to be silently listening on. Furthermore, backed by references to some of the earlier research work, undertaken with the same white

framings of the issue, this senior academic's particular framing of the problem powerfully shaped the ensuing discussion at the meeting. Consequently, a white gaze was directed exclusively upon the 'cultures' and perceived 'cultural deficits' of minority ethnic people, which silenced the introduction of any alternative perspectives on the issue. In the discussion that follows, I will elaborate further on this white framing of the issue, along with its implications for minority ethnicities and for knowledge production, social justice and social change.

De-politicised cultural framings of 'ethnicity' and its harms

Dementia research relating to minority ethnicities predominantly employs a discourse of 'culture' and 'cultural difference', whereby the barriers to minority ethnic people's access to dementia diagnosis and formal care are identified mainly in cultural terms. This includes culturally specific conceptualisations of dementia (Berwald et al., 2016; Giebel et al., 2016; Mukadam et al., 2015); culturally defined stigma around a dementia diagnosis and/ or accepting formal support (Berwald et al., 2016; Hailstone et al., 2017; Mackenzie, 2006); culturally determined norms, expectations and requirements around care (Bowes and Wilkinson, 2003; Duran-Kiraç et al., 2022; Sagbakken et al., 2020); and so on. Driven by an expressed concern for improving minority ethnic access to dementia diagnosis and support, this research is fundamentally defined by (and reinforces) a strong, ongoing 'awareness raising' agenda focused upon minority ethnic understandings and attitudes relating to dementia. This research is not devoid of references also to the need for 'culturally sensitive' and 'culturally appropriate' service provision in terms of the implications that are drawn from the research. However, the overall focus is on describing and characterising minority ethnic cultures alone – particularly as presumed bounded, fixed and discrete entities (Zubair and Norris, 2015). This keeps the white gaze of the dementia minority ethnic research directed solely towards minority ethnic populations, and on scrutinising, defining and labelling these populations' 'cultural difference'. References to the need for 'cultural appropriateness' of services and 'cultural competency' among practitioners are, however, seldom followed through by either turning the gaze on the health and social care services and practitioners or intervening in a real sense to culturally adapt the services and/or practitioner competencies, as also revealed by a recent scoping review of the published research undertaken in the UK (Blakemore et al., 2018).

The lack of appropriate attention to the study of the service organisation and delivery context (including its potential cultural adaptation), which relates closely to the issue of minority ethnic access and engagement, however, is not the only key issue here. The culture-focused framings of the minority ethnic access and engagement issue are problematic also in terms of the particular conceptualisation of 'ethnicity'. Ethnicity is understood and represented here in a mono-dimensional manner as simply being synonymous to a presumed bounded, fixed, and homogeneous ethnic culture (Zubair and Norris, 2015). The use of such a conceptualisation of ethnicity, as well as the associated culture-focused framework of the current minority ethnic dementia research, is familiar. It works in a similar way to how the dominant discourses of (cultural) diversity and 'inclusive' multiculturalism, even when celebratory, have been shown to function as mechanisms for the de-politicisation of racialised inequalities (Ahmed, 2007b, 2007c; Bell and Hartmann, 2007; Brotman, 2003; Pitcher, 2009). In the case of dementia research as well, the framing of the minority ethnic equality-of-access issue largely in terms of minority ethnic 'culture' and 'cultural difference' involves use of a de-racialised language. This effectively silences and makes invisible the critical role of 'race' and racialised social locations and positionings in creating inequalities for minority ethnic persons (Bonilla-Silva, 2014; Brotman, 2003). Minority ethnic identities are thus detached from their experiences of historical as well as current racisms and racialised exclusions (Bonilla-Silva, 2014; Daniels and Schulz, 2006). Consequently, the racialised character of the diagnosis and dementia care access inequalities remains concealed and untouched rather than being highlighted and addressed.

It is important to note here that the culture-focused framings of the issue, as discussed above, are harmful for minority ethnic people also beyond just simply silencing 'race' and hindering appropriate intervention in relation to racialised inequalities. These framings, in essence, represent white essentialist understandings of minority ethnic cultures and peoples, who are perceived, constructed, labelled and pre-determined in negative terms as the homogeneous, undifferentiated and problematic cultural *others* (Ahmad, 1989; Brotman, 2003; Torres, 2006; Zubair and Norris, 2015). As cultural *others*, minority ethnic persons (including whole communities) have become defined within both dementia and broader health research predominantly in stigmatising terms with reference to their presumed lack of knowledge and awareness of health conditions such as dementia (see, for example, Forbes et al., 2011; Ludwig et al., 2011; Nielsen and Waldemar, 2016; Parveen et al., 2017; Patel et al., 2020; Purandare et al., 2007). These populations have thus been characterised as being largely uninformed, but also additionally as deviant populations presenting extra challenges for services due to their own separate culturally defined 'special needs' (Brotman, 2003; Ronstrom, 2002; Torres, 2006).

The lack of recognition regarding the multi-dimensional and complex character of ethnicity – which encompasses much more than just a presumed fixed and static ethnic 'culture' (Barth, 1969; Cornell and Hartmann, 1998; Ford and Harawa, 2010; Modood, 2005; Song, 2003; Zubair and Norris, 2015) – while typical of dementia research, is undoubtedly problematic. As described above, this has serious implications for knowledge production relating to minority ethnicities, and thereby for social justice and social change. Acknowledging ethnicity's close interlinks also with particular racialised identities and statuses, however, is important from a social justice perspective. This is because such an acknowledgement allows for an understanding of how, rather than merely signifying specific cultural orientations, ethnicity also represents an individual's social location and positioning within a society (Ford and Harawa, 2010). This means recognising that, for persons with a minority ethnic or racialised affiliation, ethnicity as a social location also differentially shapes their exposure to the various ethnic and/or racial penalties as well as access to the opportunities and resources in society (Anthias, 2001; Bonilla-Silva, 2014; Ford and Harawa, 2010). This includes penalties, opportunities and resources that may have a bearing on a timely consultation for dementia-related symptoms. However, with such a recognition remaining largely missing from the current dementia research literature, given its particular de-politicised conceptualisations of ethnicity, the blame for the dementia diagnosis and care access inequalities remains attached to the minority ethnic persons and communities, resulting in stigmatisation of these minority ethnicities.

Shifting the responsibility and blame for the dementia diagnosis and care access inequalities on to minority ethnic persons and communities has negative implications for these persons and communities that go further beyond purely the issue of negative representation and stigmatisation. The reinforcement of negative stereotypes relating to minority ethnicities who are constructed as problematic, and these minorities' stigmatisation, through such blame-shifting further reinforces the minority ethnic persons' and communities' marginalised social positioning, affecting these peoples' health and life chances. Within some of the broader health research literature, such marginalisation (including that owing to identities that are racialised and/or stigmatised within healthcare contexts) has been shown to also have a negative impact on minority ethnic persons' trust in healthcare services and professionals. Often, this results in health-seeking delays and lower levels of healthcare utilisation among these groups (Allen et al., 2014; Gamlin, 2013; Lee et al., 2009; Martinez-Hume et al., 2017; Mclean et al., 2003; Progovac et al., 2020; Smith and Ruston, 2013; Tang and Browne, 2008).

It may then be argued that culture-focused framings of ethnicity could create a negative reinforcing feedback loop of ever-widening ethnic health inequalities. This is especially so when ethnic minority health and healthcare access inequalities are presented as grounded mainly in people's presumed cultural orientations and the disadvantages that these cultural orientations are seen to present. Culture-focused framings of ethnicity – which problematise minority ethnic cultures by presenting these as the main 'barrier' to minority ethnic engagement – are thereby likely to reinforce rather than counter racialised inequalities in dementia diagnosis and care access. This is because the reinforcement of negative cultural stereotypes, which also often represent and influence healthcare practitioners' own dominant white cultural frames of understanding, may often affect these practitioners' attitudes towards minority ethnic patients along with the character of their interactions with these patients (Holmes, 2012; Mclean et al., 2003; Tang and Browne, 2008). This, in turn, is likely to negatively affect the quality of the minority ethnic healthcare experience and these patients' future engagement with healthcare services (Aronson et al., 2013; Holmes, 2012; Lee et al., 2009; Mclean et al., 2003; Progovac et al., 2020). Arguably, this is particularly so for conditions such as dementia that may also be more widely stigmatised. However, while the current minority ethnic dementia research is preoccupied largely with the 'culture' of minority ethnic persons, it does little to understand or address the likely effects of perceived and experienced racism. Or, for that matter, the effects of racialised social locations and positionings (including those relating to healthcare contexts) on the dementia-related health-seeking practices within minority ethnic communities.

Un-silencing 'race' and racialisation through anti-racist research approaches

The harms associated with the outward-facing, essentialist, white gaze of dementia research on minority ethnicities raise a critical need to identify ways of countering this white gaze. This might include identifying ways of doing research that would unsettle the silence around 'race', racialisation and racism that is currently imposed by this white gaze. The biased, non-neutral, hierarchical and oppressive character of Western white research has long been recognised by decolonial scholars (see, for example, Mignolo, 2009; Smith, 1999, 2005). Much of this work identifies detrimental impacts in terms of representation and emancipation of peoples and communities who are not Western and/or white. Noting the positionality of indigenous or non-Western people vis-à-vis Western research, Smith (1999: 39), for instance, observes:

> As a site of struggle research has a significance for indigenous peoples that is embedded in our history under the gaze of Western imperialism and Western science. It is framed by our attempts to escape the penetration and surveillance of that gaze ..... Research has not been neutral in its objectification of the Other. Objectification is a process of dehumanization. In its clear links to Western knowledge, research has generated a particular relationship to indigenous peoples which continues to be problematic.

An important task with respect to the dementia research relating to minority ethnicities is therefore to re-direct the Western, white and also largely clinically informed gaze of the research back onto its own whiteness as well as that of the white clinical context of dementia diagnosis. This gaze has been shaped primarily by an overriding clinical concern around identifying dementia patients, labelling the condition and enforcing a diagnosis. Such shifting of the research gaze, in turn, needs to constitute not merely a decolonisation of the research but also adoption of approaches to knowledge production that are consciously anti-racist. In being anti-racist, these approaches should help to explicitly acknowledge, articulate, challenge and counter the racism and/or racial bias within the current research and its agendas and frameworks.

There are three key aspects of dementia research that need to be addressed in terms of acknowledging and making visible the likely role of 'race' and racialised social locations and positionings in creating dementia diagnosis and care access inequalities for minority ethnic persons. First, while minority ethnic communities (and their cultural understandings and attitudes) have been disproportionately positioned and viewed within this existing research as appropriate targets for change, there is a need to move beyond such *othering* culture-focused frameworks (Zubair and Norris, 2015). It would be more fruitful instead to interrogate why such presumably fixed and unchanging cultural understandings and/or attitudes may continue to persist for people from minority ethnicities. From an anti-racist research perspective, this would involve contributing to a new research agenda. Such an agenda would counter current constructions of minority ethnicities and cultures as problematic in themselves and, in doing so, point to the racism or bias underlying the current research frameworks and approaches. An anti-racist research agenda would also involve a significant move away from relying on oversimplified culture-focused explanations of lower engagement by minority ethnicities, which at present tend to form both the starting and end points of many research investigations. The anti-racist agenda would, instead, focus upon developing a nuanced, contextual understanding of the dementia-related knowledge and health-seeking practices within racialised and minority ethnic communities. It would take into account (and clearly articulate) the likely intertwining role of wider racialised inequalities, exclusions, racial discrimination and racialised subject positions (see, for example, Gamlin, 2013; Pullen et al., 2014; Smith and Ruston, 2013) in the creation of the diagnosis and care access inequalities.

Second, it is important to recognise the bias introduced with respect to knowledge production, through a sole focus of the white research gaze on the minority ethnic community context alone. This is a significant bias given that the structures, cultures and practices of the white health and social care institutions, services and/or professionals have largely escaped the scrutiny of this white gaze so far (see, for example, Blakemore et al., 2018). This is despite such structures and practices being critical to the experience, engagement and access of racialised and minority ethnic groups (Lee et al., 2009; Mclean et al., 2003; Progovac et al., 2020; Tang and Browne, 2008). Adopting an anti-racist approach to knowledge production therefore also requires turning the research gaze onto the whiteness of the dementia health and care context. There is a need, in particular, for developing a detailed understanding of how this context is perceived and experienced by racialised and minority ethnic persons. This means identifying health and social care institutions and settings, including the whiteness of these spaces and settings (and not exclusively the minority ethnic communities), as appropriate targets for potential intervention and change in the future.

Finally, the adoption of a research agenda that emanates from a commitment towards racial equity and justice requires the use of appropriate research methodologies, frameworks and processes that help counter and challenge the social hierarchies and inequalities traditionally imposed and/ or fostered (within and) via research itself (see Chapter 19 for further discussion of the importance of critical methodologies). Developing nuanced understandings of minority ethnic experiences, as well as shifting the research gaze onto the cultures and practices within healthcare settings is likely to be more fruitful in terms of a racial equity agenda if undertaken using appropriate research frameworks and methodologies. These need to be compatible, in turn, with a racial equity agenda in terms of supporting and encouraging an explicit acknowledgement and articulation of issues relating to 'race', racialisation and racism. This also means prioritising the perspectives of racialised and minority ethnic groups as the central axis around which the discourse on inequalities in access revolves (Ford and Airhihenbuwa, 2010a, 2010b; see also Chapter 16 by Hulko who explores the practice implications of doing this).

Conclusions: Shifting the gaze towards the whiteness of dementia research

In this chapter, I have argued that current dementia research relating to minority ethnicities is predominantly a white project of knowledge production. This is so, since a largely unmarked academic research whiteness has cohered to foster and promote a specific dominant white worldview in relation to its racialised others. My argument regarding the whiteness of this research relates to its two key aspects. First, the specific structures of academic research development and organisation mean that different racialised bodies (and institutions) are placed differentially. This is in terms of the power dynamics within the conduct and control of the research. Second, I argue that the implicit white conceptual, ideological and political underpinnings of this research reinforce and legitimise the racial status quo at the expense of racialised others. I take issue here specifically with the conceptualisations of 'ethnicity' within this sub-field of dementia research. The framing of the minority ethnic equality-of-access issue largely in terms of minority ethnic 'culture' and 'cultural difference' involves the use of a de-racialised language. This silences and makes invisible the critical role of 'race' and racialised social locations and positionings in creating inequalities for minority ethnic persons. I have also sought to highlight the harms of such de-politicised cultural framings of 'ethnicity' for minority ethnic persons and communities. Furthermore, I have argued that an important task is to re-direct the white gaze of this research back onto its own whiteness as well as that of the white clinical context of dementia diagnosis. Finally, I have identified some of the ways in which anti-racist approaches to knowledge production may be deployed within dementia research. The challenge here is to counter the racialised character of current knowledge production, thus paving the way for inclusive dementia research concerned with positive social change.

Note

1 I use the term 'whiteness' here, in the same way as Ahmed (2007a) does, to refer to a form of social and bodily orientation that is not reducible simply to white skin. Furthermore, this orientation may be habitual, unnoticed and/or taken for granted rather than necessarily conscious.

References

Adamson, J. (2001) 'Awareness and Understanding of Dementia in African/ Caribbean and South Asian Families', *Health and Social Care in the Community*, 9:6, 391–396.

Ahmad, W.I.U. (1989) 'Policies, Pills, and Political Will: A Critique of Policies to Improve the Health Status of Ethnic Minorities', *The Lancet*, 21:1, 148–150.

Ahmed, S. (2007a) 'A Phenomenology of Whiteness', *Feminist Theory*, 8:2, 149–168.

Ahmed, S. (2007b) 'The Language of Diversity', *Ethnic and Racial Studies*, 30:2, 235–256.

Ahmed, S. (2007c) '"You End Up Doing the Document Rather than Doing the Doing": Diversity, Race Equality and the Politics of Documentation', *Ethnic and Racial Studies*, 30:4, 590–609.

Allen, H., Wright, B.J., Harding, K. and Broffman, L. (2014) 'The Role of Stigma in Access to Health Care for the Poor', *The Milbank Quarterly*, 92:2, 289–318.

Anthias, F. (2001) 'The Concept of "Social Division" and Theorising Social Stratification: Looking at Ethnicity and Class', *Sociology*, 35:4, 835–854.

Aronson, J., Burgess, D., Phelan, S.M. and Juarez, L. (2013) 'Unhealthy Interactions: The Role of Stereotype Threat in Health Disparities', *American Journal of Public Health*, 103:1, 50–56.

Barth, F. (1969) 'Introduction', in F. Barth (eds.), *Ethnic Groups and Boundaries: The Social Organization of Culture Difference*. Long Grove: Waveland Press, 9–38.

Bell, J.M. and Hartmann, D. (2007) 'Diversity in Everyday Discourse: The Cultural Ambiguities and Consequences of "Happy Talk"', *American Sociological Review*, 72:6, 895–914.

Berwald, S., Roche, M., Adelman, S., Mukadam, N. and Livingston G. (2016) 'Black African and Caribbean British Communities' Perceptions of Memory Problems: "We Don't Do Dementia"', *PLoS ONE*, 11:4, e0151878.

Bhambra, G.K. (2017) 'Brexit, Trump, and "Methodological Whiteness": On the Misrecognition of Race and Class', *The British Journal of Sociology*, 68:S1, 214–232.

Blakemore, A., Kenning, C., Mirza, N., Daker-White, G., Panagioti, M. and Waheed, W. (2018) 'Dementia in UK South Asians: A Scoping Review of the Literature', *BMJ Open*, 8:4, e020290.

Bonilla-Silva, E. (2014) *Racism Without Racists: Colorblind Racism and the Persistence of Racial Inequality in America.* Lanham: Rowman & Littlefield.

Bowes, A. and Wilkinson, H. (2003) '"We Didn't Know It Would Get that Bad": South Asian Experiences of Dementia and the Service Response', *Health and Social Care in the Community*, 11:5, 387–396.

Brotman, S. (2003) 'The Limits of Multiculturalism in Elder Care Services', *Journal of Aging Studies*, 17:2, 209–229.

Burman, A. (2012) 'Places to Think with, Books to Think about: Words, Experience and the Decolonization of Knowledge in the Bolivian Andes', *Human Architecture: Journal of the Sociology of Self-Knowledge*, 10:1, 101–119.

Cornell, S. and Hartmann, D. (1998) *Ethnicity and Race: Making Identities in a Changing World.* London: Sage Publications.

Daniels, J. and Schulz, A.J. (2006) 'Constructing Whiteness in Health Disparities Research', in A.J. Schulz and L. Mullings (eds.), *Health and Illness at the Intersections of Gender, Race and Class.* San Francisco: Jossey-Bass Publishing, 89–127.

Department of Health (2015) *Prime Minister's Challenge on Dementia 2020.* https://www.gov.uk/government/publications/prime-ministers-challenge-on-dementia-2020 (accessed 2 July 2022).

Duran-Kiraç, G., Uysal-Bozkir, O., Uittenbroek, R., Hout, H. and Groenou, M.I.B. (2022) 'Accessibility of Health Care Experienced by Persons with Dementia from Ethnic Minority Groups and Formal and Informal Caregivers: A Scoping Review of European Literature', *Dementia*, 21:2, 677–700.

Dyer, R. (1997) *White.* London: Routledge.

Fanon, F. (1963) *The Wretched of the Earth.* New York: Grove Press.

Fanon, F. (1986) *Black Skin, White Masks.* London: Pluto Press.

Forbes, L.J.L., Atkins, L., Thurnham, A., Layburn, J., Haste, F. and Ramirez, A.J. (2011) 'Breast Cancer Awareness and Barriers to Symptomatic Presentation Among Women from Different Ethnic Groups in East London', *British Journal of Cancer*, 105:10, 1474–1479.

Ford, C.L. and Airhihenbuwa, C.O. (2010a) 'Critical Race Theory, Race Equity, and Public Health: Toward Antiracism Praxis', *American Journal of Public Health*, 100:S1, S30–S35.

Ford, C.L. and Airhihenbuwa, C.O. (2010b) 'The Public Health Critical Race Methodology: Praxis for Antiracism Research', *Social Science & Medicine*, 71:8, 1390–1398.

Ford, C.L. and Harawa, N.T. (2010) 'A New Conceptualization of Ethnicity for Social Epidemiologic and Health Equity Research', *Social Science & Medicine*, 71:2, 251–258.

Frankenberg, R. (1993) *White Women, Race Matters: The Social Construction of Whiteness.* Minneapolis: University of Minnesota Press.

Gamlin, J.B. (2013) 'Shame as a Barrier to Health Seeking among Indigenous Huichol Migrant Labourers: An Interpretive Approach of the "Violence Continuum" and "Authoritative Knowledge"', *Social Science & Medicine*, 97, 75–81.

Giebel, C.M., Jolley, D., Zubair, M., Bhui, K.S., Challis, D., Purandare, N. and Worden, A. (2016) 'Adaptation of the Barts Explanatory Model Inventory to

Dementia Understanding in South Asian Ethnic Minorities', *Aging & Mental Health*, 20:6, 594–602.

Hailstone, J., Mukadam, N., Owen, T., Cooper, C. and Livingston, G. (2017) 'The Development of Attitudes of People from Ethnic Minorities to Help-Seeking for Dementia (APEND): A Questionnaire to Measure Attitudes to Help-Seeking for Dementia in People from South Asian Backgrounds in the UK', *International Journal of Geriatric Psychiatry*, 32:3, 288–296.

Hall, S. (1992) 'The West and the Rest: Discourse of Power', in S. Hall and B. Gieben (eds.), *Formations of Modernity*. Cambridge: Polity Press, 275–320.

Headley, C. (2004) 'Delegitimizing the Normativity of "Whiteness": A Critical Africana Philosophical Study of the Metaphoricity of "Whiteness"', in G. Yancey (eds.), *What White Looks Like: African American Philosophers on the Whiteness Question*. New York: Routledge, 107–142.

Holmes, S.M. (2012) 'The Clinical Gaze in the Practice of Migrant Health: Mexican Migrants in the United States', *Social Science & Medicine*, 74:6, 873–881.

Lee, C., Ayers, S.L. and Kronenfeld, J.J. (2009) 'The Association between Perceived Provider Discrimination, Health Care Utilization, and Health Status in Racial and Ethnic Minorities', *Ethnicity & Disease*, 19:3, 330–337.

Ludwig, A.F., Cox, P. and Ellahi, B. (2011) 'Social and Cultural Construction of Obesity among Pakistani Muslim Women in North West England', *Public Health Nutrition*, 14:10, 1842–1850.

Mackenzie, J. (2006) 'Stigma and Dementia: East European and South Asian Family Carers Negotiating Stigma in the UK', *Dementia*, 5:2, 233–247.

Martinez-Hume, A.C., Baker, A.M., Bell, H.S., Montemayor, I., Elwell, K. and Hunt, L.M. (2017) '"They Treat You a Different Way": Public Insurance, Stigma, and the Challenge to Quality Health Care', *Culture, Medicine, and Psychiatry*, 41:1, 161–180.

Mclean, C., Campbell, C. and Cornish, F. (2003) 'African-Caribbean Interactions with Mental Health Services in the UK: Experiences and Expectations of Exclusion as (Re)productive of Health Inequalities', *Social Science & Medicine*, 56:3, 657–669.

Mignolo, W.D. (2009) 'Epistemic Disobedience, Independent Thought and Decolonial Freedom', *Theory, Culture & Society*, 26:7–8, 159–181.

Modood, T. (2005) *Multicultural Politics: Racism, Ethnicity and Muslims in Britain*. Edinburgh: Edinburgh University Press.

Mukadam, N., Waugh, A., Cooper, C. and Livingston, G. (2015) 'What Would Encourage Help-Seeking for Memory Problems among UK-based South Asians? A Qualitative Study', *BMJ Open*, 5:9, e007990.

Nielsen, T.R. and Waldemar, G. (2016) 'Knowledge and Perceptions of Dementia and Alzheimer's Disease in Four Ethnic Groups in Copenhagen, Denmark', *International Journal of Geriatric Psychiatry*, 31:3, 222–230.

Nimako, K. (2012) 'About Them, but Without Them: Race and Ethnic Relations Studies in Dutch Universities', *Human Architecture: Journal of the Sociology of Self-Knowledge*, 10:1, 45–52.

Parveen, S., Peltier, C. and Oyebode, J.R. (2017) 'Perceptions of Dementia and Use of Services in Minority Ethnic Communities: A Scoping Exercise', *Health and Social Care in the Community*, 25:2, 734–742.

Patel, H., Sherman, S.M., Tincello, D. and Moss, E.L. (2020) 'Awareness of and Attitudes towards Cervical Cancer Prevention among Migrant Eastern European Women in England', *Journal of Medical Screening*, 27:1, 40–47.

Pitcher, B. (2009) *The Politics of Multiculturalism: Race and Racism in Contemporary Britain*. Basingstoke: Palgrave Macmillan.

Progovac, A.M., Cortés, D.E., Chambers, V., Delman, J., Delman, D., McCormick, D., Lee, E., Castro, S.D., Román, M.J.S., Kaushal, N.A., Creedon, T.B., Sonik, R.A., Quinerly, C.R., Rodgers, C.R.R., Adams, L.B., Nakash, O., Moradi, A., Abolaban, H., Flomenhoft, T., Nabisere, R., Mann, Z., Hou, S.S.Y., Shaikh, F.N., Flores, M., Jordan, D., Carson, N.J., Carle, A.C., Lu, F., Tran, N.M., Moyer, M. and Cook, B.L. (2020) 'Understanding the Role of Past Health Care Discrimination in Help-Seeking and Shared Decision-Making for Depression Treatment Preferences', *Qualitative Health Research*, 30:12, 1833–1850.

Pullen, E., Perry, B. and Oser, C. (2014) 'African American Women's Preventative Care Usage: The Role of Social Support and Racial Experiences and Attitudes', *Sociology of Health & Illness*, 36:7, 1037–1053.

Purandare, N., Luthra, V., Swarbrick, C. and Burns, A. (2007) 'Knowledge of Dementia among South Asian (Indian) Older People in Manchester, UK', *International Journal of Geriatric Psychiatry*, 22:8, 777–781.

Ronstrom, O. (2002) 'The Making of Older Immigrants in Sweden: Identification, Categorisation and Discrimination', in L. Andersson (ed.), *Cultural Gerontology*. Westport: Auburn House, 129–138.

Sagbakken, M., Ingebretsen, R. and Spilker, R.S. (2020) 'How to Adapt Caring Services to Migration-Driven Diversity? A Qualitative Study Exploring Challenges and Possible Adjustments in the Care of People Living with Dementia', *PLoS ONE*, 15:12, e0243803.

Said, E. (1978) *Orientalism*. New York: Pantheon.

Smith, D. and Ruston, A. (2013) '"If You Feel that Nobody Wants You You'll Withdraw into Your Own": Gypsies/Travellers, Networks and Healthcare Utilisation', *Sociology of Health & Illness*, 35:8, 1196–1210.

Smith, L.T. (1999) *Decolonizing Methodologies: Research and Indigenous Peoples*. London: Zed Books.

Smith, L.T. (2005) 'On Tricky Ground: Researching the Native in the Age of Uncertainty', in N.K. Denzin and Y.S. Lincoln (eds.), *The SAGE Handbook of Qualitative Research*. London: Sage Publications, 85–107.

Song, M. (2003) *Choosing Ethnic Identity*. Cambridge: Polity Press.

Spivak, G.C. (1988) 'Can the Subaltern Speak?', in C. Nelson and L. Grossberg (eds.), *Marxism and the Interpretation of Culture*. Chicago: University of Illinois Press, 271–313.

Spivak, G.C. (1993) 'Subaltern Talk: Interview with the Editors', in D. Landry and G. MacLean (eds.), *The Spivak Reader: Selected Works of Gayatri Chakravorty Spivak*. London: Routledge, 287–308.

Tamdgidi, M.H. (2012) 'Editor's Note: To Be *of* But Not in the University', *Human Architecture: Journal of the Sociology of Self-Knowledge*, 10:1, vii–xiv.

Tang, S.Y. and Browne, A.J. (2008) '"Race" Matters: Racialization and Egalitarian Discourses Involving Aboriginal People in the Canadian Health Care Context', *Ethnicity & Health*, 13:2, 109–127.

Torres, S. (2006) 'Elderly Immigrants in Sweden: "Otherness" under Construction', *Journal of Ethnic and Migration Studies*, 32:8, 1341–1358.

Torres, S. (2015) 'Expanding the Gerontological Imagination on Ethnicity: Conceptual and Theoretical Perspectives', *Ageing & Society*, 35:5, 935–960.

Torres, S. (2019) *Ethnicity and Old Age: Expanding our Imagination.* Bristol: Policy Press.

Zubair, M. and Norris, M. (2015) 'Perspectives on Ageing, Later Life and Ethnicity: Ageing Research in Ethnic Minority Contexts', *Ageing & Society*, 35:5, 897–916.

Zubair, M. and Victor, C. (2015) 'Exploring Gender, Age, Time and Space in Research with Older Pakistani Muslims in the United Kingdom: Formalised Research 'Ethics' and Performances of the Public/Private Divide in 'The Field', *Ageing & Society*, 35:5, 961–985.

9 Frames of dementia, grieving otherwise in *The Father, Relic* and *Supernova*

Representing dementia in recent film

Sadie Wearing

In a particularly affecting moment in the 2021 BBC/BFI film *Supernova*, Tusker, a writer contemplating ending his life following a diagnosis of dementia, comments that his partner (Sam) is suffering, because 'you're not supposed to mourn someone while they're still alive'. He goes on to announce sardonically that 'he must be because I am'. This scene does a lot of work in the film's elaboration of the ethics of ending one's own life when faced with a diagnosis of 'dementia', and I start here because the film's focus on attempting, however imperfectly, to reflect on the experiences of living and dying with dementia from the perspective of the person with the condition (rather than those around them) might, at least initially, be understood, even applauded, as a characteristic of some of the more recent portrayals of dementia on film. These lines also establish one of the mainstays of critical commentary on the three films I discuss here – namely the idea that the condition is especially traumatising in its upsetting of the proper chronologies of grief. The focus on 'grieving for the living', which enacts a failure of recognition of the validity of the life that is evidently ongoing, is a trope only too familiar to critical accounts of dementia across the social sciences and the humanities. The equation of a dementia diagnosis as heralding the advent of an inevitable 'social' or 'living death' of the subject has been a feature of the ways that dementia is culturally and socially imagined, storied, and reproduced revealing, as Hannah Zeilig has pointed out, the 'underlying assumptions that infuse the political, social, and medical narratives that are told about these conditions' (Zeilig, 2014, see also Peel, 2014).

This chapter is not an exhaustive account of dementia on film, rather I am concerned here to note some recent iterations of the representation of dementia in mainstream narrative film, and to question whether these are evidence of new patterns of critical awareness emerging over the dilemmas of representation that dementia poses. In recent years, the number of 'critically acclaimed' films in Europe, the UK and the US about dementia has continued to flourish. There was perhaps evidence of the 'zeitgeist' nature of the condition in the first decades of the 21st century (Parker et al., 2021). Rather than attempting to tackle the breadth of this cultural production[1] which includes a range of types of films, from fiction to documentary to

DOI: 10.4324/9781003221982-12

workshops organised by and for people who have dementia, this chapter will analyse just three films, all released in the UK in 2020–2021: *The Father* (Dir. Florian Zeller), *Relic* (Dir. Natalie Erika James) and *Supernova* (Dir. Harry MacQueen). Whilst they are all English language 'mainstream' narrative feature films, they differ in important ways. Two are set in the UK and one is set in Australia and, more significantly, they cover a range of genres, from the family melodrama to horror. Such genre differences produce a wide range of 'feeling tones' (Ngai, 2007), with the potential to elicit a range of affective responses in the viewer. The circulation of these 'public feelings' (Berlant, 2011) may, in turn, have an impact on how the condition is understood culturally, socially and politically. But how far do these recent films challenge the problems that have already been identified as key questions for thinking through representations of this condition? (Or, more accurately, range of conditions.) Namely, the dangers of entrenching stigma, fear and denial and the production of 'epistemic injustice' (Capstick et al., 2015,) that ultimately dehumanises and renders abject the character (and, by implication, anyone else) who is identified with dementia?

These films raise a range of potentially productive issues for critical accounts of the portrayals of dementia on film. For example, has the perspectival shift, widely reported in press reactions to *The Father*, answered the critique of cinema that it has too often focused on the traumas of the caregiver and failed to attempt to represent the embodied experiences of those with dementia? (Basting, 2009, Chivers, 2011, Swinnen, 2012) If so, to what extent does this shift reflect a more progressive cultural narrative? Does *Supernova*'s elegy for a same-sex couple's relationship in the wake of dementia rearticulate the gendered dimensions of dementia and care that have interested critics or does it merely provide a homonormative gloss on what is essentially a powerfully 'affecting' argument for self-annihilation? And, finally, what shape does the cultural imaginary of dementia take in *Relic* when dementia is inflected through the horror genre? What might this offer to critical accounts concerned with questions of personhood and the ethics of representation? Whilst there is not enough space here to consider all these questions in detail, this chapter takes the opportunity afforded by this cluster of films all released within a year of each other to produce a 'snapshot' of the range of mainstream representations currently circulating in the light of some contemporary critical approaches to the representation of dementia on film.

For any critical account of dementia, an analysis of how narratives and images of the condition circulate is crucial. E. Ann Kaplan and Sally Chivers have succinctly summed up many of the issues raised over time about how dementia is represented. They argue, in their discussion of age panic in media discourses on dementia and care, that 'overwhelmingly negative images' are foremost, and these images, in turn, generate a range of 'powerful affects' in which fear dominates. The images are medicalising, ageist, highly racialised and socially limited often featuring care given to class privileged subjects by 'heroic family members' whilst 'racialised care workers' are 'backgrounded'. Kaplan and Chivers argue that the negative ways that Alzheimer's disease is 'visualised and conceptualised' have crucially important implications for practice and that improving care is dependent on recognising and challenging the meanings generated in cultural understandings of the disease. They conclude that critical analyses of the discourses surrounding dementia are therefore vital (Kaplan and Chivers, 2018).

Readings of cultural representations are an important aspect of a critical engagement with dementia because engaging with such representations enables both reflection on existing, circulating understandings of the condition and also an opportunity for interrogation of and challenge to these understandings. Representations are powerful agents in the world, often responsible for normalising and reinforcing dominant, negative, understandings of and attitudes towards 'otherised' people, including those with dementia. However, they are also complex and can operate in contradictory ways, challenging viewers to rethink their assumptions. Critical responses to dementia, and dementia studies as a field which seeks to challenge socially damaging understandings and to rethink the meanings generated around the condition, therefore need to engage with the 'powerful affects' generated through media representations and framings.

Frames of dementia, when is life greivable?

Before offering my own brief readings of these films, I want to return to the idea of 'grieving for the living' with which I began. One instantly notable aspect of the critical reception of these films was the emphasis laid on this notion. Many have noted that this is a consistent feature of public and media discourses on what it is like to negotiate the condition as a family member, loved one or carer. Mark Kermode reviewing *Relic* for *The Guardian* quotes the director of the film as explaining the film's concern to show 'the true terrors' of 'grieving for the loss of someone while they're still alive' (Kermode, 2020, NP). Peter Bradshaw echoed the sentiment in his review of *The Father*, where he finishes his piece with the same sentiment almost word for word: 'It is a film about grief and what it means to grieve for someone who is still alive' (Bradshaw, 2021, NP).

In framing dementia in terms of a temporal dysfunction in the processes of grieving the texts, and their reception, stress how loss functions as a structure in the narration of dementia. I have argued elsewhere that it is possible, often in unexpected quarters, to find popular narratives of dementia that complicate this and indeed offer much more nuanced accounts of *living* with dementia (Wearing, 2013, 2015, 2017). Nonetheless, the idea that the person with dementia is to be grieved for because they've been, euphemistically speaking, 'lost' whilst actually still alive is a powerful instance of dominant narratives of dementia that suggest it resembles a zombie-like state of living death (Behuniak, 2011). At the same time, it raises a series of ethical questions about the status of the person that remains, and is familiar in critical accounts of the social and cultural construction of dementia. My specific concerns here, however, focus on the perhaps slightly less familiar questions raised by the notions of grief and its relationship to recognition, and are influenced by Judith Butler's reflections on the powers of mourning and violence (2004, 2009). Mourning, it is argued, operates by designating some lives as more grievable than others and thus differentially allocates the status of human according to norms and frames, assigning value through discursive and cultural means.[2]

Butler's work, in asking 'when is life grievable?', illuminates the processes of exclusion and differentiation, of casting some lives as liveable and others as abject through a mediation on whether life is grievable and by extension how 'power functions differentially, to target and manage certain populations, to de-realise the humanity of subjects' (Butler, 2004, p. 68). Suggestively (given the metaphorical link Zeilig (2014) notes between dementia and the stealthy dangers of 'terrorism'), Butler points out how the US's opponents in the 'War on Terror' are figured as 'spectrally human, the deconstituted' (p. 91), placed outside of the conceptualisation of the human and through their 'ungrievability' linked to their status as 'like' the mentally ill.

> The terrorists are *like* the mentally ill because their mind set is unfathomable, because they are outside of reason, because they are outside of 'civilisation', if we understand that term to be the catchword of a self-defined Western perspective that considers itself bound to certain versions of rationality and the claims that arise from them.
>
> (2004, p. 72)

Whilst Butler is concerned here with the effects of state power enacted on Otherised populations, this is provocative for considering the ways that dehumanisation works in relation to (as Butler terms it) 'the mentally ill', who are by inference **already** designated as the 'spectrally human' in this analysis. Moreover, the links Butler makes to the question of grievability here are also worth pursuing since the specific attachment to the formulae 'grieving for the living' in relation to dementia does not deny that the life is grievable; rather, it confirms that the grief is firmly attached to the subject **but** only on condition that the subject remains recognisable as a subject of recollection. Hence, in these films the stress is given on whether the character recognises or importantly 'will recognise' in the future a loved one or carer. This constitutes an ironic contrast with the sense of recognition that Butler refers to, where it involves a much fuller cognisance of the 'ethical call' that recognition *of* rather than *by* the other affords. In *Frames of War*, Butler pursues this question of recognition via the philosopher Levinas to consider the ways in which the critical imperative is to learn to read the 'frames' that establish the 'norms' that encompass the human. The human in this analysis is always a contested category and one that needs to be constantly negotiated through the framings which operate as gatekeepers to who is included and excluded. The human is understood as 'a value and a morphology that may be allocated and retracted, aggrandized, personified, degraded and disavowed, elevated and affirmed' (2009, p. 76). Tellingly in relation to thinking about film and visual media, Butler suggests:

> If as …Levinas claims, it is the face of the other that demands from us an ethical response, then it would seem that the norms that allocate who is and who is not human arrive in visual form. These norms work to *give face* and to *efface*. Accordingly, our capacity to respond with outrage, opposition and critique will depend in part on how the differential norm of the human is communicated through visual and discursive frames. There are ways of framing that will bring the human in to view in its frailty and precariousness, that will allow it to stand for the value and dignity of human life, to react with outrage when lives are degraded or eviscerated without regard for their value as lives. And there are the frames that foreclose responsiveness.
>
> (2009, p. 77)

In this chapter I am interested in thinking with Butler's work to consider how recent films and the discourses within them 'frame' dementia and the lives of people who have it, paying particular attention to the cultural politics of mourning and grievability. It is difficult to ignore the politics of mourning in these films and the commentary on them; Butler's work highlights the question of *when* life is grievable and how the temporality of this relates to the conceptualisation of life as considered liveable. Examining ideas around appropriate modes and times of mourning raises questions that have been important for critical accounts of dementia, which, like Butler, have considered the processes of abjection and dehumanisation (see also Chapter 11 in this volume). For example, the 'ableism and sanism' that 'work in concert with each other, abjecting bodies as less than' (Thornycroft, 2020, p. 92), which, as Shakespeare, Zeilig and Mittler point out, limits the 'articulation of the rights of people with dementia and thus their ability to retain their humanity to the ends of their lives' (2019, p. 10).

Supernova, elegy for the living

As indicated at the outset of this chapter, Tusker is living, to use Sarah Lachlan Jain's expression in 'Prognosis Time' (Jain, 2007, see also Puar, 2009). Having received a diagnosis of dementia, the film follows Tusker and his partner Sam, as they take what is revealed as a very final road trip together. Sam learns on the journey that Tusker is planning to end his life as a result of his diagnosis. The film follows the genre conventions of both the family melodrama and the road trip. Tusker and Sam wrestle with the decision that Tusker has taken to kill himself, having gathered family and friends for a final party and having found a suitably beautiful and deserted cottage away from their shared home in which to die. Sam is a concert pianist, and the film ends with his performance of Elgar's Samut D'Amour, as if the film has not already sufficiently firmly set its tone as one of elegy and grief. Indeed, the film's tone is dominated by memorialising and elegy; the pair are returning to places that have significance for them, the landscape of the lake district literally enabling reflection on the permanence of the view over the inexorable changes that are occurring in Tusker.

Tusker's plan to end his life is a demonstration of his relentless commitment to a defence of his autonomy but it is also presented as a sign of his love and commitment to his partner, and what the caring role would mean for him. Sam's resistance to the suicide takes the form of both an acknowledgement of his own fear for the future and a refusal to enter into the debate: 'we're going to pretend this never happened', he insists, and 'we are not having this conversation', and whilst he claims he will care until the end, the outcome of their argument is never really in any doubt. The film increasingly frames Tusker as an isolated figure, pictured at one point alone in the very background of the frame, when he has 'wandered' down a lane panicking Sam. Despite being both materially comfortable and in a loving and supportive relationship, Tusker offers an eloquent defence of his right to die at the time of his choosing, whilst he is still able to recognise himself and his partner. Prognosis time here is time marked by dread, knowing the inevitability of the progress of the condition and that as Tusker puts it: 'there will be a time when I'll forget who is doing the forgetting'. Tusker is preoccupied by the imminent loss of what he considers to be his self; he declares both that the self is already fading, that he 'just looks like him', and that he is determined to 'be remembered for who I was not for who I'm about to become'. Ending his life before this fate literally worse than death occurs is, he says, 'the only thing I can control'.

The film then conforms to Anne Basting's 'tightly told tragedy' (2009), which she identified as typical of the ways that narrative feature films often story the condition. Such stories, it has been suggested, do nothing to challenge the stigma and fear surrounding the condition. Indeed, one might go further and suggest that the eloquence with which Tusker argues for his own annihilation, the beautiful backdrop against which he chooses to die, and the love and compassion with which he is surrounded render any other possible outcome unthinkable and intolerable, or, as Butler puts it, foreclosed. It is particularly significant that the scenes which end the film take place away from the couple's real home, their domestic space. The fantasy that is enacted here is one in which a retreat from the domestic space of relationality and care is represented as not only possible but commendable; Tusker literally finds a place to die that will obfuscate the need for care. In having Tusker articulate his desire to die, the film establishes the lucidity of the subject who is able to apprehend their own 'social death'. The implications of this are clear: this is a person whose ability to clearly see his own diminishment through progressive incapacity and to grieve for themselves makes sense of the decision to end his own life before what remains of his autonomy is lost forever. It is all the more moving because it is delivered with a certain knowing archness – the formulae of grieving for the living generally stress the pain and loss for the person 'left behind', usually in cinema the partner or child. In this film, however the expectation that the central focus of the narrative will be that of the person who has not been diagnosed with dementia is interrupted – and the narrative stays with the couple who are *both* 'grieving for the living'. This scene and the film more generally are both moving and troubling. In all the films I look at here, considerable screen time, attention and care are taken to register, even honour, however imperfectly, the experience of dementia of the person who has it as well as those that love them, but whether this attempt actually shifts the representations to a more critical analysis of the ways that dementia narratives operate to instil dread, horror and fear of the condition remains highly questionable.

Further, the living or social death that is understood here as particular to those with dementia has been challenged by Michael Banner (2013) who argues that assisted dying or euthanasia arguments are constructed as if the social has no material effect on the questions raised by 'late modern dying'. Specifically, the horror of social death imagined as specific to dementia in general and Alzheimer's in particular, Banner argues, is actually on a spectrum with 'long dying', which is much more typical for many, even most – with or without dementia – also include elements of such a social death. Extended and extensive isolation is common for the majority of the population who do not have economic and social capital.[3] Banner suggests that, given the links between social conditions and the losses of selfhood that accompany the end of life in a range of circumstances, it is crucial to track the specific aspects of selfhood and subjectivity that are at risk for those who are dying with Alzheimer's. This in turn would enable a better understanding of how practices of care and sociality might compound or ameliorate the experience. Careful study of people's lived experience, such as that enabled by ethnographic methods in social anthropology, he suggests, is needed in order to gain insights which would enable ethical practices. He calls attention in this discussion to the question of the 'horror' of dementia and the loss of care practices for the dying, which have accompanied increased longevity in the population at large.

In *Supernova*, though it seems too obvious to even note, the equation of the loss of cognition and memory equating to the total loss of selfhood that Tusker, ironically, manages so effectively to communicate has been challenged by those working with people with dementia. For example, Pia Kontos (2004) has advocated for an 'alternative vision' to the 'assumed loss of selfhood in the current construction of Alzheimer's disease' through a reconceptualisation of selfhood as 'embodied and reproduced through our practical and corporeal actions' (p. 846). The possibility of something meaningful continuing to exist between Tusker and Sam, perhaps through practices of care, and the possibility of, however altered, forms of subjectivity and selfhood surviving cognitive decline and increased incapacity and debility remain outside the film's field of intelligibility, outside the frame. The point here is not to claim that Tusker's insistence on exercising his agency and 'choice' whilst he still can is ethically wrong or incomprehensible; it is demonstrably rational within the framing offered. Rather it is to think about how this figuration of dementia sits alongside a pattern of representation within which *only* this course of action makes any sense.

'There's something doesn't make sense about this': The domestic uncanny[4] in *The Father*

If *Supernova* literally cannot imagine a future which would involve the actual practice of care for its central loving couple and instead provides the protagonist with a beautiful place and an appropriate time to die, *The Father* is far more interested in the practices and practicalities of caring and living with dementia. The tone of *Supernova* is elegiac and mournful, and it encourages the viewer to take solace from the sadness of its story in its expressions of love and tenderness and in its evocation of beautiful landscapes and classical music. However, the tone of *The Father* is quite different. Predominantly marked by the 'ugly feelings' (Ngai, 2009) of anxiety and dislocation, *The Father*, as many reviewers noted, subjects the viewer to an unrelentingly confusing and disorienting worldview, where the spectator repeatedly shares with the protagonist, Anthony, what appear to be certainties as to where and when we are, only to have these certainties whipped away in vertiginous betrayals of the norms of narration and cinematic time, space and conventional editing.

The opening of the film can serve as an example of how the film repeatedly sets up the viewer's alignment with the perspective of Anthony, and all that this restricted narration will induce, but without signalling this, leaving the viewer unsure and unsettled. The opening credits and opening scene are of a woman striding down a street of mansion blocks (situating the milieu of the film as that of well-heeled, wealthy London). Over these images is a soundtrack of classical music with insistent, staccato strings, which builds to an operatic aria that seems to be building to some kind of dramatic climax. We cut to the interior, the hall of a mansion flat with a large front door centre frame through which the woman enters calling 'Dad, it's me', the operatic score keeps building, the woman enters a room where she says, somewhat exasperatedly, 'there you are'. The man who has been sitting with headphones takes them off and the audience realise that the anxiety inducing soundtrack is not signalling the imminent dramatic expose of, perhaps, a dead body (it's not that film, though the Morse-like invocation of opera might be preparing viewers for something of the sort), rather the music is being played by the man himself through his headphones, 'what are you doing here?' He asks. In the ensuing scene they argue about how he's behaved towards a carer and whether the carer has stolen his watch. The awareness that we have been experiencing Anthony's sensations via the music foreshadows how the film will continue throughout to disorientate the viewer. This is achieved primarily by changes in the décor of the flat; it takes some time to understand that what seem to be the usual flashback structures of cinematic representations of time passing and actual memory are not this at all but are instead instances of Anthony's experiences of reality where 'doubles' of his family are found, 'new' characters appear, a son in law, a carer, who patiently or impatiently try to correct his understanding or behaviour. Doors, windows, fireplaces and corridors unexpectedly alter, whilst remaining uncannily familiar. Indeed, Freud's rendering of the 'uncanny' as, famously in German, the 'unhomely' or unheimlich is highly resonant here, because for Freud, ultimately, it is the proximity, the 'likeness' to what is familiar whilst remaining strange that induces the sensation of the uncanny. Anthony's experiences and by extension the viewer's are resonant of Freud's descriptions, as in the characters appearing as 'doubles'. At the beginning of his essay Freud seems to dismiss the idea that 'intellectual uncertainty' is necessarily constitutive of the uncanny, though he later admits not only that it may be but also that it is in contemplating another's altered state that may induce sensations of the uncanny (which has implications of the affective force of representations of dementia which, as so many reviewers note, 'haunt'). He is interested, too, in the way the uncanny is related to 'something repressed that recurs' and in the negotiation of spaces which are both familiar and strange:

> An involuntary return to the same situation, but which differ radically from it in other respects, also result in the same feeling of helplessness and of something uncanny …Or when one wanders about in a dark, strange room, looking for a door or the electric switch, and collides for the hundredth time with the same piece of furniture.
>
> (Freud, 1919, p. 237)

In *The Father's* interiors, we are repeatedly 'involuntarily returned' to the same situation with radical differences: kitchen cabinets are replaced seemingly randomly, a beloved picture is above a fireplace until it isn't, tables and layouts shift, and finally doors open onto entirely new spaces. From the hall we have become familiar with, we are taken through a door which opens onto a hospital ward where Anthony's 'other' daughter is hooked up to machines, and Anthony momentarily has to re-reckon with the grief of her death. Finally, the space 'resolves' one last time into that of another kind of 'home'. The film ends with Anthony in a care home, left overwhelmed by confusion and grief, not only for his daughter but also for himself: 'what about me, who exactly am I?' he asks and the audiences 'confusions' are resolved, with the devastating insight that he is entirely at the mercy of the figures of nurses who, it is intimated have, or may at any time, subject him to abuse.

In this reading of *The Father*, I've tried to account for the disorientating 'uncanny' experience of watching the film through an interpretation which mirrors the film's devices for offering a perspective on dementia which attempts to imaginatively reproduce experiences of the condition. In his review of the film Peter Bradshaw rightly notes that 'the universe is gaslighting Anthony with these people' and that in so doing it produces 'genuine fear' akin to watching a traditional horror film. The review in the *New York Times* also likens the experience as 'shockingly close to horror'. As so many have noted, when fear is the dominant affect associated with dementia, the social and cultural implications are concerning (Low and Purwaningrum, 2020) but does this film's stress on Anthony's complex ongoing humanity and vulnerability, briefly experienced, in however mediated a form, by the audience, complicate the negativity of the representation? How distinct is this from *Supernova*'s framing of dementia as the unliveable life?

Body horrors: Care, relationality and ethical responsiveness in *Relic*

If *The Father* was read as 'shockingly close' to horror, *Relic*, the final film under consideration here, is a genuine horror film, complete with traditional horror tropes such as spooky woods with intimations of flyblown corpses, supernatural manifestations in a house that seems determined to entrap its inhabitants within its shifting walls and a black mould-like growth which appears to infect not only the house but also the three generations of women who are struggling to exist within it, and, intermittently, to escape from it. The eldest of the three women, Edna, the grandmother figure, has dementia, and the film starts with her daughter Kay and granddaughter Sam returning to the family home because she has gone missing. During the course of the film the horrors of the house and what is happening to the grandmother are gradually revealed, as the younger women attempt to care for her and to persuade her to leave. The film ends with the house and its ambiguous mould-like substance 'winning', keeping the three women within its walls, with ambiguous effects.

David Thomson has noted that *Relic* was one amongst a rash of dementia-themed horror films in the last few years, and he questions their cultural function, 'maybe the genre metaphor is a way of not going deeper in human examination that's where my worry surfaces – that horror can be a strategy for diverting proper fear' (Thomson, 2020, p. 40). This 'proper fear' refers to the failures of taking responsibility for upholding 'decency' to others in our 'refusal to face reality' (p. 41), not least in the politics of immigration in the US that Thomson goes on to discuss. The implication is also, however, that the genre uses horror tropes to distract the viewer from dementia and death. Fear is invoked but only as a distraction. This perspective contrasts with many of the critical accounts of dementia narratives where the concern is that eliciting fear in relation to dementia produces epistemic injustices to people with the condition and stigmatises them and their carers. None-theless, Thomson's comments do alert us to think further about what these screen horrors are screening from view and what, conversely, a reparative (Sedgwick, 2002) reading of *Relic* might offer.

Eve Sedgwick uses the term 'reparative reading' to counter the tendency, or even orthodoxy, in critical thinking to indulge in 'paranoid' responses to culture. Paranoid readings are predicated on revealing supposedly hid-den truths of harms, as if exposure and suspicion are enough to counter a political reality where such aggression is often far from hidden. Reparative readings and impulses stem from a desire that is 'additive and accretive…it wants to confer plenitude on an object that will then have resources to offer' (Sedgwick, 2002, p. 149). For marginalised groups, this is particularly cru-cial, in order that they may be able to 'extract sustenance from the objects of culture – even of a culture whose avowed desire has often been not to sustain them' (pp. 150–151). Offering a 'reparative' reading of the films that depict dementia therefore includes the recognition that the lives of people with the condition are not 'sustained' by existing social formations and cultural production but hopes that critical engagement can also entail elements of reparation.[5] Such an orientation also follows Lisa Folkmarson Käll's lead. Käll suggests that the act of 'productive reading' of films is 'not only possi-ble but also of significant importance for rethinking conceptualizations of Alzheimer's disease and other conditions of dementia as leading to a loss of selfhood and identity' (2015, p. 269). She reminds us that

> cultural representations are not in any way simply given for a neutral spectator. Instead, they are continuously reproduced through per-ception, interpretation and analysis. Not only how characters with Alzheimer's disease are depicted but also how these characters are per-ceived and interpreted will matter for the ways in which stereotypical views of persons with Alzheimer's disease are reinforced, challenged, and transformed.
>
> (pp. 269–270)

Käll's discussion of two films about dementia, *Away from Her* and *En Sång För Martin*, is concerned with bringing 'to light how a constitutive inter-corporeal connection between embodied subjects forms individual expres-sions and ways of being in the world'. A graphic and frightening horror film might not seem likely ground for a similar expression of 'constitutive inter-corporeal connection' but I want to suggest that *Relic*'s concerns with the relations between carers and cared for, and generations closely related to embodied and radically altering subjects does, like the films Käll considers, 'offer encounters with existential and ethical dilemmas that do not afford easy solutions but instead demonstrate the continuously unfinished task of reflection, questioning and re-evaluation' (Käll, 2015, p. 270).

Unlike the realist dramas *Supernova* and *The Father*, and indeed the films Käll analyses, in *Relic* the fear is the point. The horror genre confronts dread and makes it explicit, enabling in this case, I suggest, an opportunity for reflection on questions of care, relationality and ethical responsiveness. In *Relic* the house, which behaves as a living, if decaying, breathing thing, is a domestic space encompassing memories not only of a family's growth but also of its traumatic relationship to past failings of care, generational haunt-ings of neglect. The house includes a stained-glass window, preserved from another property, in the vicinity, in which, it would seem, a relative was left to die alone and uncared for. More recently, Edna, or perhaps the house, appears to have been responsible for the entrapment of another vulnerable subject, Jamie, a neighbour who has Down's syndrome (a helpful reminder that other groups are subject to the stigmatisations and aggressive projec-tions of others due to their cognitive differences[6]). Some form of retribution for this failing seems to be enacted here when the house and the growths of black hair like 'mould' spread through walls and into Edna and, eventually, her daughter and granddaughter.

One reading of the film might note the 'monsterisation' of the grand-mother, whose dementia is represented as 'contagious', thus reproducing precisely those harmful and stigmatising tropes so often reproduced in representations. However, another reading is possible. Perhaps more tell-ing than the Alice in Wonderland-like shrinking of walls which entrap the younger generation 'with' the grandmother (which might be conventionally read as a crude and cruel 'allegory' of what it means to care for someone) is the final scene of the film where, despite the terrifying horrors they have lived through in the house, the younger women choose to stay and care for what is left of their mother/grandmother. In this final scene, layers of encrusted gore are carefully and lovingly removed by Kay from her mother's body, and she is gradually revealed as an entirely altered being, almost a new-born, clean and 'new' a child-like or perhaps alien-like being, 'unrecognisable' perhaps but still responded and related to, 'I can't leave her' insists Kay, and her daughter also cannot leave her own mother. The soundscape here is of an eerie wheezing, almost but not a death rattle. Kay and her daughter lay down with 'relic', three generations of women repudiating the legacy of abandonment and neglect.

Conclusion: New directions or more of the same?

Critical analysis of film reveals the cultural meanings which accrue to the various conditions that make up the term 'dementia'. Tracking even subtle shifts in the ways that the condition is imagined is an important part of a wider critical project to interrogate understandings of the term, and the ways that it can operate in stigmatising, and ultimately dehumanising, ways.

Countering these tendencies requires a critical approach which is attentive to the work that representation does in 'framing' dementia and the human subjects connected to it. The three films I have analysed here do signal a shift towards a perspective that puts the person with the condition rather than their partner or family at the centre. They highlight the specific form of vulnerability that the condition produces, and they stress the need to find accommodations with a common circumstance of life. However, they also reproduce longstanding tropes that equate the loss of memory with a catastrophic loss of selfhood and autonomy. Films about people who have dementia matter because they participate in, reproduce and challenge public understandings and feelings about the condition and its effects on those who live with it.

The three films here offer a variety of perspectives on the condition and the ethical questions its representation raises in terms of recognition, responsibility and understandings of subjectivity. In *Supernova*, the melancholic attachment to the sovereign self, autonomous and relentlessly rational, envisages relationality as circumscribed to literal self-sacrifice and provides a fantasy of the good death which literally cannot include or envisage the ravages of the condition. Whilst within the framing of the film this is, of course, entirely intelligible, like Michael Haneke's *Amour* its equation of love with death raises difficult questions over the recognition of life in 'prognosis time'. Tusker's articulate defence of his right to control the timing of his death and the loss of the self he is grieving is hard to resist. Not least because Sam has no vocabulary with which to counter this claim to autonomy, given his own fears that he won't be able to cope with the care required and that indeed his own selfhood is at risk. In the logic of their understandings of their subjectivity there does indeed seem no viable option to recognise a value in continuing a life beyond memory, no concept of living and staying in the present is available to either character. Most disturbingly the film offers the compensatory fairy tale sop of conceptualising death as offering eternal life as stardust (hence the title of the film).

The Father, by contrast, refuses any such compensatory schema and instead, for much of the film, 'gaslights' the viewer into experiences which are designed to put the spectator into Anthony's psychological state, to experience with him the dislocations and traumas of living with dementia. Whilst this film conforms to many of the most fear-inducing capacities of representations of people with dementia, the film's insistence on maintaining its focus on Anthony, rather than his daughter, and the emphasis that is placed on his perspective and vulnerability opens up space to think through the specific forms of vulnerability and violence that some people with dementia are subject to – not least because of the dehumanising tropes with which the condition is so often associated.

Finally, *Relic* uses the most evidently grotesque and disgusting imagery to, ironically, tell a tale of redemption, care and shared vulnerability. One way to consider these films might be to consider how someone newly diagnosed with dementia or someone caring for someone newly diagnosed might respond. In what ways do these representations lift the 'heavy weight of negative cultural representations [which] clouds the collective vision of the person living with dementia'? (Shakespeare et al., 2019). Whilst I have endeavoured here to offer reparative or positive readings of these films, these questions remain both pertinent and fraught.

Notes

1 I'm using the term 'mainstream' quite loosely here to describe films which are both commercially oriented and widely screened in cinemas and across major streaming platforms and reviewed in both broadsheet newspapers and specialist film journals and which don't announce themselves as 'oppositional' or 'activist' cinema.
2 It is important to note that these reflections, particularly in *Precarious Life* and *Frames of War*, come out of the context of the US's post-9/11 wars. Butler's concern is with the ways in which the US's targets and detained subjects are, through the suspension of their status as legal subjects, conceptualised as outside of the norms of the human. As such the work is concerned with the operations of state power in the management of otherised peoples and populations. The racialised and cultural contours of these arguments are key and I am cognizant of the dangers of suggesting that representations of the privileged white subjects who dominate the films I am concerned with here are directly comparable to the victims of the US in Abu Ghraib or Guantanamo Bay.
3 This economic reality is provocative when considering how many of the films about dementia in the US and the UK feature highly educated, middle-class well off protagonists. Sam and Tusker in *Supernova* and Anthony in *The Father* are typical in this regard.
4 I'm indebted to Amber Jacobs for this term which she used when curating a series of film screenings which had the domestic uncanny as a highly generative theme.
5 See also Heather Love (2010).
6 See Shakespeare et al. (2019) for a discussion of the links between struggles for rights for people with learning disabilities and those with dementia. For an exploration of the necessary re-evaluation of 'slow life' in relation to people with learning disabilities see Hickey-Moody (2015).

References

Banner, M. (2013) 'Dying and "Death before Death": On Hospices, Euthenasia, Alzheimer's and on (not) Knowing How to Dwindle', in *The Ethics of Everyday Life*. Oxford: Oxford University Press, pp. 107–134.

Basting, A. (2009) *Forget Memory*. Baltimore: John Hopkins University Press.

Behuniak, S.M. (2011) 'The Living Dead? The Construction of People with Alzheimer's Disease as Zombies', *Ageing & Society* 31, pp. 70–92.

Berlant, L., 2011. 'Cruel optimism', in *Cruel Optimism*. Durham: Duke University Press pp. 23–49.

Bradshaw, P. (2021) '*The Father* Review: Anthony Hopkins Superb in Unbearably Heartbreaking film', *The Guardian*, 10 June 2021.

Butler, J. (2004) *Precarious Life, the Powers of Mourning and Violence*. London: Verso.

Butler, J. (2009) *Frames of War, When Is Life Grievable?* London: Verso.

Capstick, A., Chatwin, J. and Ludwin, K. (2015) 'Challenging Representations of Dementia in Contemporary Western Fiction Film: from Epistemic Injustice to Social Participation', in A. Swinnen and M. Schweda (eds.), *Popularizing Dementia, Public Expressions and Representations of Forgetfulness*. Bielefeld: Transcript Verlag, pp. 229–251.

Chivers, S. (2011) *Old Age and Disability in Cinema*. Toronto: University of Toronto Press.

Freud, S. (1919) 'The "Uncanny"', in J. Strachey (ed.), *The Complete Standard Edition of the Works of Freud*, Volume XVII. London: Hogarth Press, pp. 219–233.

Hickey-Moody, A. (2015) 'Slow Life and Ecologies of Sensation', *Feminist Review* 111, pp. 140–148.

Jain, S. (2007) 'Living in Prognosis: Toward an Elegiac Politics', *Representations* 98(1), pp. 77–92.

Käll, L.F. (2015) 'Intercorporeal Relations and Ethical Perception', in A. Swinnen and M. Schweda (eds.), *Popularizing Dementia: Public Expressions and Representations of Forgetfulness*. Bielefeld: Transcript Verlag, pp. 253–274.

Kaplan, E. and Chivers, S. (2018) 'Alzheimer's, Age Panic, Neuroscience: Media Discourses of Dementia and Care', Oxford Research Encyclopaedia of Communication. Retrieved 10 February 2022, from: https://oxfordre.com/communication/view/10.1093/acrefore/9780190228613.001.0001/acrefore-9780190228613-e-765.

Kermode, M. (2020) '*Relic* Review: Heart-Breaking Horror about Alzheimer's', *The Guardian*, 1 November 2020.

Kontos, P. (2004) 'Ethnographic Reflections on Selfhood, Embodiment and Alzheimer's Disease', *Ageing and Society* 24, pp. 829–849.

Love, H. (2010) 'Truth and Consequences: On Paranoid Reading and Reparative Reading' *Criticism* 52(2), pp. 235–241.

Low, L.F. and Purwaningrum, F. (2020) 'Negative Stereotypes, Fear and Social Distance a Systematic Review of Depictions of Dementia in the Context of Stigma', *BMC Geriatrics* 20, p. 477.

Ngai, S. (2007) *Ugly Feelings*. Cambridge and London: Harvard University Press.

Parker, J., Cutler, C. and Heaslip, V. (2021) 'Dementia as Zeitgeist: Social Problem Construction and the Role of a Contemporary Distraction', *Sociological Research Online* 26(2), pp. 309–325.

Peel, E. (2014) 'The Living Death of Alzheimer's versus 'Take a Walk to Keep Dementia at Bay: The Metaphor of Dementia in Print Media and Carer Discourse', *Sociology of Health & Illness* 36(6), pp. 885–901.

Puar, J.K. (2009) 'Prognosis Time: Towards a Geopolitics of Affect, Debility and Capacity', *Women and Performance a Journal of Feminist Theory* 19(2), pp. 161–172.

Sedgwick, E. (2003) 'Paranoid Reading and Reparative Reading, or, You're So Paranoid, You Probably Think This Essay Is About You', in *Touching Feeling*, Affect, Pedagogy, Performativity. Durham and London: Duke University Press, pp.123–151.

Shakespeare, T., Zeilig, H. and Mittler, P. (2019) 'Rights in Mind: Thinking Differently about Dementia and Disability', *Dementia* 18(3), pp. 1075–1088.

Swinnen, A. (2012) "Everyone is Romeo and Juliet!" Staging Dementia in Wellkåmm to Verona by Suzanne Osten. *Journal of Aging Studies* 26(3), pp. 309–318.

Thomson, D. (2020) 'Who's Afraid of Fear?' *Sight and Sound*, November 2020, pp. 38–41.

Thornycroft, R. (2020) 'Crip Theory and Mad Studies: Intersections and Points of Departure', *Canadian Journal of Disability Studies* 9(1), pp. 91–121.

Wearing, S. (2013) 'Dementia and the Biopolitics of the Biopic: From *Iris* to *The Iron Lady*', *Dementia* 12(3), pp. 315–325.

Wearing, S. (2015) 'Deconstructing the American Family. Figures of Parents with Dementia in Jonathan Franzen's *The Corrections* and A.M. Homes' *May We Be Forgiven*', in A. Swinnen and M. Schweda (eds.), *Popularizing Dementia, Public Expressions and Representations of Forgetfulness*. Bielefeld: Transcript Verlag, pp. 43–67.

Wearing, S. (2017) 'Troubled Men: Ageing, Dementia and Masculinity in Contemporary British Crime Drama', *Journal of British Cinema and Television* 14(2), pp. 125–142.

Zeilig, H. (2014) 'Dementia as a Cultural Metaphor', *The Gerontologist* 54(2), pp. 258–267.

Part III
Care and control

Part II

Care and control

10 Precarity and dementia

Amanda Grenier and Chris Phillipson

Introduction

Ideas and assumptions about cognitive impairment, combined with approaches to ageing organised around productivity, success, and activity, have contributed to views of dementia as an unsuccessful, 'failed', or 'frailed' old age. Dominant frameworks on ageing and late life often configure frailty and dementia as the opposite of a 'healthy' or 'active' late life, and at the socio-cultural level, frailty and dementia signal a fall into the 'fourth age', typically associated with decline and dependency (see Baltes and Smith, 2003; Gilleard and Higgs, 2015; Grenier, 2012; Laslett, 1991). Public discourses on dementia often convey disease-led definitions accompanied by notions of fear and the end of life. Dementia has been represented as a dreaded disease and 'horrific' end to life (Gilleard and Higgs, 2010), a 'social death' (Mulkay and Ernst, 1991), and 'ageing without agency' (Gilleard and Higgs, 2015). Consider the 2013 statement 'Dementia steals lives' (UK Department of Health, 2013) and the proposed response of finding 'a cure or disease modifying therapy by 2025' (see World Dementia Council). As noted by George (2010: 586), this everyday language shapes social perceptions, aligning dementia with enmity and fear, and leads to dementia being seen 'as something external to us'.

Ideas about dementia as 'failure' and 'deterioration' seep into health and social care practices and everyday encounters, with organisations and institutions arranged in ways which reflect and further enact these realities both through treatment and spatial formations. Institutional practices mark the boundaries of health and illness, with frailty and dementia configured as locations of risk, and targets for particular types of treatments. For example, the provision of care for people with dementia reveals an intricate relationship between care, the economy, and private interests (e.g. the pharmaceutical industry and nursing home sector) (Estes, 1979; Polivka and Luo, 2019); evidence and enactments of biomedical interpretations of ageing (Estes and Binney, 1989); and moments where dementia may collide with a loss of rights and citizen entitlements (Phillipson, 2015). They also result in spatial dimensions where people with frailty tend to live at home

DOI: 10.4324/9781003221982-14

(often alone), and people with dementia live with members of their family or in long-term care (Portacolone, 2013). Further, within long-term care, responses to frailty or dementia take place on different wards, floors, or sections of the facility. Whether taken for granted, or 'imagined', ideas about frailty and dementia as decline, and the segregation to particular places, re-enforce stigma, and the marginalisation/exclusion of people living with the diagnosis. Dementia and living in long-term care present us with the need to examine responses to dementia and vulnerability, how these configure older people with dementia as devalued subjects, and the subsequent failures of state that arise with regard to care in times of crisis.

This chapter considers dementia through the lens of precarity, examining the structured and lived experiences of people with dementia living in long-term care. In earlier work, we have suggested that older people living with dementia experience exclusion and precarity, and that agency in dementia may be differently expressed and/or recognised (Grenier and Phillipson, 2013; Grenier et al., 2017). This chapter extends this analysis, drawing on ideas about precarity to think through exclusion, biomedicalisation, and the failure to adequately respond to the needs of older people with dementia, with particular reference to older people living in residential care and/or nursing homes. We begin by outlining what we mean by precarity and situating precarious ageing as a new phase in the social construction of later life. We then explore how the intersecting features of the biomedicalisation of ageing, financialised care structures, and the construction of people with dementia in need of care as devalued subjects contributed to experiences of abandonment and suffering. The discussion gives particular attention to the impact of COVID-19, the results of which have powerfully illustrated the devaluation of people living in care homes in general, and those with dementia in particular.

Precarious ageing as a new configuration of late life

Our interpretation of precarity and dementia is rooted in critical gerontology which draws attention to power dynamics, and the relationship between social structures and experiences, particularly as enacted through institutional and organisational practices (Dannefer, 2021). The concept of precarity highlights insecurities, unwanted risks, and costly hazards of contemporary life that result from global change, declining social protection, and new forms of discrimination (Gallie et al., 2003; Grenier et al., 2017; Schram, 2015). Historically, the concept of precarity has been applied to labour force conditions and working age adults. A central tenet is that neo-liberal capitalism has created a precariat class characterised by a lack of job security, including intermittent or underemployment (Standing, 2011, 2021). As emphasised by Grenier et al. (2017: 12):

> Precarity draws attention to the implications of neo-liberal practices
> that have altered late life through the combined impact of …short-term

contracts, falling trade union membership, and declining forms of social protection that include a reliance on family/kin or market care, and private market pensions.

More generally, the concept of precarity has been used to understand how shifting social and political contexts create insecure and challenging conditions and circumstances for many older people (see Grenier et al., 2020). These include those brought about by anxieties related to changes in function or cognition, and/or the need for care (Grenier et al., 2017).

Although insecurity and inequality have long been embedded in the lives of older people, the idea of precarity suggests a distinctive shift in mechanisms of institutional support with regard to care. In the case of the Global North, three types of changes may be observed with regard to formal care systems to assist people through the life course. The first, developed over the decades from the 1950s to the 1980s, was characterised by the consolidation of a *welfare state* marked by (age-based) features such as mandatory retirement, state pensions, and occupational benefits of various kinds (Phillipson, 2013). This initial phase, while offering universal supports and measures to lift older people out of poverty, was criticised for constructing older people as a dependent group, and characterised by paternalistic structures and relationships, and rigid age-based and normative interpretations of the life course (Estes, 1979; Townsend, 1979).

The second phase, characteristic of the period from 1990 to 2020, was dominated by a focus on so-called *'active ageing'*, with measures to extend working life and promote what was termed a 'successful' and 'healthy' later life (Calasanti and King, 2021; Timonen, 2016). Such frameworks challenged age-based and decline-centred models, but in a way that gave primacy to healthy and youth-driven versions of ageing. In this response, divisions emerged between older people deemed to be in the *third age* and thus representing success, and groups of older people relegated to the *fourth age* as a result of impairment and/or disability, and thus denied access to the attributes of active, healthy, and successful ageing. Ageing became dichotomised into self-reliance and individual strength, or the failure thereof, as marked by dependence, deterioration, and a need for care. This polarisation between healthy ageing and frailty reverberated into the dividing practices of service eligibility whereby older people were depicted and classified as either independent and self-reliant or vulnerable targets of service (Grenier, 2007). In doing so, the production and reproduction of unequal ageing through service systems and structures was overlooked.

The argument developed here is that a third phase of ageing is now underway, with the period of 'active ageing' replaced by one more accurately defined as *'precarious ageing'*, reflected in the weakening of institutional supports provided through the labour market and the welfare state, and reinforced by the impact of COVID-19 (Christakis, 2020; Tooze, 2021) and emergencies created by uncontrolled fires and flooding associated with climate change (Vince, 2022). This new phase is unique with regard to thinking about ageing because it suggests not only how changes occurring through the life course influence later life to shape ageing in particular ways, but also how what appears as individual or social relationships result from political choices, financialised priorities, and the constructions of valued/ devalued subjects. This period of precarious ageing reveals the impacts of social change, and how inequality accumulates in later life, thereby affecting certain groups of people more than others. Our argument is that older people with dementia, especially those who live in long-term care, are one such group who are particularly affected by this new phase of precarious ageing. For people living with dementia, precarious ageing can be seen to take place at the intersection of biomedical definitions of disease and need (and being in need), the structure of care systems, and being cast as a devalued subject. In the next section, we explore each of these forces as contributing to precarious ageing.

Biomedicalisation of ageing

COVID-19 has prompted us to reconsider the biomedicalisation of ageing as a means to further understand various forms and iterations of precarity, and to explain the pandemic responses to people living in care homes, the majority of whom are likely to have some form of dementia. Estes and Binney, in an influential essay, outlined how the '"biomedicalisation of ageing" socially constructs old age as a process of decremental physical decline and places ageing under the domain and control of biomedicine' (1989: 587). Our argument is that the emergency conditions of the pandemic served to increase the power of biomedicine and its influence over the lives of older people. The experiences of older people who require access to health and care were already heavily medicalised through assessments of function and/ or cognition, and in particular, the categorisations and spatial configurations of frailty and dementia. It is thus not surprising that a group that was already dominated by disease-based models and health practices of functional and cognitive assessment has found these reinforced as a result of the conditions imposed by COVID-19.

COVID-19 has intensified the biomedical reach over the lives of older people with functional and cognitive impairments, and particularly those living in long-term care, where there have been multiple violations of human rights (for evidence in the UK see Amnesty International, 2020; Calvert and Arbuthnot, 2021). Drawing on Estes and Binney, COVID-19 revealed the two inter-twined aspects of biomedicalisation:

> (1) the social construction of ageing as a medical problem (thinking of ageing in terms of a medical problem) and (2) the praxis (or practices) of ageing as a medical problem (behaviors and policies growing out of thinking of ageing as a medical problem).
>
> (1989: 587)

Decisions about responses to COVID-19 and policy became a contested terrain between government, medicine, and public health, with the role of sociological analysis often marginalised. Yet, within these debates, medical and health responses have given authority to the exclusion of other perspectives and been enacted with little attention to the social implications that such measures of isolation and restricted social contact would entail (see also Chapters 11 and 12 for further discussion of these conditions).

The situation of older people in residential care homes is illustrative of the failure to address the social dimensions of the pandemic. This has happened across a number of institutional settings, including our respective locations of Canada and the UK. In the UK, this has to be seen in the context of 39,017 people living in residential and nursing homes in England whose deaths certificates involved COVID-19 (for the period from April 10, 2020 to March 31, 2021). Along with this catastrophic toll came the mental anguish of people locked away from family and friends during the period of lockdown, with the majority of homes imposing severe restrictions on the movement of residents within homes (Alzheimer's Society, 2020).

In Toronto, Canada, the location purported to have one of the longest early periods of global lockdown, older people experienced up to 66 consecutive days of isolation in one stretch (many being confined to their rooms), with practices only shifting to mirror broader community approaches to isolating close contacts late in the pandemic[1] (Seniors Services and Long Term Care, 2020). Such practices of power exercised by public health and medical professionals illustrate precisely the sets of social relations noted in Estes and Binney's (1989: 587) work on biomedicalisation, where the power of medicine combined with other features relating to industry and the economy. What the pandemic brought to the surface was how thinking about issues such as COVID-19 exclusively as *medical problem* ignores the cultural, economic, and social processes which underpin both the distribution of illnesses and deaths and the conditions under which daily life is experienced (see, further, Marya and Patel, 2021).

The impact of biomedicalisation during the pandemic has been to reveal the way in which older people were simultaneously *'protected'* (quarantined at home and in care homes) and *'abandoned'* (in some cases with the complete withdrawal of staff in countries such as Italy and Spain).[1,2] This was especially so in relation to residential and nursing home care, where in the case of the UK, untested hospital patients were discharged into care homes with inadequate supplies of personal protection equipment (PPE), and agency staff working across multiple homes, thereby increasing the chance of infection, and a lack of oversight from government and statutory agencies (Amnesty International, 2020; Calvert and Arbuthnot, 2021). Similar responses took place in Canada, where the military was called in to assess conditions in long-term care, producing a damning report which documented 'Patients observed crying for help with staff not responding for (30 min to over 2 hours)', 'Inadequate nutrition due to significant staffing issues, most residents were reported to not having received 3 meals per day and there was a significant delay in meals', and whereby 'at the time of arrival many of the residents had been bed bound for several weeks; No evidence of residents being moved to wheelchair for part of day, repositioned in bed, or washed properly' (Mialkowski, 2020).

Precarity: Structures of need and care

One of the foundations of our argument and interest in precarity and ageing is that the need for care is the crucial pivot for definitions and responses to older people. Transitions into care invariably have transforming effects, whether in respect of self-image, status, and/or identity. However, rather than being grounded in discussions of care, such transitions often become overshadowed by a focus on age itself. From this perspective, welfare state responses can be seen to be triggered by attention to age, but further articulated through notions of protection and dependence, as well as ideas about shared risks and the social contract. As responses to ageing moved to approaches centred around 'activity' and 'success', the emphasis shifted towards the importance of self-reliance, and a retreat from models of protection, as illustrated by ideas such as 'living well with dementia' and an emphasis on self-management and peer support. This corresponds with both the cultural imperative of independence and the neoliberal emphasis and retrenchment of the welfare state. Indeed, the valorisation of the third age resulted in a denial of seeing or witnessing the needs of those in the so-called fourth age. Older people and their families were expected to take responsibility for care, and care provision increasingly moved into the market through managed care and for-profit care homes (see Fine, 2020; Polivka and Luo, 2019; Simmonds, 2021). Older people with care needs were relegated to the fourth age, both socially and culturally, and through care practices which divided and relegated the classifications of need and the spaces within which older people in need would receive care.

What we see in the latest phase through which ageing is managed is a deeper entrenchment of the medical and spatial configurations of needing care in late life combined with the political economy of marketised care across various national contexts of the West, and even in Nordic countries that are often assumed to have the best models of welfare state public provisions of care (Meagher and Szebehely, 2013). Our suggestion is precarious ageing can be seen to elongate the risks and negative social constructions that have come to be associated with the fourth age, albeit in a slightly different way. Two iterations seem to be happening in this regard. First is that this fourth age is not only representative of a social or cultural construct (Gilleard and Higgs, 2015) but also illustrative of a set of practices that abandon and neglect older people with care needs, most of whom have dementia or are deemed to be frail. Second, and related, is how these sets of practices are inter-twined with the political economy of care (see Armstrong and Armstrong, 1996). For example, high costs of market system care create divisions between those who can afford private care and those who cannot, thereby reconfiguring 'deservedness' into an individual and familial responsibility for risk. In such models, care for older people plays out slightly differently within public and private care system models.

The relationship between need and care became acutely visible in responses to COVID-19. Biomedicalisation, along with the emphasis on independence and the evolution of care as a market-based issue, drastically diminished the quality of life of older people living with dementia in care homes. COVID-19 exposed what political economists of care and social gerontologists have argued for some time, in particular the extent to which care is configured as a profitable industry, the financial instability of the public care home sector (its own precariousness reflecting that of its clientele), chronic shortages of staff, and the marginalisation of 'social' over 'health' care needs (Armstrong and Armstrong, 1996; Estes, 1979; Simmonds, 2021). COVID-19 rendered the fault lines of care glaringly and publicly visible through the pressures facing low-paid staff, shortages of protective equipment, and the lack of support from statutory providers (Calvert and Arbuthnot, 2021).

The pandemic revealed the shift towards responses of care characterised by *precarious forms of ageing*. Precarity draws attention to the politics of care and creates the conceptual capacity to link understanding of the structures which produce particular social relations, whether medical, institutional, or political, with the ontological experiences which accompany these locations. The challenges within existing care structures, and priorities of care, thus not only created greater exposure of older people to the risks of COVID-19, but did so in a way that reveals the intricate power relations between systems, structures, and devalued subjects who need care. Older people's social needs and lived experiences became marginalised to interventions carried out under the rhetoric of protection. And yet, the ways in which care was enacted in institutional contexts multiplied risks as a result of structures of care characterised by congregate spaces with shared bathrooms, labour distribution patterns of part-time work that had emerged as part of managed care, and the reliance on family models. Indeed, features of private and market care were found to increase the risks of older people living in these settings. For example, in Canada, and in some of the large conglomerates in the United States, care homes which subscribed to part-time labour contracts where workers moved across multiple sites and locations per day (primarily private homes) had higher levels of infection than facilities that employed full-time unionised workers (Wallace and Winsa, 2021).

As Butler (2009: 25) poignantly notes, precarity is a 'politically induced condition in which certain populations suffer from failing social and economic networks of support and become differentially exposed to injury, violence, and death'. Our argument is that the current response to care that we characterise as *precarious ageing* extends and deepens the risks and negative impacts experienced by older people, because responses are not only about the structures (biomedical and otherwise) and economic configurations of care, but also about how choices are bolstered and sustained by 'politically induced conditions' that are interconnected with whether or not one is viewed to have a life deemed to be 'worth living' and, as argued by Butler, 'worth preserving' (Butler, 2009; see further Grenier et al., 2020).

Precarity: Impact on and through devalued lives

Care responses to, and provision for, older people cannot be separated from the social, cultural, political, and economic contexts within which they occur. Precarity and dementia viewed through a lens of precarity, and as part of a broader transition to responses of *precarious ageing*, offer a location to unpack how the symbolic and actual exclusion of older people with dementia is intricately linked with the intersection of biomedicalisation, financialised care markets, and ideas about devalued subjects (Simmonds, 2021). Standing (2011, 2021) defines a 'precarious life' as characterised by a chronic state of uncertainty and instability. The consequences can lead to a 'truncated status' associated with a loss of basic rights (civil, political, economic, social, cultural) for some groups (e.g. certain medical conditions, migrants, the homeless).

Throughout the pandemic, older people living in care homes (many of whom had dementia) experienced a restriction of movement, limited social interaction, and likely also possible confusion and social isolation (Mialkowski, 2020; Seniors Services and Longterm Care, 2020). It is here that the relationship between the structures and everyday life is profoundly revealing. In Butler's (2006, 2009) work on precariousness, she develops the argument that we all experience 'precariousness' in our lives, that 'interdependence' is a feature of the human condition—that '[...] precariousness implies living socially, that is, the fact that one's life is always in some sense in the hands of the other' (Butler, 2009: 14). The lives of older people in care homes were without question entirely in the hands of others, but with minimal levels of social protection.

As a result, there was an acceleration in the transition to *precarious ageing* which had been underway before the pandemic. Older people in the time of COVID-19 came under the control of medical and health professionals as well as institutional spaces, and, in doing so, crystalised a new phase of precarious ageing in which social selves, needs, and relationships were neither recognised nor permitted. Responses of care were overlooked—reconfigured around neglect and abandonment that we describe as precarious ageing. In this sense, older people with dementia became yet another example of what Povinelli (2011) terms 'economies of abandonment', where the emphasis on liberal economies causes groups to suffer neglect and abandonment, and systems permit devalued subjects to suffer and 'let die' (see Grenier, 2021). Where older people differ is that this suffering is also legitimated by dually powerful forces of biomedicine and the political economy. As such, our analysis as critical gerontologists should not only focus on the social exclusion of people living with dementia but also on the transition to a more politically induced precarity that is characterised by suffering and abandonment.

Discussion

The example of people living with dementia in care homes reveals the movement to a new phase of precarious ageing with an intensification in the extent of unmet needs. To date, our attention to precarity and ageing has focused on more material examples, related to poverty and deprivation witnessed in urban centres, migration, or late life homelessness (see Grenier et al., 2020). The analysis of precarity, as it is experienced from within the location of dementia, provides a specific illustration that links more closely with two longstanding areas of biomedical critique within critical gerontology, and the financial marketisation of care (Polivka and Luo, 2020). It exposes the extent to which the dominance of the biomedical discourse, combined with the privatisation of care systems, and devalued subjects in the case of the pandemic, obscured social needs for interaction, citizenship, and human rights.

Responses to older people with dementia in the context of the pandemic reveal the existence and entrenchment of *precarious ageing* at the intersections of biomedical dominance, private care markets, and a widening politics of neglect. Early contributions to critical gerontology revealed how the biomedicalisation of ageing resulted in undue focus on the medical and functional needs of older people (Estes, 1979). Over time, we have witnessed how the biomedicalisation of ageing has come to dominate and shape care responses to older people, particularly through functional assessments of frailty and cognitive impairment (dementia), and altered responses to care. In each, the dividing practices of being frail (or not) or having dementia (or not) are used to assess impairment and allocate and ration services that are medical and rehabilitative. Practices thus prioritise care needs that are biomedical/functional in nature, leaving the social dimensions of ageing, care needs, and life course transitions outside of what is deemed 'medically necessary', and thus an individual/familial responsibility. Further, when carried out in the context of a financialised care market, divisions emerge between those who can afford to make 'choices' about care and those who must receive their care within rationed public contexts, offering uneven opportunities to circumvent the systems most heavily weighted with standardised medical practices and the stigma of needing care.

Care needs within the context of financialised care markets and understood and responded to via biomedical practices also configure the spaces between home, family, and institution. Models of care organised around individual and family responsibility, and the shortage of services to support people living with dementia at home and in the community (Simmonds, 2021), have resulted in public services being heavily rationed. As the bar for eligibility for limited services continues to rise, the ranks of home care services and long-term care facilities are increasingly populated by people with high level needs that require heavy levels of nursing care, with the majority of older people living in care facilities having dementia and/or frailty. This relegates older people with frailty or dementia to particular spaces and, symbolically, to the status of 'others', with those who live in care facilities removed from the public view and often located in former forensic or medical institutions (Achenbaum, 1995; Katz, 1996). Once in long-term care, often by means of having few other options, or needing 24-hour support, this group is structured outside public view, social boundaries, and regular social interactions. Such configurations produce not only exclusion based on residence, but social relations and imaginaries that solidify *precarious ageing*. This includes, for example, the within institution social and spatial divisions between older people with frailty and dementia, who often occupy separate floors or sections of the facility according to their diagnosis. The power and politics of the spatial configurations based on biomedical assessments, devalued subjects, and care markets become crucial to understanding the response to older people living with dementia in care homes during COVID-19, and as we argue, responses to care that are reflective of precarious ageing.

Critical gerontologists have drawn attention to the problematic sociocultural interpretations of living with dementia as a 'lost life', a 'fate worse than death', and of long-term care as a last resort (Gilleard and Higgs, 2010; Kontos and Naglie, 2007). The suggestion we make in this chapter is that living with dementia is a particular location of precarity related to needing care, and one which demonstrates the perfect storm of conditions which produced a non-response to care based on abandonment and neglect. There are a number of features that can be seen to contribute to the devaluation of subjects, and responses which overlook the experiences of older people living with dementia who need care. In addition to the fear and stigma associated with dementia, older people with dementia are more likely to live in long-term care facilities and have high care needs that increase over time (Bartlett and O'Connor, 2007). The interactions of people living with dementia thus become limited to the particular institutional sphere—with contacts often comprised of care workers and families (where available). Further, communication may be limited, both by means of the number of contacts and by impairments of speech or memory that mean the stories and accounts of people living with dementia in care settings are discounted. The features of the need for care, institutional location, and heightened potential for exclusion create conditions of risk and vulnerability. Attention to the analysis of precarity and precariousness, however, reminds us how devalued lives are pushed to the margins of society, abandoned or neglected by means of not being deemed worthy of care, and subject to cruel and unnecessary punishment (see Povinelli, 2011; Sassen, 2014). It is precisely these conditions that fostered responses to institutionalised older people in COVID-19, demonstrating how precarity and precariousness can affect (and legitimise) social abandonment and neglect (Calvert and Arbuthnot, 2021).

COVID-19 produced the conditions for the phase of precarious ageing, as witnessed in the lives of people living with dementia in institutional care settings. Older people with dementia were viewed as devalued subjects, and conditions of suffering were permitted to take hold (see also Introduction and Chapter 11). People living with dementia in care homes have a need for medical, instrumental, and social interaction/support. Yet, pandemic responses left basic needs unmet and ignored (Mialkowski, 2020). In many cases across a range of international settings, older people were locked in, abandoned, and denied (in-person) interaction of their families and supports. Their lives became limited to health encounters enacted by medical professionals and personal care workers (Tapper, 2021). Many older people died in long-term care facilities, sometimes in dreadful conditions. While some older people managed to survive, their 'social selves' were re-located to the margins of everyday life. Their subjectivity became entirely characterised by risk, and the only recognised self was that which could be medically assessed and protected (or not). Such conditions meant that it was also difficult to understand the experiences of people living with dementia because everyday interactions with families (where available) and research on social conditions were also shut down (see also Chapter 12). While we expect to hear stories from families as societies open up, it is likely that such stories will be stifled by official narratives of necessity and protection.

In the case of the pandemic, we argue that the combined biomedicalisation of ageing and dementia, the configurations of institutional care within a financialised market, social and cultural ideas of dementia as a devalued location, and an emergency situation intersected to produce precarity and suffering among older people. Arguably, older people living in a range of situations were negatively impacted by the pandemic, and particularly those diagnosed with dementia and/or frailty in institutional settings. Amnesty International declared that the human rights of older people had been violated in the case of dementia, and the Canadian military produced a scathing report on the experiences of neglect of older people (Mialkowski, 2020). At this point, it remains to be seen what action will be taken. However, the parallels with research on precarity among migrants or persons without status are striking (see Chapter 11 in this volume), and may suggest a further entrenchment of precarious ageing whereby the historical protection of older people is eroding, and being replaced by responses characterised by abandonment and neglect (see Grenier, 2021). Of course, this is not the first analysis of neglect and the absence of care. Estes and colleagues (1993) wrote about how the financialised care market created 'zones of no care' in the context of the United States. Estes work took a structural analysis, and 30 years later, we witness how such structures have combined with social and cultural ideas of devaluing, and mechanisms of biomedical dominance and functional health assessments to ration services within financialised care markets, resulting in the abandonment, neglect, and violation of human rights of older people. COVID-19 not only publicly revealed the existing fault lines in care services, but acutely demonstrated how the vulnerabilities experienced from within the location of dementia and care could easily tip older people from precariousness into despair, cause people to endure suffering, and permit the violation of human rights (see Chapter 12).

A number of ironies and contradictions exist where protection and care are concerned. Older people with dementia are often considered a vulnerable group. They are 'protected' by research ethics (many of whom configure them as too vulnerable to speak on their own behalf) and spoken for by medical professionals and families. While a counter approach has been to endorse attributes of personhood, inclusion, and agency, responses and social relations during the pandemic revealed the extent to which these measures failed to protect people in the context of COVID-19. In the case of older people living with dementia in long-term care facilities, being deemed to have a devalued or expendable life allowed a failure of care to occur. The fragments that have emerged from military reports, media images, and exposées suggest that older people living with dementia during COVID-19 have been viewed as an expendable group—confirmed by the death toll in care homes across most Western countries (Anand et al., 2021). It is this movement to the margins that requires a critical response from gerontology, heeding the lessons and possible moment of change that the pandemic affords (if recognised), and re-building supports and care for older people to ensure well-being of older people. We conclude with the statement that

> If we see pandemics purely as a function of biological details….we may be lulled into thinking that there is nothing we can do to prevent or arrest such events. But if we see pandemics as sociological phenomena as well, we can more clearly recognise the role of human agency. And the more we see our own role in shaping the emergence and unfolding of pandemic disease, the more proactive and effective our response can be.
> (Christakis, 2020: 316)

Viewing pandemic responses as a consolidation of biomedical interpretations, financialised care markets, and devalued subjects reveals the extent to which precarious ageing is taking hold.

Conclusion

The suggestion made throughout the chapter is that a shift is taking place to *precarious ageing*, and that older people living with dementia in care homes are particularly affected. The location of living with dementia in care homes reflects conditions of precarity at the intersections of the need for care, bio-medicalised understandings and approaches, a financialised care market, and the construction of devalued subjects. Further, the precarity of dementia and needing care, particularly among those living in long-term care, was exacerbated by the COVID-19 pandemic because it secluded older people in institutional contexts, removed them from social contact with their families and friends, and made them entirely reliant on medical and health care systems and staff. While this chapter is conceptual and does not yet have research-based evidence from the perspective of people living with dementia in the time of COVID-19, the conditions of life in a pandemic reveal the vulnerabilities that come with the onset of dementia and ongoing care needs, and the configurations of care which relegate people with dementia to particular spaces or conditions (either living alone with few supports or in long-term care). A critical perspective on precarity and dementia also reveals how the constructions of subjects with dementia and the responses to older people are inherently political—they are a product of biomedicalised views, financialised care, and devalued subjects. And from this view, reveal how responses have exposed older people living with dementia to risk, violence, and abandonment—a reality that became prominent in emergency times during COVID-19.

At this point, we can only guess at how it may have felt to experience the pandemic for people living with dementia in long-term care. The social and cultural devaluation and/or depictions of cognitive impairment may have played some role in both the decisions made (or justification thereof) and the experiences of the pandemic. Imagine going from one day of having visitors to solitary existence: the stoppage of all social programmes; all encounters experienced through masks, Plexiglas, and protective suits (where available); confinement to one's room; and being deprived of (or virtual only) interactions with one's immediate network of health care professionals. What precarity reveals is that responses to dementia are configured in ways that prioritise biomedical needs, create and sustain zones of no care, and reinforce the exclusion and abandonment of older people who are deemed to have devalued lives. It also, however, suggests a more disturbing possibility that the culmination of the construct of a devalued life has shifted the response from one of exclusion to allowing older people to languish and/or worse perish (see Sassen, 2014). It is this reading that emerges where the UN statement of the violation of human rights and the Canadian military report are concerned. Caregivers and families are considered an important voice to draw attention to problems in practice, and to advocate for the needs of older people. Without these voices being given access to witness or speak on behalf of older people with dementia, we were left without direct accounts of living with dementia in a long-term care home during the pandemic. Yet, at the same time, questions can also be posed about the relative silence of regulators, advocates, and charities. Where were these voices? And how were such responses permitted to occur?

The analysis of precarity and precariousness, however, also offers solutions to address the issues identified through this analysis by developing and fostering shared humanity and shared vulnerability (Fineman, 2013). Such views on care are typically linked with human rights or social justice frameworks. One of our concerns, however, is the extent to which such frameworks prompt a response, and the pandemic is arguably evidence that they failed to do so. Adapting a perspective focused on shared humanity through culture, society, and care systems is a substantial (but worthwhile) social project. Indeed, arguments have been made that the COVID pandemic may bring about the recognition of a renewed social network of protection and the re-instatement of programs that have been dismantled over the years. However, what is clear with regard to older people living with dementia is that there is also a need for a fundamental shift from disease-based models and views of older people with dementia as 'other'. Such models have been advocated as part of the need for cultural change (Dupuis et al., 2016). Our suggestion is to link this analysis with the analysis of precarity as it is created and sustained through medical and care systems, and as it configures spaces and approaches that lead to exclusion, and worse abandonment or suffering. It involves the need for systemic change in care and the political economy of care as a commodity, as well as relational transitions that view dementia as part of the life course in relation to ourselves and as part of a larger commitment to care for those in need of care.

Acknowledgements

Thank you to Daphne Imahori for her assistance with referencing and formatting.

Notes

1 https://www.ctvnews.ca/health/coronavirus/like-being-in-solitary-confinement-residents-families-angry-at-return-of-strict-lockdowns-in-long-term-care-1.573099[9.]
2 For relevant reports, see https://www.politico.eu/article/the-silent-coronavirus-covid19-massacre-in-italy-milan-lombardy-nursing-care-homes-elderly/; https://www.bbc.co.uk/news/world-europe-52014023;https://ageingissues.wordpress.com/2020/04/08/covid-19-and-the-crisis-in-residential-and-nursing-home-car[e]/.

References

Achenbaum, W.A., 1995. *Crossing Frontiers: Gerontology Emerges as a Science.* Cambridge: Cambridge University Press.
Alzheimer's Society, 2020. *The Impact of COVID-19 on People Affected by Dementia* [online]. Available at: https://www.alzheimers.org.uk/sites/default/files/2020-08/The_Impact_of_COVID-19_on_People_Affected_By_Dementia.pdf [Accessed: 31 January 2022].
Amnesty International, 2020. *UK: Older People in Care Homes Abandoned to Die Amid Government Failures during COVID-19 Pandemic* [online]. Available at: https://www.amnesty.org/en/latest/news/2020/10/uk-older-people-in-care-homes-abandoned-to-die-amid-government-failures-during-covid-19-pandemic/ [Accessed: 31 January 2022].

Anand, J., Donnelly, S., Milne, A., Nelson-Becker, H., Vingare, E.L., Deusdad, B., Cellini, G., Kinni, R.-L. and Pregno, C., 2021. The Covid-19 Pandemic and Care Homes for Older People in Europe - Deaths, Damage and Violations of Human Rights. *European Journal of Social Work*. DOI: 10.1080/13691457.2021.1954886.

Armstrong, P. and Armstrong, H., 1996. *Wasting Away: The Undermining of Canadian Health care*. Toronto: Oxford University Press.

Baltes, P. and Smith, J., 2006. New Frontiers in the Future of Aging: From Successful Aging of the Old to the Dilemmas of the Fourth Age. *Gerontology*, 49(2), pp. 123–135. DOI: 10.1159/000067946.

Bartlett, R. and O'Connor, D., 2007. From Personhood to Citizenship: Broadening the Lens for Dementia Practice and Research. *Journal of Aging Studies*, 21(2), pp. 107–118.

Butler, J., 2006. *Precarious Life: The Powers of Mourning and Violence*. London: Verso.

Butler, J., 2009. *Frames of War: When Is Life Grievable?* London: Verso.

Calasanti, T. and King, N., 2021. Beyond Successful Aging 2.0: Inequality, Ageism, and the Course of Normal Old Ages. *The Journals of Gerontology: Series B*, 76(9), pp. 1817–1827. DOI: 10.1093/geronb/gbaa037.

Calvert, J. and Arbuthnott, G. 2021. *Failures of State: The Inside Story of Britain's Battle with Coronavirus*. London: Mudlark Books.

Christakis, N., 2020. *Apollo's Arrow: The Profound and Enduring Impact of COVID-19 on the Way We Live*. New York: Little, Brown Spark.

Dannefer, D., 2021. *Age and the Reach of the Sociological Imagination: Power, Ideology and the Life Course*. New York: Routledge.

Department of Health, 2013. *Dementia: A State of the Nation Report on Dementia Care and Support in England*, London: DoH. Available at: https://assets.publishing.service.gov.uk/government/uploads/system/uploads/attachment_data/file/262139/Dementia.pdf.

Dupuis, S., McAiney, C.A., Fortune, D., Ploeg, J. and Witt, L.D., 2016. Theoretical Foundations Guiding Culture Change: The Work of the Partnerships in Dementia Care Alliance. *Dementia*, 15(1), pp. 85–105. DOI: 10.1177/1471301213518935.

Estes, C., 1979. *The Aging Enterprise*. San Francisco, CA: Jossey Bass.

Estes, C. and Binney, E., 1989. The Biomedicalization of Aging: Dangers and Dilemmas. *The Gerontologist*, 29(5), pp. 587–596. DOI: 10.1093/geront/29.5.587.

Estes, C., Phillipson, C. and Biggs, S., 1993 *Social Theory and Ageing: Sociological and Policy Perspectives*. Buckingham: Open University Press

Fine, M., 2020. 'Reconstructing Dependency: Precarity, Precariousness and Care in Old Age', in A. Grenier, C. Phillipson, and R. A. Settersten, eds. *Precarity and Ageing: Understanding Insecurity and Risk in Later Life*. Bristol, UK: Policy Press, Chapter 8.

Fineman, M.A., ed., 2013. *Vulnerability: Reflections on a New Ethical Foundation for Law and Politics*. Surrey: Ashgate Publishing.

Gallie, D., Paugam, S. and Jacobs, S., 2003. Unemployment, Poverty and Social Isolation: Is There a Vicious Circle of Social Exclusion? *European Societies*, 1(5), pp. 1–32. DOI: 10.1080/1461669032000057668.

George, D., 2010. Overcoming the Social Death of Dementia through Language. *The Lancet*, 376, pp. 586–587. DOI: 10.1016/S0140–6736(10)61286-X.

Gilleard, C. and Higgs, P., 2010. Aging without Agency: Theorizing the Fourth Age. *Ageing and Mental Health*, 14(2), pp. 121–128. DOI: 10.1080/13607860903228762.

Gilleard, C. and Higgs, P., 2015. Social Death and the Moral Identity of the Fourth Age. *Contemporary Social Science: Journal of the Academy of Social Sciences*, 10(3), pp. 262–271. DOI: 10.1080/21582041.2015.1075328.

Grenier, A., 2007. Constructions of Frailty in the English Language, Care Practice and the Lived Experience. *Ageing & Society*, 27(3), pp. 424–445. DOI: 10.1017/S0144686X06005782.

Grenier, A., 2012. *Transitions and the Life Course: Challenging the constructions of growing old*. Bristol: Policy Press.

Grenier, A., 2021. *Late Life Homelessness: Experiences of Disadvantage and Unequal Aging*. Montréal: McGill Queens University Press.

Grenier, A., Lloyd, L. and Phillipson, C., 2017. Precarity in Late Life: Rethinking Dementia as a 'Frailed' Old Age. *Sociology of Health and Illness*, 39(2), pp. 318–330. DOI: 10.1111/1467–9566.12476.

Grenier, A. and Phillipson, C., 2013. Rethinking Agency: Structural and Interpretive Approaches. In: J. Baars, J. Dohmen, A. Grenier and C. Phillipson, eds. *Ageing, Meaning and Social Structure: Connecting Critical and Humanistic Gerontology*. Bristol: Policy Press. Ch. 4.

Grenier, A., Phillipson, C. and Settersten, R.A., eds., 2020. *Precarity and Ageing: Understanding Insecurity and Risk in Later Life*. Bristol, UK: Policy Press.

Katz, S., 1996. *Disciplining Old Age: The Formation of Gerontological Knowledge*. Charlottesville: University of Virginia Press.

Kontos, P.C. and Naglie, G., 2007. Bridging Theory and Practice: Imagination, the Body, and Person-Centred Dementia Care. *Dementia*, 6(4), pp. 549–569.

Laslett, P., 1991. *A Fresh Map of Life: The Emergence of the Third Age*. Cambridge: Harvard University Press.

Marya, R. and Patel, R., 2021. *Inflamed: Deep Medicine and the Anatomy of Injustice*. London: Allen Lane.

Meagher, G. and Szebehely, M., 2013. *Marketisation in Nordic Eldercare: A Research Report on Legislation, Oversight, Extent and Consequences*. Stockholm: Department of Social Work, Stockholm University.

Mialkowski, C.J J., 2020. *OP Laser – JTFC Observations in Long Term Care Facilities in Ontatrio*. Toronto: Headquarters, 4th Canadian Division, Joint Task Force (Central).Mulkay, M. and Ernst, J., 1991. The Changing Profile of Social Death. *European Journal of Sociology/Archives européennes de sociologie*, 32(1), pp. 172–196. DOI: 10.1017/S0003975600006214.

Phillipson, C., 2013. *Ageing*. Cambridge: Polity Press.

Phillipson, C., 2015. The Political Economy of Longevity: Developing New Forms of Solidarity. *Sociological Quarterly*, 56(1), pp. 80–100. DOI: 10.1111/tsq.12082.

Polivka, L. and Luo, B., 2015. The Neoliberal Political Economy and Erosion of Retirement Security. *The Gerontologist*, 55(2), pp. 183–190. DOI: 10.1093/geront/gnv006.

Polivka, L. and Luo, B., 2017. Neoliberal Long-term Care: From Community to Corporate Control. *The Gerontologist*, 59(2), pp. 222–229. doi:10.1093/geront/gnx139.

Polivka, L. and Luo, B., 2020. From precarious employment to precarious retirement: neoliberal health and long-term care in the United States. In A. Grenier, C. Phillipson and R.A. Settersten Jnr. (eds.) *Precarity and ageing* (pp. 191–214). Bristol: Policy Press.

Portacolone, E., 2013. The Notion of Precariousness among Older Adults Living Alone in the U.S. *Journal of Aging Studies*, 27(2), pp. 166–174. DOI: 10.1016/j.jaging.2013.01.001.

Povinelli, E., 2011. *Economies of Abandonment: Social Belonging and Endurance in Late Liberalism*. Durham, NC: Duke University Press.

Sassen, S., 2014. *Expulsions*. Cambridge: Harvard University Press.

Schram, S.F., 2015. *The Return of Ordinary Capitalism: Neoliberalism, Precarity, Occupy*. New York: Oxford University Press.

Seniors Services and Long Term Care, 2020. *COVID-19 Pandemic in City of Toronto Longer-Term Care Homes: Submission to the Independent LTC Commission*. Toronto: Seniors Services and Long Term Care. Available at: https://www.toronto.ca/wp-content/uploads/2021/03/8e2f-SSLTCCommissionReportOct8.pdf [Accessed 17 February 2022].

Simmonds, B., 2021. *Ageing and the Crisis in Health and Social Care*. Bristol: Policy Press.

Standing, G., 2011. *The Precariat: The New Dangerous Class*. London: Bloomsbury Press.

Standing, G., 2021. *The Precariat: The New Dangerous Class. Special COVID-19 Edition*. London: Bloomsbury Press.

Tapper, J., 2021. 'This is an attack on Human Rights': UK Care Homes Still Denying Family Visits to Residents. *The Guardian*, [online], 20 November. Available at: https://www.theguardian.com/society/2021/nov/20/uk-care-homes-deny-family-visits-human-rights [Accessed 15 January 2022].

Timonen, V., 2016. *Beyond Active and Successful Ageing: A Theory of Model Ageing*. Bristol: Policy Press.

Tooze, A., 2021. *Shutdown: How Covid Shook the World's Economy*. London: Allen Lane.

Townsend, P., 1979. The Structured Dependence of Older People. *Ageing & Society*, 1(1), pp. 5–28. DOI: 1017/S0144686X81000020.

Vince, G., 2022. *Nomad Century: How Climate Migration Will Reshape Our World*. London: Penguin Books.

Wallace, K. and Winsa, P., 2021. Doctors Point to Staffing Issues as Second Wave of COVID-19 Rips through Ontario's Nursing Homes. *Toronto Star*, [online] 4 January. Available at: https://www.thestar.com/news/gta/2021/01/04/doctors-point-to-staffing-issues-as-second-wave-of-covid-19-rips-through-ontarios-nursing-homes.html [Accessed 17 February 2022].

Walsh, K., Scharf, T., Van Regenmortal, S. and Wanka, A., 2021. *Social Exclusion in Later Life: Interdisciplinary and Policy Perspectives*. Cham, Switzerland: Springer.

11 An emerging necropolitics of the dementias

Hamish Robertson and Joanne Travaglia

Introduction

The year 2020 saw two key issues for societies in the 21st century intersect with unanticipated speed and intensity. The first was the emergence of COVID-19, a viral (SARS variant) pandemic that has affected every country on the planet in some degree, with ongoing effects in many societies. It is important to note that pandemics may be seen as 'natural' events, but their effects may be heavily influenced by social conditions as well as political and cultural responses. The other issue is the growing demographic trend of global population ageing. While ageism was already well-entrenched in many societies (Chang et al., 2021), the impact of COVID-19 has only served to heighten both an awareness of ageism and its profound impacts on the lives of older people during moments of crisis (Maxfield et al., 2021; McDonald, 2021; Monahan et al., 2020). The major demographic group to experience unequal outcomes in both morbidity and mortality has been the older part of many populations and the associated framing of those who are already unwell as being 'disposable'. This has had quite profound effects for those with a dementia and associated health problems. Our position here is that these established processes have intensified during the pandemic in ways that have important implications for the future of population ageing and the continuing treatment of people with a dementia. While the clinical medical paradigm of the dementias is problematic enough, lacking effective treatments and cures, the socio-political dimension becomes more problematic still.

This chapter explores these issues, with a particular focus on the dementias, by adopting and extending Mbembe's (2003, 2019) necropolitical concept. Necropolitics in Mbembe's work addresses how 'to kill or to allow to live constitute the limits of sovereignty' (Mbembe, 2003, p. 11). The central question Mbembe seeks to address is 'under what practical conditions is the right to kill, to allow to live, or to expose to death exercised?' (Mbembe, 2003, p. 12). We will use the concept to analyse how ageing and the dementias are framed as threats, subject to coercive state identification, surveillance, regulation and action. Our premise here is that the dementias

DOI: 10.4324/9781003221982-15

are 'provoking' a particular kind of necropolitics that have implications for a rapidly growing number of older people and especially those with a dementia. The conceptualisation of the dementias as pathology needs to be examined in more than purely medical or clinico-pathological terms. The dementias, as a site of intervention for the healthcare establishment, constitute a growing socio-political domain of influence and action. That domain and its 'governance' have significant implications for people diagnosed with a dementia, their carers and communities more broadly.

In this chapter, we expand on some of our previous writing in this area and extend it using the concept of necropolitics developed by Mbembe (2003, 2019) to examine the more specific case of dementia. Mbembe's (2003) concept of 'necropolitics' emerged from the intersection of Foucault's scholarship on the biopolitical with his own work on colonialism, including racism, and its consequences. The key emphasis of Mbembe has been on the role of sovereignty and the role of the state in deciding who *may* live and who *must* die (our emphasis). Coming as health researchers with experience in both aged care and patient safety, this central idea has considerable resonance. In particular, we have modified or extended that idea to consider *where and how* people (especially when classified as patients) may live and die (Mbembe, 2019). We do so in the belief that this not only helps extend the utility of Mbembe's concept to different domains of practice but also extends its value in examining key issues and concerns such as the rhetoric adopted in society towards people with a dementia.

In addition, the dementias are obviously closely correlated with the ageing process and, consequently, they tend to develop in association with other health-related problems. This makes the utility of the necropolitical concept variously useful in that it permits an explicit focus on the dementias and how they, and those diagnosed with a dementia, are treated, as well as being a viable tool for unpacking the complexities of people with dementia living with various other health conditions and how these are treated from the clinical to the socio-political levels. We have written elsewhere that medicine is a territorial undertaking (Robertson and Travaglia, 2022). This territorialisation of health and illness (and dying and death), also considered by Foucault and others (Foucault, 1978) for example, constitutes specific *sites* that can be seen as distinctly necropolitical. The diversion of acutely unwell older people from hospitals to residential aged care facilities is, in the Australian context from which we write, able to be seen as a necropolitical process – the concentration of medically unwell people with a dementia in facilities from which they are unlikely to emerge alive and where their modes of living and dying are effectively managed through a necropolitical lens.

A key feature of this process is that the diagnosis of a dementia in situ has become an essential part of this necropolitical processing of this patient group. The framing of dementia as a chronic and incurable condition shifts the focus from the treatment and curative modalities favoured by medicine to a *disease management* strategy in which the inevitable outcome is assumed to be progressive decline and eventual death. The problem here is the how, where and when of those processes and the associated care received by such persons along their trajectories. The lack of effective treatments is problematic for medicine in many contexts because it negates the capabilities of medicine as an interventional form of practice. It also leads to the potential for rationing care because 'the dementing person' is framed as being on an inevitable pathway which dehumanises them due to its effects on their memory and behaviour. We have seen this during the COVID-19 pandemic more starkly than previously as patients with dementia were often abandoned or discharged, in some cases, to residential care to die while infected with the disease. Much of this was wrapped in an equally problematic discussion of 'co-morbidities' that, while we lack the space to discuss it here, awaits a closer and more critical analysis than has been undertaken to date. In addition, the COVID-19 pandemic permitted a more open rhetoric about whose lives mattered in relation to the potential for treatment and cure of the disease under which the triage concept often flagged older people and those with chronic conditions, including the dementias, as less deserving of interventions and care (see also Grenier and Phillipson's reflection on this in Chapter 10).

A further argument around 'palliative care', which we have recently examined elsewhere (Robertson and Travaglia, 2022), emerged in this context as part of this narrower necropolitical conception in which various sub-elements of the 'who may live and who must die' focus of Mbembe's framing emerged. What we saw was a variety of existing tools, in the science and technology studies sense, adjusted to the moment and adapted for people with dementia. The specific location of more advanced cases in residential care facilities added to this locational aspect of necropolitical practice in that such places became less about living what remained of patients' lives and more about normalising them as places of imminent death from COVID.

The value here lies in seeing beyond the rather obvious fact of ageism, and its effects, to understand how a necropolitical analysis can inform our understanding of the positioning of older age, older people with a dementia and population ageing at a systemic level. In particular, we develop the idea that health and aged care environments reflect a variety of necropolitical assumptions around *who may live and who must die* that are both pervasive and multi-layered with the dementias illustrating this framing of ageing and illness as a locus for necropolitical interventions. We also develop our own interpretation of Mbembe's concept to inquire how state power is exercised in relation to the positioning of older people in terms of how they may (be permitted to) live and how they (may be permitted/encouraged and even made to) die. These are always important issues but in the context of progressive population ageing, we believe their importance for both theorists and practitioners can only grow in significance. A failure to examine these issues will, in effect, normalise the prevailing necropolitics of our time and have potentially immense consequences for older people themselves and those who care for them.

Population health and necropolitical consequences

More explicitly the concept of 'population' became a foundation stone of the 19th century state which has remained entwined with the concepts of 'health' and 'illness' ever since. We now even have 'population health' as a distinct, albeit often confused, concept distinct from public health and other more generic conceptualisations (Kindig and Stoddart, 2003; Lantz, 2019). Others, including Nancy Krieger (2012), have also examined how complex and contradictory the idea of 'population' is, and its complicated relationship with 'health'. Kunitz (2007) discussed some elements of this conceptual landscape in his work *The Health of Populations* where he explored distinctions between knowledge that was generalisable and that which remained specific and even local. The problematic issue from our interpretation is that the state formation has become embodied; therefore, ageing and associated dementias being framed as pathology can reinforce the 'disposability' of unwell older people. This includes a more general approach via healthcare rationing and associated consequences during the pandemic in which medically unwell older people in aged care facilities were framed as less deserving of care and/or protection from COVID. Indeed, at the time of writing, deaths amongst aged care residents in Australia continued to be the main component of COVID-related mortality. There has been a decline in interest in the pandemic and yet the necropolitical dimension continues unabated since to lose interest in a vulnerable group and its mortality is precisely the kind of necropolitical form we propose in this chapter.

A 'web' of intersecting ideas (population, disposable categories, the older person) continues to inform public perception, medical practice and political theorising in the representation of ageing and the dementias. Such representations intersect with a variety of forms of necropolitical framing because they position individuals as having more or less value as human beings due to their status as 'dementing'. The implicit assumption that, for example, the possession of memory (often very loosely defined) versus the loss of memory in Alzheimer's disease makes a person less than they were, is also a necropolitical positioning of the ageing process and its correlates.

We take issue with this positioning here because COVID-19 has shown that disease transitions may not be linear and that they rely on ideological and practical pre-commitments that may in fact not be consistently present in the richer countries. Instead, we have seen a variety of failures and missteps in the responses of the 'developed' countries to various pandemics over the past several decades, including the HIV epidemic, SARS and the current COVID-19 scenario (e.g. Lewis, 2021). Many lives were lost not only due to the severity and complexity of these diseases but also due to a lack of preparedness, in some cases, and prevailing social prejudices that were backed by political power, as in the case of HIV/AIDS (Von Collani et al., 2010). The additional or particular risk faced by certain individuals and groups, most notably older people, people with disabilities and people from 'ethnic minorities', came to the fore quite early on in the emergence of the COVID-19 pandemic. As with HIV/AIDS, the risks which may have been associated with health status were magnified by the responses of health systems, services, practitioners and governments. As Scully (2020) argues: 'Pandemics such as COVID-19 place everyone at risk, but certain kinds of risk are differentially severe for groups already made vulnerable by pre-existing forms of social injustice and discrimination'. She goes on to show how in the UK, disablism in relation to triage guidance for the allocation of care was based on

> ... disablist assumptions about disability and health status, quality of life, and social utility, that unjustly and potentially catastrophically disadvantage people with disability in COVID-19 and other global health emergencies.
>
> (2020)

Similar arguments have been made about the treatment (or lack of treatment) for people from different 'racial'/ethnic groups (including refugees), genders and socio-economic status (Bowleg, 2020; Chakraborty, 2021; Daher-Nashif, 2022; Sandset, 2021). The situation for older people, concluded Donnelly (2020, p. 453), came down to a choice by governments, societies and/or health systems/services of either 'cocooning' (that is employing additional resources to keep older people safe during the pandemic) or 'culling' (seeing the death of older people as potentially providing a benefit to 'society'). In examining COVID responses in three countries, Australia, the UK and the US, Lichtenstein (2021) found evidence of ageism, including:

> Public responses to lockdowns and other measures [which] cast older adults as a problem to be ignored or solved through segregation. Name-calling, blame, and "so-be-it" reactions toward age vulnerability [which] were commonplace ... Indefinite isolation for older adults [which] was widely accepted, especially as a vehicle to end public lockdowns and economic crises.
>
> (2021, e2006)

Thus, in our analysis, COVID-19 affirms the existence of a necropolitics of dementia in a specific, and also extended, 'moment' as the pandemic has emerged and progressed. The socio-political responses have not only included conventional arguments around the rationing of care for those 'more likely' to survive but also produced a rhetoric of value and utility. This has been used against already vulnerable groups, including those with a dementia (in the clinical biomedical sense) but also people who possess impairments more broadly. The impact of COVID-19 and its associated loss of life has been especially significant in aged care facilities in many countries where responses to protect residents were often slow and inadequate. In the

US, in particular, hospital patients with COVID were often discharged to aged care facilities which, in turn, spread the disease amongst older people not previously infected. This process was, in our analysis, an iterative one because medically unwell people, often with a dementia, were taken to acute care environments and then, if they survived, discharged back to aged care facilities where they could potentially infect the other residents and staff. Thus, the necropolitical element can also be seen as applying to both older people and those whose role it is to care for them. In effect, both become potentially disposable and thus subject to a regime in which the aged care environment itself becomes a necropolitical one – whether or not it might have been so prior to the pandemic.

The relationship between aged care and the dementias is an intimate one. Many older people with a milder dementia are living in the community with varying access to services (e.g. Kalisch et al., 2020). However, aged care facilities have increasingly become sites for the management of older people who cannot safely live in the community or for whom current systems of care are inadequate. While this often includes physical impairments and chronic diseases such as heart, lung and vascular conditions, a major and growing factor in admission to aged care facilities is the diagnosis and progression of a dementing illness – often in addition to other 'co-morbidities' (Bunn et al., 2014). This makes aged care facilities sites of *concentration* for people with a dementia, even, as some observers have commented, carceral sites for those with a dementia as can be seen in the debate around 'secure' dementia units and the like (e.g. Repo, 2019, see also Chapter 12 in this volume).

This creation of sites which concentrate on medically unwell older people with progressive health conditions, including dementia, helps to position them as the objects of necropolitical rhetoric and action or inaction. This lack of 'capacity' in effect marks them as not simply incapable of defending their own interests directly but reliant on the way they are *represented* to ensure that they receive appropriate care during 'business as usual' but, even more so, in a crisis such as that represented by COVID-19. Such representation assumes a lack of voice on the part of people with dementia and, even when that voice is acknowledged, a diminution of its value.

Ageing as pathology, pathology as weakness

One of the long-standing problems with the pathological view of illness discourse is that it is all too often invested in the individual, marking an implicit moral claim as to who gets ill and who does not, and from or with what condition (Gunderman, 2000). This is especially problematic in the content of *chronic* conditions where the original aetiology may be difficult to identify and the progressive and, usually, incurable nature of the condition makes claims on current and future needs and resources. This level of actual and assumed dependency is problematic for the contemporary state formation and for structures built around or influenced by capitalist modes of thought (Sell and Williams, 2020). In these sorts of constructions, disease seems to be couched as a secular punishment for personal failures just as poverty has been framed for several hundred years in much of European thought (Lundahl et al., 2020).

For those older people relying on public and community support, the analysis differs quite markedly. Here, chronic disease is frequently framed as a failure of informed decision-making, 'lifestyle choices' and associated poor behaviours (e.g. Adler and Stewart, 2009; Egger and Dixon, 2014). The dementias, difficult to predict as they are, do not blend well with this 'bad behaviour' model but efforts continue to be made to make that happen (Rosenberg et al., 2020). More than this, the life expectancy of an individual with a progressive dementia diagnosis (of whatever type or mix) can be considerable.

This produces an open-ended concern with both high dependency and life expectancy in the person with a dementia, such as how long will their 'suffering' continue. One consequence is that the dementias are often represented as 'dehumanising' and, effectively, a state worse than death itself in some cases – especially end-stage dementia – and especially in the media (Peel, 2014). An element in this relies on the myth of memory as the signal identifier of what it means to be a functional human being. Such constructions suggest that for the person with a progressive dementia there is or will be a stage at which their humanity ceases and that life itself also ceases to have 'meaning'. Not only is this a highly problematic interpretation but it brings us to the focus of this chapter, an essential necropolitical analysis of ageing, age-related disease and, in particular, the dementias.

Necropolitical strategies and the state

Here we briefly outline three specific ways in which the modern state has produced and continues to produce an on-going pattern of necropolitical consequences through its actions on categories of persons, specific demographic groups and individuals. The first is the power of the state to elevate or *diminish* the quality of life of the living through direct and indirect actions as well as through inaction, such that some people may even actually choose death as an 'option'. The second is where the power of the state is used to *produce,* directly or indirectly, death as a deliberate outcome. And third, there is a history of the emergent modern state *punishing* people in and after death through the abuse of their bodily remains and deliberately making them invisible in death (e.g. Nystrom, 2014). Let us briefly discuss each of these in turn as constituting a broader framework for our necropolitics of ageing and dementia.

The modern state has a long history of development that has generally included some very conditional ideas around the nature of citizenship and belonging. One idea that persists in the aged care and disability sectors, for example, is the importance of a healthy population, free from disease, disability and deformity. This idea has for more than a century framed the state as corporeal entity in its own right (Porter, 2003). More than this, state ideology has frequently, via eugenics and 'population planning' strategies for example, promoted very particular ideas of what the 'healthy state' is composed of and looks like (inclusions and exclusions abound but tend to be remarkably similar) (Reilly, 2015). Historically, this has often involved a moralising or virtuous aspect alongside the structural applications of medical power and public health interventions (Porter, 2011). The 'healthy' state is one in which the population tends to be homogenous on multiple levels (language, ethnicity and even religion) and which worked to free itself from unhealthy groups and individuals. Historical revisionist discourses often suggest this process somehow ceased with the end of the Second World War and the associated atrocities witnessed during this period and that we have since become more enlightened. However, in our analysis, this process is both contemporary and ongoing (e.g. the treatment of 'minorities' in many countries).

The groups and individuals targeted by state violence have almost always involved social categories of people perceived as threats to this idealised state 'body' including the 'promiscuous', those with sexually transmitted diseases, the mentally ill, the indigent poor and so on. Even in the 21st century we can see the inculcation of aspirational health as a state-informed strategy with systemic and capitalist consequences, such as trying to buy good health, the pervasive use of language such as 'self-management' and 'lifestyle choices', and even access to healthy environments, including green spaces (e.g. Rojas-Rueda et al., 2019).

Such groups have often been the targets of social policies that divested them of power, agency and even the usual 'rights' of *citizens*, reducing them to lesser versions of the healthy, conformist citizen idealised by the state (e.g. Lanoix, 2007). The conditions of life for such outsiders have often been marginal at best and frequently reduced in both quality and quantity (e.g. Indigenous peoples and their life expectancies in the settler states). Even now, in 21st century nation states, many such groups continue to experience state interventions that have negative consequences for them (e.g. the sterilisation of women with disability or in prison) (Fofana, 2021; Frohmader and Meekosha, 2012). The presumed universality of human rights touted in the shadow of the Second World War has frequently been and continues to be subverted in many such contexts.

In the second scenario, we can observe a variety of state actions as having direct and indirect consequences for 'unhealthy' groups and individuals. While older age is an obvious scenario in which public and state-sanctioned discourse readily talks of 'unproductive lives' without any irony or even awareness of where such language originates, other examples also exist. Thus, we can observe the exclusion of Indigenous peoples in Australia and elsewhere as a form of excision from the healthy nation state. Such scenarios are frequently enforced through state-directed or state-sanctioned forms of violence, including incarceration rates out of all proportion to population levels and direct abuses by state players, including police, prison and even health authorities. Indeed, depending on how broadly we define state violence, this could be extended to include many other areas of social policy (e.g. access to, exclusion from and treatment in educational systems, for example).

A necropolitics of ageing

As we have discussed elsewhere (Robertson and Travaglia, 2020), there is a substantive necropolitical dimension to population ageing in the post-industrial countries of the 21st century. Ageing is viewed nominally as a success (longer life expectancies), as a failure (low consumers, high care needs, etc.) and as an existential economic threat (costs of care, labour force issues, production issues, etc.). In Marxist terms, the theory of enduring crisis is thus intrinsic to demographic theory and societal responses. There is no positive outcome because young populations have been posed as problematic for decades (especially on the basis of racialised thinking in relation to low- to middle-income countries) and, likewise, population ageing has been framed as threat at least since the 1920s (Thane, 1990). Thus, each demographic change is framed as an emergent crisis that threatens current modes of funding, service design and delivery – as though these were somehow fixed in time and perfected in form.

Our experience includes substantive work in the patient safety arena with particular reference to patient safety inquiries (see Hindle et al., 2006). Vulnerable groups, including older people, have always been a focus for negative outcomes in health and social care environments (Braithwaite et al., 2007). In other words, the responses to older people during the COVID-19 pandemic are not new in any way. Rather, they reflect persistent ageism and institutional violence towards the weak and vulnerable in our societies (see Chapters 10 and 12 in this volume for further discussion of alternative interpretations of institutionalised care).

A necropolitical analysis of the dementias

The framing of many older people's deaths as 'unavoidable' during the pandemic, especially by politicians, clearly illustrates how persistent ageism is in 21st century society. Scenarios in which some care staff left their patients to die, in countries including Italy and Spain, also showed how the intersectionality of ageing and illness can be both devalued and poorly managed concurrently. These two are amongst the oldest societies in Europe, with Spain tipped to have the highest European life expectancy in a few years' time (Troya, 2021) and yet the desertion of those residents was the first response of some providers in a crisis event (McDonald, 2021). We anticipate that further analysis of this particular phenomenon will show how extensive this response was and the post hoc rationalisations that will emerge in an effort to normalise such deaths and the lack of preparedness that underpinned them.

One of the emerging issues in a COVID-19 long-view world is the ongoing, and possibly expanding, neurological impacts of the pandemic (Prasad et al., 2021; Wood, 2020). Already, the issue of ongoing neurological effects has been raised, and not for the first time, with some COVID-19 patients experiencing specific neurological symptoms including loss of smell, taste and emotional distancing (Liou et al., 2021). A sub-set of 'recovering' COVID-19 patients have also been shown to experience longer-term (long COVID), persistent symptoms that impact on their health and well-being, including their capacity for full recovery (in this context a return to their pre-COVID health status and capacities) (e.g. Mendelson et al., 2021). This early-stage data suggest that there will be a group of people who experience potentially life-long effects from the disease as they age. In addition, some of these neurological effects are consistent with age-related pathologies, such as the dementias (Ferrucci et al., 2021; Miners et al., 2020). The necropolitics of this scenario are yet to be fully evidenced, but this suggests that, for example, COVID-related dementia may yet be an emergent aspect of a necropolitical inquiry.

We suggest that the necropolitical dimensions of COVID-19, already enmeshed in societal norms and prejudices around the ageing process and towards older people more generally, will continue to develop and play out as the pandemic and responses to it develop. Especially concerning examples include the use and abuse of do-not-resuscitate orders (DNR and any associated terminologies and euphemisms) in the United Kingdom. During the early stages of the COVID-19 pandemic, the use of DNRs appears to have been scaled up as part of the 'clinical benefit' terminology used in relation to a lack of resources, including ICU beds, to properly respond to demands for treatment and care (Milam et al., 2020). Amnesty International (2020) had already collected evidence to support its concerns about this, with more information accumulating since. Even as we write, there is evidence to suggest that several thousand people in the UK were placed on DNR orders during the pandemic (to date), with several hundred of these being down without discussion with or consent by either patients or family members (CQC, 2021). The consequences of this kind of 'blanket' application continue to play out in lives lost and some truly disturbing experiences for both patients and their families (e.g. CQC, 2021). Here too, the kinds of institutional formations and technologies associated with the contemporary state illustrate the *generativity* of necropolitical outcomes through state and agency decision-making processes. The creation of particular places for aged care, then dementia care, then secure dementia care and so on has its own particular effects. Our own work in patient safety research illustrates this all too well in that these categories have effects on the person categorised and their subsequent treatment and care (Robertson and Travaglia, 2022; Travaglia, 2018). The pandemic has, in our estimation, made this much more obvious in that the necropolitical dimension was evident early on in the care of insitutionalised older people and equally so now, as the pandemic recedes, in the reduction in attention to COVID-related deaths in aged care.

Even without this crisis event scenario, our position is that ageing and the dementias are largely framed within a broader, extensive and prevailing necropolitics. The dementias resist, at this time, many effective treatments. This makes them antipathetic to medical myths of treatment and cure, with associated cost implications for *care*. The existence of so many people with conditions that, in much prevailing discourse, make them less human is a rebuke to the ideology of the contemporary state, its structures and mechanisms. The need that such people have for actual care, especially in neoliberal states, is doubly confronting because the dominant position is one of individualised support in a rational needs-based system. Lastly, we flag the potential loss of personhood that often accompanies a diagnosis of a dementia, as though without memory or 'acceptable' behaviours, the person loses their fundamental humanity (the empty shell, etc.). While there is an established literature on this issue, it also represents a necropolitical stance in which access to care and the attribution (and thus withdrawal) of personhood are indelibly linked (Harrison, 1993). The value here, we suggest, in exploring this from a necropolitical position is that we can examine dementia specifically, ageing more generally, and vulnerable groups and their experiences more broadly still – all while maintaining a consistent theoretical focus.

Conclusion

In this chapter, we have attempted to illustrate how long-standing ideas about the nature of the state, of health and populations have developed in parallel with social prejudices about and towards older people with dementia (amongst others). The specific consequences have included institutional prejudices towards and actions against older people in a variety of contexts, including numerous patient safety inquiry outcomes in the United Kingdom and elsewhere. The COVID-19 pandemic has illustrated that these problems are structural and exacerbated during crisis events due to the lack of preparedness of many contemporary systems, and a willingness to sacrifice older people when time and resources are limited. Many other examples exist, including events we saw during the Katrina disaster (e.g. Fink, 2013) but there is a clear and consistent pattern in many such events in which vulnerable groups and individuals are the most likely to be placed at risk and even harmed (Travaglia et al., 2019). One of those groups has always been and remains the unwell older person, especially those with a dementia. This chapter has taken this observation and extended it using the necropolitical concept as an explanatory mechanism for why and how those conditions exist and persist.

There is a tendency to see each disaster event as singular, unique and even natural. This is not our analysis. Rather, we suggest that there is a key necropolitical dimension in play under which such harmful decisions are rationalised, institutionalised and normalised because many such lives are already devalued in many contemporary societies. The idea that the state, its agencies and employees have the right to exclude some socially manufactured categories of person such that their deaths result is a fundamentally necropolitical act. To designate some groups as fundamentally expendable is a necropolitical act, and the COVID pandemic, in our analysis, affirmed this analysis yet again. Finally, the progressive nature of global population ageing and the anticipated scale of the dementias mean that the potential human cost of a sustained necropolitical posture towards the dementias, as explored here, has huge potential for continuing harms against an already vulnerable group.

References

Adler, N. E., & Stewart, J. (2009). Reducing Obesity: Motivating Action While Not Blaming the Victim, *Milbank Quarterly, 87*(1), 49–70.

Amnesty International (2020). *As If Expendable*, Amnesty International Inc., London. https://www.amnesty.org.uk/files/2020-10/Care%20Homes%20Report.pdf?kd5Z8e Wzj8Q6ryzHkcaUnxfCtqe5Ddg6=.

Bowleg, L. (2020). We're not All in this Together: On COVID-19, Intersectionality, and Structural Inequality. *American journal of public health, 110*(7), 917–917.

Braithwaite, J., Travaglia, J., & Nugus, P. (2007). *Giving a Voice to Patient Safety in New South Wales*. Sydney: Clinical Excellence Commission and Centre for Clinical Governance Research UNSW.

Bunn, F., Burn, A.-M., Goodman, C., Rait, G., Norton, S., Robinson, L., et al. (2014). Comorbidity and Dementia: A Scoping Review of the Literature. *BMC Medicine, 12*(1), 1–15.

Chakraborty, D. (2021). The "living dead" within "death-worlds": Gender Crisis and Covid-19 in India. *Gender, Work and Organization, 28*(S2), 330–339.

Chang, E.-S., Monin, J.K., Zelterman, D., & Levy, B.R. (2021). Impact of Structural Ageism on Greater Violence against Older Persons: A Cross-national Study of 56 Countries. *BMJ Open, 11*(5), e042580.

CQC (2021). *Protect, Respect, Connect – Decisions about Living and Dying Well during COVID-19 – Final Report*, Care Quality Commission. https://www.cqc.org.uk/sites/default/files/20210318_dnacpr_printer-version.pdf.

Daher-Nashif, S. (2022). In Sickness and in Health: The Politics of Public Health and their Implications during the COVID-19 Pandemic. *Sociology Compass, 16*(1), e12949.

Donnelly, S. (2020). The elderly and COVID-19: Cocooning or culling—the choice is ours. *QJM: An International Journal of Medicine, 113*(7), 453–454.

Egger, G., & Dixon, J. (2014). Beyond Obesity and Lifestyle: A Review of 21st Century Chronic Disease Determinants. *BioMed Research International*, 731685.

Ferrucci, R., Dini, M., Groppo, E., Rosci, C., Reitano, M. R., Bai, F., et al. (2021). Long-lasting Cognitive Abnormalities after COVID-19. *Brain Sciences, 11*(2), 235.

Fink, S. (2013). *Five Days at Memorial Hospital.* London: Atlantic Books.

Fofana, M.O. (2022). Time and Time Again: The Reincarnations of Coerced Sterilisation. *Journal of Medical Ethics, 48*, 805–809.

Foucault, M. (1978). *The History of Sexuality.* London: Allen and Unwin.

Frohmader, C., & Meekosha, H. (2012). Recognition, Respect and Rights: Women with Disabilities in a Globalised World. In D. Goodley, B. Hughes, & L. Davis (Eds.), *Disability and Social Theory* (pp. 287–307). London: Palgrave Macmillan.

Gunderman, R. (2000). Illness as Failure: Blaming Patients. *Hastings Center Report, 30*(4), 7–11.

Harrison, C. (1993). Personhood, Dementia and the Integrity of a Life. *Canadian Journal on Aging/La revue canadienne du vieillissement, 12*(4), 428–440.

Hindle, D., Braithwaite, J., Iedema, R., & Travaglia, J. (2006). *Patient Safety: A Comparative Analysis of Eight Inquiries in Six Countries.* Sydney: Centre for Clinical Governance, University of New South Wales.

Kalisch Ellett, L.M., Pratt, N.L., Nguyen, T.A., & Roughead, E.E. (2020). Use of Health and Support Services by People Living with Dementia in the Community Setting. *Australasian Journal on Ageing, 39*(4), 341–349.

Kindig, D., & Stoddart, G. (2003). What Is Population Health? *American Journal of Public Health, 93*(3), 380–383.

Krieger, N. (2012). Who and What Is a "Population"? Historical Debates, Current Controversies, and Implications for Understanding "Population Health" and Rectifying Health Inequities. *The Milbank Quarterly, 90*(4), 634–681.

Kunitz, S.J. (2007). *The Health of Populations: General Theories and Particular Realities.* New York: Oxford University Press, USA.

Lanoix, M. (2007). The Citizen in Question. *Hypatia, 22*(4), 113–129.

Lantz, P.M. (2019). The Medicalization of Population Health: Who Will Stay Upstream? *The Milbank Quarterly, 97*(1), 36.

Lewis, D.E. (2021). Is the Failed Pandemic Response a Symptom of a Diseased Administrative State?. *Dædalus, 150*(3), 66–88.

Lichtenstein, B. (2021). From "Coffin Dodger" to "Boomer Remover": Outbreaks of Ageism in Three Countries with Divergent Approaches to Coronavirus Control. *The Journals of Gerontology: Series B, 76*(4), e206–e212.

Liou, J.M., Chen, M.J., Hong, T.C., & Wu, M.S. (2021). Alteration of Taste or Smell as a Predictor of COVID-19. *Gut, 70*(4), 806–807.

Lundahl, M., Rauhut, D., & Hatti, N. (2020). *Poverty in the History of Economic Thought.* Abingdon: Routledge.

Maxfield, M., Peckham, A., Guest, M.A., & Pituch, K.A. (2021). Age-Based Healthcare Stereotype Threat during the COVID-19 Pandemic. *Journal of Gerontological Social Work, 64*(6), 571–584.

Mbembe, A. (2003). Necropolitics. *Public Culture, 15*(1), 11–40.

Mbembe, A. (2019). *Necropolitics.* Durham, NC: Duke University Press.

McDonald, T. (2021). Lethal Ageism in the Shadow of Pandemic Response Tactics. *International Nursing Review.* https://doi.org/10.1111/inr.12700.

Mendelson, M., Nel, J., Blumberg, L., Madhi, S.A., Dryden, M., Stevens, W., & Venter, F.W.D. (2021). Long-COVID: An Evolving Problem with an Extensive Impact. *SAMJ: South African Medical Journal, 111*(1), 10–12.

Milam, A. J., Furr-Holden, D., Edwards-Johnson, J., Webb, B., Patton III, J. W., Ezekwemba, N. C., et al. (2020). Are Clinicians Contributing to Excess African

American COVID-19 Deaths? Unbeknownst to Them, They may Be. *Health Equity, 4*(1), 139–141.

Miners, S., Kehoe, P. G., & Love, S. J. A. s. r. (2020). Cognitive Impact of COVID-19: Looking Beyond the Short term. *Alzheimer's Research & Therapy, 12*(1), 1–16.

Monahan, C., Macdonald, J., Lytle, A., Apriceno, M., & Levy, S.R. (2020). COVID-19 and Ageism: How Positive and Negative Responses Impact Older Adults and Society. *American Psychologist, 75*(7), 887.

Nystrom, K.C. (2014). The Bioarchaeology of Structural Violence and Dissection in the 19th-Century United States. *American Anthropologist, 116*(4), 765–779.

Peel, E. (2014). 'The living death of Alzheimer's' versus 'Take a walk to keep dementia at bay': Representations of Dementia in Print Media and Carer Discourse. *Sociology of Health & Illness, 36*(6), 885–901.Porter, D. (2003). Municipal Medicine: Public Health in Twentieth-Century Britain, and Body and City: Histories of Urban Public Health. *Bulletin of the History of Medicine, 77*(3), 732–736.

Porter, D. (2011). *Health Citizenship: Essays in Social Medicine and Biomedical Politics.* Berkeley: University of California Medical Humanities Press.

Prasad, K., Al Omar, S.Y., Alqahtani, S.A.M., Malik, M.Z., & Kumar, V. (2021). Brain Disease Network Analysis to Elucidate the Neurological Manifestations of COVID-19. *Molecular Neurobiology, 58*(5), 1875–1893.

Reilly, P. R. (2015). Eugenics and Involuntary Sterilization: 1907–2015. *Annual review of genomics and human genetics, 16*, 351–368.

Repo, V. (2019). Carceral Layers in a Geropsychiatric Unit in Finland. *Geografiska Annaler: Series B, Human Geography, 101*(3), 187–201.

Robertson, H., & Travaglia, J. (2020). The Necropolitics of COVID-19: Will the COVID-19 Pandemic Reshape National Healthcare Systems? *Impact of Social Sciences Blog.*

Robertson, H., & Travaglia, J. (2022). Palliative Care as a Necropolitical Technology. In D.J. Fleming & D.J. Carter (Eds.), *Voluntary Assisted Dying: Law? Health? Justice?* (1st ed., pp. 31–48). Canberra: ANU Press.

Rojas-Rueda, D., Nieuwenhuijsen, M.J., Gascon, M., Perez-Leon, D., & Mudu, P. (2019). Green Spaces and Mortality: A Systematic Review and Meta-Analysis of Cohort Studies. *The Lancet Planetary Health, 3*(11), e469–e477.

Rosenberg, A., Mangialasche, F., Ngandu, T., Solomon, A., & Kivipelto, M. (2020). Multidomain Interventions to Prevent Cognitive Impairment, Alzheimer's Disease, and Dementia: From FINGER to World-Wide FINGERS. *The Journal of Prevention of Alzheimer's Disease, 7*(1), 29–36.

Sandset, T. (2021). The Necropolitics of COVID-19: Race, Class and Slow Death in an Ongoing Pandemic. *Global Public Health, 16*(8–9), 1411–1423.

Scully, J. L. (2020). Disability, Disablism, and COVID-19 Pandemic Triage. *Journal of Bioethical Inquiry, 17*(4), 601–605.

Sell, S.K., & Williams, O.D. (2020). Health under Capitalism: A Global Political Economy of Structural Pathogenesis. *Review of International Political Economy, 27*(1), 1–25.

Thane, P. (1990). The Debate on the Declining Birth-Rate in Britain: The 'Menace of an Ageing Population, 1920s-50s. *Continuity and Change, 5*(2), 283–305.

The Necropolitics of COVID-19: Will the COVID-19 Pandemic Reshape National Healthcare Systems? | Impact of Social Sciences (lse.ac.uk).

Travaglia, J. (2018). Disturbing the Doxa of Patient Safety: Comment on "False Dawns and New Horizons in Patient Safety Research and Practice". *International Journal of Health Policy and Management, 7*(9), 867.

Travaglia, J., Debono, D., Robertson, H., Debono, G., Rossiter, C., Dean, S., et al. (2019). *Patient Safety and Vulnerability: Overview Report.* Sydney: Centre for Health Services Research, University of Technology Sydney.

Troya, M.S. (2021). Spain's Aging Population: Four Provinces Will Have the Highest Average Age in Europe by 2050, *El Pais*, 13th May. https://english.elpais.com/society/2021-05-13/spains-aging-population-four-provinces-will-have-the-highest-average-age-in-europe-by-2050.html.

Von Collani, G., Grumm, M., & Streicher, K. (2010). An Investigation of the Determinants of Stigmatization and Prejudice toward People Living with HIV/AIDS. *Journal of Applied Social Psychology, 40*(7), 1747–1766.

Wood, H. (2020). New Insights into the Neurological Effects of COVID-19. *Nature Reviews Neurology, 16*(8), 403

12 Segregation and incarceration of people living with dementia in care homes

Critical disability and human rights approaches

Linda Steele, Lyn Phillipson, Kate Swaffer and Richard Fleming

Introduction

For people living with dementia, the COVID-19 pandemic highlights the pre-existing deep-rooted ageism and ableism, persistent social inequalities and precarity, and systemic problems of incarceration, violence, neglect and social isolation in care homes (Anand 2021; Dehm et al. 2021; Kontos et al. 2021; Peisah et al. 2020; Robertson and Travaglia 2020). These dire circumstances have been exemplified by media stories of people in care homes in nations such as Canada (Olson 2020) and Spain (Parra 2020) dying of COVID-19 or neglect after being abandoned by staff during the early months of the pandemic in 2020. The longer term neglect that has surfaced in the 'shadow' of COVID-19 (Sedensky and Condon 2020) has prompted renewed calls for recognition of human rights of people living with dementia and deinstitutionalisation of the aged care system, including through the provision of community-based housing, support and resources for people living with dementia (Herron et al. 2021; Knapp et al. 2021; Quinn 2021). These calls follow the longstanding leadership of dementia rights activists in the movement for greater recognition of equality, liberty and inclusion of people living with dementia (Dementia Alliance International 2016; Swaffer 2018) and increasing engagement with dementia human rights over the past decade by United Nations bodies (Devandas 2019b), civil society (Brown 2019; Flamm 2018) and scholars (Byrnes 2020; Cahill 2018; Green et al. 2022; Grenfell et al. 2022; Meenan et al. 2015; Mitchell 2018; Mitchell et al. 2021; Steele et al. 2019, 2021; Verbeek et al. 2021).

This chapter introduces lived experiences, critical disability studies scholarship and human rights as vital resources in understanding and challenging injustices associated with people living with dementia in care homes. We focus on challenging common, mundane and often invisible and taken-for-granted dimensions of care homes. Common features in the environmental design of care homes – dementia care units, locked doors and gates – give rise to confinement of residents with dementia and their separation from other residents and the broader community. These design features are compounded with negative and ambivalent staff and family attitudes

DOI: 10.4324/9781003221982-16

towards people living with dementia and their rights, lack of resources and supports available to people living with dementia, substituted decision-making laws to limit the movement, expression, autonomy, social experiences and well-being of people living with dementia in care homes, and government policies and funding structures that provide structural support and legitimacy to these arrangements (Steele et al. 2020, 2021). On the one hand, generally, these conditions are accepted as necessary and benevolent means of protecting people living with dementia, other residents and the general public (Dreyfus et al. 2018; Steele et al. 2020). However, on the other hand, human rights activism (Brown 2019; Devandas 2019b; Flamm 2018; Swaffer 2018) and scholarship (Green et al. 2022; Steele et al. 2019, 2020) have reframed the material, attitudinal, relational and legal dynamics of care homes as amounting to discrimination, segregation and incarceration that violate human rights to equality, legal capacity, liberty, and independent living and community inclusion. These two positions are often dialectically opposed, and the dominance of the former in government policy and dementia care provision makes it difficult to gain widespread support for human rights as a tool to guide transformation of the political conditions and everyday lives of people living with dementia.

This chapter begins with one of the authors (Kate Swaffer) discussing the lived experiences of people living with dementia of incarceration and segregation and their acts of everyday and organised resistance to these circumstances. It then draws on analytical tools from critical disability studies scholarship that support an alternative way of understanding care homes in terms of dehumanisation, segregation and incarceration. Critical disability studies scholarship is the focus of discussion because it has directly engaged with institutionalisation, coercion and control and is situated in radical anti-oppression politics. Next, the chapter explores human rights as providing transformative tools to address the segregation and incarceration in care homes that we illuminated through lived experiences and critical disability theory. This exploration centres on four dialectics presenting the conventional and human rights approaches to: (1) inequality and segregation of people living with dementia, (2) decision-making on incarcerating people living with dementia in care homes, (3) conditions of people living with dementia in care homes and (4) community living as an alternative to care homes. The UN Convention on the Rights of Persons with Disabilities (CRPD) is the focus of the discussion in this section because dementia is a condition giving rise to cognitive and other disability and the CRPD is the international human rights instrument specifically for disabled people. We conclude by reflecting on possibilities for engaging human rights to bring about transformational change.

People living with dementia in care homes – Experiences and activism

The lived experiences and activism of people living with dementia are the impetus for this chapter's exploration of injustices of care homes. In this section, one of the authors (Kate Swaffer) shares her personal reflections – as an aged care nurse, family member and person living with dementia.

In 1977, in Australia, while working in an aged care facility (then referred to as a nursing home), Swaffer's professional experience as a qualified nurse was that people living with dementia were segregated in four-bed wards within a nursing home, and if mobile, they were strapped or shackled to beds or chairs. The design of nursing homes then, now referred to in Australia as residential aged care facilities (RACFs), was based on a hospital design, with long corridors leading to wards, and few if any single rooms. For Swaffer, this RACF was the first in Adelaide that she knew of, to build a designated locked unit for people with more advanced dementia. At the time, Swaffer believed it to be an advance in dementia care, as it meant the restrictive shackles and harnesses were removed, and confinement was reduced as the residents had some liberties to move around freely within the locked unit.

Years later, Swaffer was faced with being a legal guardian for three people in her close circle living with dementia requiring assisted living, and with the best of intentions found placement for each person in a RACF. Each person she was responsible for placing into 'care' consistently complained about having been 'locked in jail'. Her father-in-law asked every time Swaffer visited, which was daily, from day one of placement and up until he died, 'why have you put me in jail; you promised me this would be my home?'. He also regularly asked for his own key to his new home. The three people living with dementia in Swaffer's close circle complained about the poor quality of the food; they complained about the lack of access to the garden or to the outside in general; they complained about the lack of allied health services such as physiotherapy or dental care; they complained about the way they were forced into a routine that was clearly for the benefit of staff, and not respectful of their own preferences and pre-entry RACF routines, not aligned with the information provided about their personal preferences. They also complained often about the restrictive visiting hours, the lack of meaningful and personalised activities and the lack of exercise of any kind.

As their legal guardian, Swaffer had promised and was legally obliged to support these three family members, and to ensure they were being well cared for with respect and dignity. However, it was evident that those under her guardianship were being physically and chemically restrained and restricted in their individual freedoms, within an institutional setting which equated to incarceration.

It remains easy for families and guardians to fall into the ruse of believing a person's safety is more important than their autonomy, and more important than their legal and human right to be supported to live in their community. To deal with the many breaches of human rights, it has been necessary to take a rights-based approach to residential care, especially for people living with dementia. The stigma and myths surrounding people living with dementia mean they are automatically deemed to have limited capacity to make their own decisions, and it is deemed acceptable to incarcerate them, leaving their care to inadequately trained staff.

Dementia Alliance International (DAI) is a charitable organisation run by and for people living with dementia. Founded in 2014 it has members in 49 countries. DAI is the first organisation in the history of the Conference of State Parties Conference (CoSP) on the Convention on the Rights of Persons with Disabilities (CRPD) to have hosted a side event specifically focused on dementia, and in particular dementia as a major cause of disability. This was done not only to highlight dementia as a disability, but to emphasise the many violations of the rights of people living with dementia.

In a statement made at this conference (Dementia Alliance International 2019), Swaffer who herself lives with younger onset dementia and is a leading international dementia rights activist stated:

> Approximately 7 years ago the Dementia Envoy for the World Dementia Council Dr Gillings said people with dementia may need to take to the streets and march on the steps of parliaments. This is the beginning of that march, so that people with dementia are not left behind in the 2030 Agenda [for Sustainable Development Goals].

Critical disability studies scholarship and people living with dementia in care homes

Informed by the lived experiences of people living with dementia just discussed, in this section we draw on threads from critical disability studies scholarship to reconceptualise the circumstances of people living with dementia in care homes in terms of ableism, dehumanisation, segregation and incarceration, and the CRPD.

Critical disability studies scholarship challenges the conventional approach to disability as an individual, natural, medical lack and instead explores how disability is constructed as undesirable because it is contingent on social, political and economic norms (Goodley 2017, see also Chapter 14). Ableism is premised on the political rather than medical causes of difference along dis/ability lines, serving to hierarchise people and populations on the basis of their relative 'fitness' and the benefit or burden of the individual to the overall well-being and prosperity of the nation. This conceptual hierarchy of 'fitness' means only some people in society – rarely those who are disabled – are considered deserving of access to property, resources, and legal protections to sustain life and flourish, and ultimately to recognition as full humans. Ableism gives rise to ontological violence – denying to people with disability a legitimate right to be recognised as humans and to exist (Steele and Frohmader 2021). Material violence and injustice against disabled people are justified on the basis that they do not have what Judith Butler refers to as 'grievable' lives (Butler 2004). They are ungrievable because 'disability is an unwanted existence [...] Their pain cannot be comprehended because their disability renders their bodies and lives devalued and, hence, incapable of eliciting grief' (Steele et al. 2020; see also Spivakovsky 2018).

Bringing the concept of ableism to the dementia context illuminates how people living with dementia are profoundly dehumanised in society and through care homes. They are viewed as not meeting cognitive social norms which is sometimes referred to as cognonormativity (or able-mindedness by Kafer 2013). This failure to meet these norms is associated with continuity over the adult life course of memory, comprehension, communication and personality, and age-related social norms of youthfulness, independence and productivity. When people living with dementia are perceived as failing to meet these norms, they are viewed as unproductive, nearly dead and an economic, emotional and physical burden on others (Aubrecht and Boafo 2020). They are dehumanised in a very particular way: by being associated with waste and death (Steele et al. 2021, p. 322).

In a neoliberal context, disabled people are seen as economically unproductive and dependent on others (Erevelles 2011; Goodley 2017). Their bodies instead become sources of economic extraction through warehousing in congregate residential and service settings (Ben-Moshe and Stewart 2016). Applying these ideas to the dementia context, we become alert to how the framing of people living with dementia as unproductive and a burden on families and the community is subverted into a source of economic gain through cost-efficient neglectful care and warehousing in care homes.

In being cast outside full humanness and political and legal subjectivity, disabled people are denied status as 'legitimate knowers' who can give meaning to themselves and their experiences (Liegghio 2013, p. 123). This is compounded even further when dementia occurs in older age, and intersects with ageism to compound stigma and discrimination (Werner and Kim 2021). This denial can be understood as violence in two respects. First, disabled people are seen as non-agential, vulnerable and in need of protection and are denied the status as political actors, capable of exercising resistance to legal and medical authority and their living circumstances (Beaupert 2018). Second, others are legally and socially authorised to decide on what happens to disabled people's bodies and lives, giving rise to non-consensual interventions such as medical treatment and institutionalisation. These interventions are understood as legal and non-violent, where they would otherwise be considered illegal and violent if done against a full (non-disabled) human (Steele 2014). Bringing these insights to the dementia context, ageing, chronic and mental illness and disability intersect to produce a particularly intense brand of epistemic exclusion (Matthews 2016; Young et al. 2019). Non-consensual confinement and physical and chemical restraints in care homes are accepted as non-violent and just, and as necessary responses to people living with dementia's expressions of distress, boredom and resistance which are pathologised as 'Behavioural and Psychological Symptoms of Dementia' or challenging behaviours. Swaffer (2019) argues that BPSD does not exist, and has been used as a form of control, against people living with dementia.

Critical disability studies scholarship provides tools to reconsider the places within which disabled people live. Disability residential centres, mental health facilities and nursing homes which are conventionally under-stood as caring, protective and therapeutic spaces are reframed as 'carceral' (i.e. prison-like) spaces because they enable control and confinement *through* discourses and practices of care, protection and treatment (Chapman et al. 2014). Throughout their lives, some individuals are confined across a number of these sites, at times with seamless legal and systems transitions between them. Chapman et al. (2014) use the term 'institutional archipelago' to refer to the networked and interconnected nature of these sites of control and confinement. Bringing these critical insights to the dementia context, care homes can be understood as involving incarceration of people living with dementia, even though care homes are conventionally presented as benign and therapeutic settings. Moreover, if situated in the archipelagic context, care homes which house people living with dementia as well as older and younger people with other disabilities can be understood as one part of the bigger picture of control and confinement of disabled people, including if particular disabled people age out of or have support needs considered too great for other institutions, or if disabled people move into nursing homes when other institutional settings in which they were living close as part of deinstitutionalisation policies (Spagnuolo 2016). Thus, care homes are an important focus of critical scholarly work in conceptualising and challeng-ing carceral control of people living with dementia *and* disabled people more broadly.

Critical disability theory also provides openings for disrupting and trans-forming these structural injustices. Liat Ben-Moshe (2013, 2020) explores the concept of abolition – a term conventionally associated with prisons – in the context of disability institutions. In popular discourse, the term 'abol-ish' means to put an end to something. In the care home context, its con-ventional meaning would suggest that abolishing care homes simply means closing down care homes, with no consideration of what comes next and of the alternative housing and support arrangements. However, in critical dis-ability studies scholarship, abolition is more complex and is a process rather than an event – it is about building more just and equitable communities so institutions (for care, punishment, whatever reason) are unnecessary. We see in this approach to abolition the possibility of addressing many of the dynamics we have introduced earlier – the material conditions of segrega-tion and incarceration as well as the cultural, legal and economic drivers that shape these material conditions.

Dialectic arguments and counter-arguments

In this section, we explore human rights as providing transformative tools that could be used to address the segregation and incarceration in care homes that we illuminated through lived experiences and critical disability the-ory. We do so with reference to the CRPD because this instrument directly addresses issues of discrimination, segregation and institutionalisation as issues of inequality and structural injustice. While people living with dementia have historically not been the focus of analysis and application of the CRPD (Steele et al. 2019), there is growing momentum in the UN (Devandas, 2019a, 2019b) and civil society (Dementia Alliance International 2016, 2019) to utilise the CRPD in relation to people living with dementia, and specifically in the context of care homes.

Inequality and segregation: Biomedical difference vs equality

The term 'dementia' is derived from the Latin prefix 'de' meaning without and 'mens' which carries the meaning of brain, intellect, faculties and understanding. A common understanding of this is simply to be 'out of your mind'. This label has informed and reflected the opinions of lay people since it was first used by Aulus Celsus who lived between 25 BC and 50 AD (Vatanabe et al. 2020). The identification of the causes of dementia as lying in identifiable and potentially understandable changes in the brain is relatively recent, dating back to the work of Alois Alzheimer in the early 20th century. The fact that this work is still far from complete and has not yet produced a cure for dementia, or a reliable means to prevent it, has left the views held by lay people relatively unchallenged. Some of the stigma surrounding dementia may in fact be informed by the biomedical view, underpinned by Cartesian thinking and the locating of personhood in the mind (Walrath and Lawlor 2019). In addition, both negative portrayals and publicity about dementia in the mainstream media have also historically contributed to public fear and a social construction of people living with dementia that is potentially both prejudicial and dehumanising (Behuniak 2011; Gerritsen et al. 2018).

One aspect of the lay view may be described as the belief that people living with dementia are so biomedically different from others that they must be obliged to accept treatment, irrespective of their wishes. A recent survey of attitudes to dementia involving interviews with 70,000 people from 155 countries (Alzheimer's Disease International 2019) showed that the general public (averaged across the 155 countries) agreed to the statement that 'It is better for people living with dementia to be forced into treatment with their doctor even if they do not want to go' (male 47.8%, female 46.2%) (Alzheimer's Disease International 2019, p. 51). Sadly, the general public's belief was supported by that of the healthcare practitioners who reported that their colleagues ignore people living with dementia: 47.8% in high-income countries, 55.8% in upper-middle income countries and 43.5% in low-/lower-middle countries (Alzheimer's Disease International 2019, p. 50).

The conventional approach to people living with dementia as naturally different reflects a medical model of dementia, which can instead be viewed as ableism and countered by the human rights argument that people living with dementia are entitled to equality and non-discrimination. Equality and non-discrimination are central to the CRPD – as a general principle, a substantive right and a thread running through all of the other substantive rights in the CRPD (UN Committee on the Rights of Persons with Disabilities 2018, pp. 1–2). Article 5(2) of the CRPD calls on States Parties to 'prohibit all discrimination on the basis of disability and guarantee to persons with disabilities equal and effective legal protection against discrimination on all grounds'. The CRPD's definition of discrimination extends to 'structural or systemic discrimination' which operates at the population level and is not reducible to the experiences of specific individuals (Pyaneandee 2019). States Parties are not only obligated to respond and prevent discrimination, but engage in positive steps at the individual and structural levels to realise equality. In particular, there is the obligation to provide reasonable accommodations.

The right to equality and non-discrimination provides a political tool to unseat the assumption of disability as a natural basis for inequality *and* gives rise to the expectation of entitlement to the resources and supports to realise equality. The UN Committee on the Rights of Persons with Disabilities refers to this as an 'inclusive equality' approach. This approach moves beyond formal legal equality to include fair redistributive, recognition, participative and accommodating dimensions (UN Committee on the Rights of Persons with Disabilities 2018, p. 3). Indeed, the former Chair of the UN Disability Committee, Theresia Degener, explains that this is grounded in human rights as universal and incapable of restriction on the basis of disability (2016, p. 4). Degener proposes that the CRPD advances a 'human rights model' of disability that is premised on 'transformative equality' (Degener 2016). Transformative equality 'targets changing these structures and systems with a variety of positive measures' (Degener 2016, p. 17). This suggests that nothing short of structural transformation of society, involving the abolition of care homes and the development of alternative living arrangements, shifts in resource allocation to ensure economic equity, and cultural shifts in how dementia is understood in society more broadly will fully realise Article 5 (Degener 2016).

Article 5 provides a political tool to challenge ableism and ageism at the core of segregation and incarceration of people living with dementia in care homes, and their subjection to violence, neglect and indifference within them. In particular, this Article supports an understanding of the systemic nature of discrimination against people living with dementia and the importance of addressing the material, legal and cultural dynamics of this. The right to equality and non-discrimination for people living with dementia provides the foundation for rights to autonomy, liberty and community living which we now turn to discuss.

Deciding about confinement: Incapacity to make decisions vs legal capacity

People living with dementia are often regarded as incapable of making decisions for themselves and thus experience discrimination in being denied legal capacity. The ADI report (Alzheimer's Disease International 2019) showed that there was widespread agreement from the general public to the statement that 'It is important to remove family responsibilities from people with dementia so as not to stress them' (M 60.4%, F 56.7%) (Alzheimer's Disease International 2019, p. 51).

It would be misleading to represent these views as universal; however, there are clear cultural differences. When asked about whether people do things for you that you could do yourself because they know you have dementia, respondents living with dementia in upper-middle-income countries (75%) (Alzheimer's Disease International 2019, p. 25) reported higher rates of others doing things for them, in comparison to high-income countries (59.1%) (Alzheimer's Disease International 2019, p. 25) and low-/lower-middle-income (50%) countries. The highest prevalence of others doing things for respondents living with dementia that they can do themselves was in the South-East Asian region (87.5%) (Alzheimer's Disease International 2019, p. 25). As the cultures in South-East Asia are known, traditionally, to have a high regard for elders, it may be that this reflects a particularly strong version of what is probably a common cultural attitude that doing things that people can do for themselves is a sign of deference towards older people. Other research also reinforces the motivations of informal carers of people living with dementia as being rooted in love, reciprocity, filial piety, duty and obligation, regardless of culture (Greenwood and Smith 2019). These also suggest that the motivation for taking over responsibilities from the person with dementia is often well intentioned.

We also see evidence of discriminatory denial of legal capacity in the involuntary placement of a person living with dementia into residential care. Evidence for this may be found in the agreement to the statement: 'If I had a family member with dementia it would be better to move them to a nursing home even if they didn't want to go'. This was the response given by 25% of people living in high-income countries (Alzheimer's Disease International 2019, p. 54). Respondents were also more likely to force someone living with dementia into a nursing home if it was not a member of their family.

This conventional position can be challenged by Article 12 of the CRPD which is about equal recognition before the law. This involves persons with disabilities having their decisions recognised on an equal basis with others and being provided with the support they require to make decisions (also referred to as 'supported decision-making') (UN Committee on the Rights of Persons with Disabilities 2014, pp. 6–7). Supported decision-making must respect the 'rights, will and preferences' of disabled people (UN Committee on the Rights of Persons with Disabilities 2014, p. 4). Supported decision-making involves diverse strategies, including 'development and recognition of diverse, non-conventional methods of communication, especially for those who use non-verbal forms of communication to express their will and preferences' and facilitating advance planning (UN Committee on the Rights of Persons with Disabilities 2014, pp. 6–7). Underpinning

Article 12 is 'universal legal capacity whereby all persons, regardless of disability or decision-making skills, inherently possess legal capacity' (UN Committee on the Rights of Persons with Disabilities 2014, p. 6). Thus, converse to assuming people living with dementia are automatically unable to make decisions because of their disability, the assumption is instead that everyone *can* make decisions with the appropriate support and there is an expectation from governments that this support will be provided when needed (De Sabbata 2020). The right to equality before the law is a 'threshold right' (UN Committee on the Rights of Persons with Disabilities 2018, p. 12) because having one's decisions legally recognised is necessary for the enjoyment of other rights, such as liberty and independent living (UN Committee on the Rights of Persons with Disabilities 2014, pp. 8–9; 2018, p. 12). A key implication of Article 12 is that people living with dementia should be given the opportunity to decide where they live, rather than others deciding for them (UN Committee on the Rights of Persons with Disabilities 2017, p. 15).

Article 12 provides a political tool to challenge the epistemic violence arising from the conventional approach to people living with dementia as incapable of making decisions about where they live and what happens to their bodies, and as requiring others to make decisions on their behalf in order to protect them.

We now turn to discuss decisions to detain people living with dementia in care homes, and then the opportunity for them to choose where they live in the community.

Conditions of confinement: Safety and security of self and other vs liberty and freedom from violence

Fear of persons living with dementia is widespread. The ADI survey revealed that the general public (averaged across the 155 countries) agreed with the statement 'A person living with dementia is impulsive and unpredictable' (M 61.2%, F 65.8%) (Alzheimer's Disease International 2019, p. 51). A substantial proportion of the general public take this further by agreeing that 'People with dementia are dangerous more often than not' (M 18.9%, F 20%) (Alzheimer's Disease International 2019, p. 51) and 'People with dementia pose a risk to their neighbours unless they are in a hospital or nursing home' (M 17.2%, F15.3%) (Alzheimer's Disease International 2019, p. 51).

The conventional understanding of people living with dementia as safe and secure through confinement in care homes can be challenged by Articles in the CRPD that centre liberty and freedom from the violence and harm associated with confinement. Article 14 of the CRPD provides for the right to liberty and security of the person. It requires that States Parties ensure that people with disabilities, on an equal basis with others, '[e]njoy the right to liberty and security of person' and '[a]re not deprived of their liberty unlawfully or arbitrarily, and that any deprivation of liberty is in conformity with the law, and that the existence of a disability shall in no case justify a deprivation of liberty'. Deprivation of liberty occurs when individuals 'are confined to a restricted space or placed in an institution or setting, not free to leave, and without free and informed consent' (Devandas 2019a, p. 10). Deprivation of liberty is unlawful where there is no legal order in place permitting their confinement, and it is arbitrary (in the sense of being 'imposed in a manner that is inappropriate, unjust, disproportionate, unpredictable, discriminatory or without due process' (Devandas 2019a, p. 10)) if confinement occurs on the basis of disability because this is discriminatory (even if pursuant to law) (Devandas 2019a, pp. 10–11; see also UN Committee on the Rights of Persons with Disabilities 2015, pp. 1–2). Detention of disabled people that is based on 'danger to self or others', 'need of care' or 'medical necessity' will also constitute arbitrary detention for the purpose of Article 14 (Devandas 2019a, p. 11).

The UN Disability Committee has identified the right to liberty and security of the person as 'one of the most precious rights to which everyone is entitled' particularly for people with cognitive disabilities (UN Committee on the Rights of Persons with Disabilities 2015, p. 1). The UN Disability Committee has stated that individuals who are deprived of their liberty in violation of Article 14 must be assisted in their release from the premises, with provision of 'access to housing, means of subsistence and other forms of economic and social support' and 'compensation, as well as other forms of reparations' (UN Committee on the Rights of Persons with Disabilities 2015, p. 7).

This right could provide a political tool to challenge the carceral nature of care homes even where that confinement is framed as purportedly benevolent, and to demand the end to the incarceration of people living with dementia. Indeed, recent reports by the UN Special Rapporteur on the Rights of Persons with Disabilities (Devandas 2019a, 2019b) have recognised deprivation of liberty in relation to older disabled people.

Article 15 on freedom from torture, inhuman and degrading treatment and Article 16 on freedom from violence provide political tools to challenge the assumption of the inherent physical and psychological safety and non-violence of care homes, including specifically in relation to use of restrictive practices. Yet, in order for people living with dementia not to be confined and segregated through care homes, we must also unseat the assumption that their inclusion in the community is burdensome, as we now turn to discuss.

An alternative future of community living and inclusion: Social and economic burden vs independent living and community inclusion

Perceiving the person living with dementia as essentially different, incapable of making decisions and potentially dangerous lays a firm foundation for seeing them as social burdens and responding by isolating and incarcerating them. This is consistent with the view of stigmatisation as a process which starts with the labelling of difference and stereotyping, both of which underpin the normalisation of both individual behaviours of 'separation' and eventually institutional forms of discrimination (Link and Phelan 2001). For example, people living with dementia responding to the ADI survey (Alzheimer's Disease International 2019) reported that being excluded from socialising, hobbies or attending events is a widespread response. Respondents living with dementia in high-income countries (38.1%), upper-middle-income countries (57.1%) and low-/lower-middle-income (50%) countries reported experiencing this form of unfair treatment because of their dementia (Alzheimer's Disease International 2019, p. 25). Respondents reported feeling 'avoided', 'ignored' and 'ostracised' in their social life due to having dementia where many of them 'no longer get invited to social gatherings' (71-year-old female from the United States of America) (Alzheimer's Disease International 2019, p. 25).

The conventional understanding of people living with dementia as a burden on the community can be challenged by Article 19 of the CRPD which provides the right to live independently and full participation in the community. 'Independent living' means that 'individuals with disabilities are provided with all necessary means to enable them to exercise choice and control over their lives and make all decisions concerning their lives' (UN Committee on the Rights of Persons with Disabilities 2017, para. 16(a)). Being 'included in the community' has been explained as having access to support in order to 'be fully included and participate in all spheres of social life' (UN Committee on the Rights of Persons with Disabilities 2017, p. 4).

In recognising the discriminatory nature of institutionalisation, the UN Disability Committee has emphasised the circumstances that can force people into 'choosing' care homes, stating: 'Institutionalization is discriminatory as it demonstrates a failure to create support and services in the community for persons with disabilities, who are forced to relinquish their participation in community life to receive treatment' (UN Committee on the Rights of Persons with Disabilities UN Disability Committee 2018, p. 14). At a structural level, realising Article 19 includes repealing laws that restrict choice about where disabled people live, implementing deinstitutionalisation policies, and reallocating resources so as to have available a range of supports and accommodations for community living and participation. At an individual level, meeting the obligations in Article 19 involves freeing people from institutions and providing support to people with disabilities to make choices as to where they live (UN Committee on the Rights of Persons with Disabilities 2017, pp. 4–5).

The significance of Article 19 should not be understated; it provides a political tool for challenging not merely the incarceration in care homes of individuals living with dementia but the entire system of care homes, the systematic warehousing of people living with dementia and the institutional archipelago more broadly. It encourages us to be ambitious in activism and critical thinking, and focus on demanding a world without care homes *and* where people living with dementia are included and supported within the community.

Conclusion

This chapter has offered some analytical and political tools to articulate and dismantle individual and structural harms experienced by people living with dementia in care homes. It has challenged the assumption that care homes are therapeutic, benevolent and benign by instead highlighting the carceral character of care homes and how they fit within broader dynamics of dehumanisation, discrimination, segregation, incarceration and violation of people living with dementia at the intersections of ableism, ageism and neoliberalism. Indeed, entry into care homes is also coercive as there are often few alternatives to institutional facilities when someone does require assisted living accommodation. By approaching dementia as a disability, the chapter explored how human rights and specifically the CRPD provide both a political framing of care homes as unjust and strategies to realise transformative change.

Perhaps for some readers the approach to dementia and care homes taken in this chapter might be confronting or unsettling and the hurdles to change the status quo might seem overwhelming or insurmountable. However, we close this chapter by reassuring readers that this is not an inevitable response. For the past 40 or so years, addressing segregation and incarceration in residential settings has been a primary focus of activism and policy development in the context of disabled people more broadly, and much can be learned from successes and failures of these experiences. Moreover, in the past decade since the coming into force of the CRPD, a rich body of theory and practice has developed around supported decision-making and deinstitutionalisation (of large and smaller disability residential settings), particularly in relation to people with intellectual disability, thus giving strategies for change that could be developed in the context of people living with dementia. Ultimately, if we approach dementia as a disability, another reality of equality, dignity and inclusion is possible.

References

Alzheimer's Disease International. (2019) *World Alzheimer Report 2019: Attitudes to Dementia*. London: Alzheimer's Disease International.

Anand, J.C., Donnelly, S., Milnec, A., Nelson-Becker, H., Vingare, E., Deusdad, B., Cellinig, G., Kinnia, R., & Pregnog, C. (2021) 'The Covid-19 Pandemic and Care Homes for Older People in Europe - Deaths, Damage and Violations of Human Rights', *European Journal of Social Work*. https://doi.org/10.1080/13691457.2021.1 954886.

Aubrecht, K., & Boafo, A. (2020) 'Deconstructing Dependency and Development in Global Dementia Policy', in K. Aubrecht, C. Kelly, & C. Rice (eds.), *The Aging/Disability Nexus*. Vancouver: University of British Columbia Press, pp. 200–217.

Beaupert, F. (2018) 'Silencing Prote(x)t: Disrupting the Scripts of Mental Health Law', *UNSW Law Journal*, vol. 41, no. 3, pp. 746–782.

Behuniak, S.M. (2011) 'The Living Dead? The Construction of People with Alzheimer's Disease as Zombies', *Ageing and Society*, vol. 31, no. 1, pp. 70–92.

Ben-Moshe, L. (2013) 'The Tension between Abolition and Reform', in M.E. Nagel & A.J. Nocella II (eds.), *The End of Prisons: Reflections from the Decarceration Movement*. Amsterdam: Rodopi pp. 83–92.

Ben-Moshe, L. (2020) *Decarcerating Disability: Deinstitutionalization and Prison Abolition*. Ann Arbor: University of Michigan Press.

Ben-Moshe, L., & Stewart, J. (2016) 'Disablement, Prison and Historical Segregation: 15 Years Later', in R. Malhotra (ed.), *Disability Politics in a Global Economy: Essays in Honour of Marta Russell*. Abingdon and New York: Routledge, pp. 87–104.

Brown, B. (2019) *Fading Away: How Aged Care Facilities in Australia Chemically Restrain Older People with Dementia*. New York: Human Rights Watch.

Butler, J. (2004) *Precarious Life: The Powers of Mourning and Violence*. London: Verso.

Byrnes, A. (2020) 'Human Rights Unbound: An Unrepentant Call for a More Complete Application of Human Rights in Relation to Older Persons—and Beyond', *Australasian Journal on Ageing*, vol. 39, pp. 91–98.

Cahill, S. 2018. *Dementia and Human Rights*. Bristol: British Policy Press.

Chapman, C., Carey, A.C., & Ben-Moshe, L. (2014) 'Reconsidering Confinement: Interlocking Locations and Logics of Incarceration', in L. Ben-Moshe, C. Chapman, & A.C.C. Carey (eds.), *Disability Incarcerated: Imprisonment and Disability in the United States and Canada*. New York: Palgrave Macmillan, pp. 3–24.

De Sabbata, K. (2020) 'Dementia, Treatment Decisions, and the UN Convention on the Rights of Persons with Disabilities. A New Framework for Old Problems', *Frontiers in Psychiatry*, vol. 11, 571722. https://doi.org/10.3389/fpsyt.2020.571722.

Degener, T. (2016) 'Disability in a Human Rights Context', *Laws*, vol. 5, no. 3. doi:10.3390/laws5030035

Dehm, S., Loughnan, C., & Steele, L. (2021) 'COVID-19 and Sites of Confinement: Public Health, Disposable Lives and Legal Accountability in Immigration Detention and Aged Care', *University of New South Wales Law Journal*, vol. 44, no. 1, pp. 59–102.

Dementia Alliance International (2016) *The Human Rights of People Living with Dementia: From Rhetoric to Reality*. Ankeny: Dementia Alliance International.

Dementia Alliance International (2019) *Statement by DAI chair Kate Swaffer #COSP12*, viewed 2 January 2022. https://dementiaallianceinternational.org/blog/statement-by-dai-chair-kate-swaffer-cosp12

Devandas, C. (2019a) *Report of the Special Rapporteur on the Rights of Persons with Disabilities: Report on the Deprivation of Liberty of Persons with Disabilities*, A/40/54, 11 January 2019.

Devandas, C. (2019b) *Report of the Special Rapporteur on the Rights of Persons with Disabilities: Report on the Rights of Older Persons with Disabilities*, A/74/186, 17 July 2019.

Dreyfus, S., Phillipson, L., & Fleming, R. (2018) 'Staff and Family Attitudes to Fences as a Means of Detaining People with Dementia in Residential Aged Care Settings: The Tension between Physical and Emotional Safety', *Australian Journal of Social Issues*, vol. 53, no. 2, pp. 107–122.

Erevelles, N. (2011) *Disability and Difference in Global Contexts: Enabling a Transformative Body Politic*. New York: Palgrave Macmillan.

Flamm, H. (2018) *"They Want Docile": How Nursing Homes in the United States Overmedicate People with Dementia*. New York: Human Rights Watch.

Gerritsen, D.L., Oyebode, J., & Gove, D. (2018) 'Ethical Implications of the Perception and Portrayal of Dementia', *Dementia*, vol. 17, no. 5, pp. 596–608.

Goodley, D. (2017) *Disability Studies: An Interdisciplinary Introduction*. Thousand Oaks: Sage Ltd.

Green, C., Tinker, A., & Manthorpe, J. (2022) 'Human Rights and Care Homes for Older People: A Typology of Approaches from Academic Literature as a Starting Point for Activist Scholarship in Human Rights and Institutional Care', *The International Journal of Human Rights*, vol. 26, no. 4, pp. 717–739.

Greenwood, N., & Smith, R. (2019) 'Motivations for Being Informal Carers of People Living with Dementia: A Systematic Review of Qualitative Literature' *BMC Geriatrics*, vol. 19, no. 1. https://bmcgeriatr.biomedcentral.com/articles/10.1186/s12877-019-1185-0

Grenfell, L., Mackay, A., & Debeljak, J. (2022) 'Human Rights Accountability and Redress for Systems of Ill-treatment in Residential Aged-Care', *Monash University Law Review*, vol. 47, no. 3, pp. 1–56.

Herron, R., Kelly, C., & Aubrecht, K. (2021) 'A Conversation about Ageism: Time to Deinstitutionalize Long-Term Care?', *University of Toronto Quarterly*, vol. 90, no. 2, pp. 183–206.

Kafer, A. (2013) *Feminist, Queer, Crip*. Bloomington: Indiana University Press.

Knapp, M., Cyhlarova, E., Comas-Herrera, A., & Lorenz-Dant, K. (2021) *Crystallising the Case for Deinstitutionalisation: COVID-19 and the Experiences of Persons with Disabilities*. London: Care and Police Evaluation Centre, LSE.

Kontos, P., Radnofsky, M.L., Fehr, P., Belleville, M.R., Bottenberg, F., Fridley, M., Massad, S., Grigorovich, A., Carson, J., Rogenski, K., Carpenter, K.S., Dupuis, S., Battalen, J., McDonagh, D., Fassbender, K., & Whitehouse, P. (2021) 'Separate and Unequal: A Time to Reimagine Dementia', *Journal of Alzheimer's Disease*, vol. 80, no. 4, pp. 1395–1399.

Liegghio, M. (2013) 'A Denial of Being: Psychiatrization as Epistemic Violence', in B. Lefrancois, R. Menzies, & G. Reaume (eds.), *Mad Matters: A Critical Reader in Canadian Mad Studies*. Toronto: Canadian Scholars Press Inc, pp. 122–129.

Link, B.G., & Phelan, J.C. (2001) 'Conceptualizing Stigma', *Annual Review of Sociology*, vol. 27, no. 1, pp. 363–385.

Matthews, N. (2016) 'Learning to Listen: Epistemic Injustice and Gothic Film in Dementia Care Education', *Feminist Media Studies*, vol. 16, no. 6, pp. 1078–1092.

Meenan, H., Rees, N., & Doron, I. (eds.) (2015) *Towards Human Rights in Residential Care for Older Persons: International Perspectives*. London: Routledge.

Mitchell, B. (2018) 'Identifying Institutional Elder Abuse in Australia through Coronial and Other Death Review Processes', *Macquarie Law Journal*, vol. 18, pp. 35–56.

Mitchell, W., Byrnes, A., Bergman, A., & Peisah, C. (2021) 'The Human Right to Justice for Older Persons with Mental Health Conditions', *The American Journal of Geriatric Psychiatry*, vol. 29, no. 10, pp. 1027–1032.

Olson, I. (2020) '"It Was So Inhumane": Conditions in Dorval Seniors' Residence Prompt Investigation', *CBC News*, 11 April 2020. https://www.cbc.ca/news/canada/montreal/west-island-staff-covid-19-1.5528956.

Parra, A. (2020) "'Didn't Give a Damn': Inside a Ravaged Spanish Nursing Home', *AP News*, 28 May 2020. https://apnews.com/article/virus-outbreak-madrid-health-spain-ap-top-news-cc24b24790f4328c7f16ea25cb496b64.

Peisah, C., Byrnes, A., Doron, I., Dark, M., & Quinn, G. (2020) 'Advocacy for the Human Rights of Older People in the COVID Pandemic and Beyond: A Call to Mental Health Professionals', *International Psychogeriatrics*, vol. 32, no. 10, pp. 1199–1204.

Pyaneandee, C. (2019) *International Disability Law: A Practical Approach to the United Nations Convention on the Rights of Persons with Disabilities.* London and New York: Routledge.

Quinn, G. (2021) 'COVID-19 and Disability: A War of Two Paradigms', in M. Kjaerum, M.F. Davis, & A. Lyons (eds.), *COVID-19 and Human Rights*. Milton: Taylor & Francis Group, pp. 116–132.

Robertson, H., & Travaglia, J. (2020) 'The Necropolitics of COVID-19: Will the COVID-19 Pandemic Reshape National Healthcare Systems?', *Impact of Social Sciences*, viewed 2 January 2022. https://blogs.lse.ac.uk/impactofsocialsciences/2020/05/18/the-necropolitics-of-covid-19-will-the-covid-19-pandemic-reshape-national-healthcare-systems/.

Sedensky, M., & Condon, B. (2020) 'Not Just COVID: Nursing Home Neglect Deaths Surge in Shadows', *AP News*, 19 November 2020. https://apnews.com/article/nursing-homes-neglect-death-surge-3b74a2202140c5a6b5cf05cdf0ea4f32.

Spagnuolo, N. (2016) 'Building Backwards in a "Post" Institutional Era: Hospital Confinement, Group Home Eviction, and Ontario's Treatment of People Labelled with Intellectual Disabilities', *Disability Studies Quarterly*, vol. 36, no. 4. https://dsq-sds.org/article/view/5279/4480

Spivakovsky, C. (2018) 'The Impossibilities of "Bearing Witness" to the Institutional Violence of Coercive Interventions in the Disability Sector', in C. Spivakovsky, K. Seear, & A. Carter (eds.), *Critical Perspectives on Coercive Interventions: Law, Medicine and Society*. London: Routledge, 97–113.

Steele, L. (2014) 'Disability, Abnormality and Criminal Law: Sterilisation as Lawful and "Good" Violence', *Griffith Law Review*, vol. 23, no. 3, pp. 467–497.

Steele, L., Carr, R., Swaffer, K., Phillipson, L., & Fleming, R. (2020) 'Human Rights and Confinement of People Living with Dementia in Care Homes', *Health and Human Rights: An International Journal*, vol. 22, no. 1, pp. 7–19.

Steele, L., & Frohmader, C. (2021) *Submission in Response to Restrictive Practices Issues Paper of the Royal Commission into Violence, Abuse, Neglect and Exploitation of People with Disability, on behalf of Women with Disabilities Australia*. Hobart: Women with Disabilities Australia.

Steele, L., Swaffer, K., Carr, R., Phillipson, L., & Fleming, R. (2021) 'Ending Confinement and Segregation: Barriers to Realising Human Rights in the Everyday Lives of People Living with Dementia in Residential Aged Care', *Australian Journal of Human Rights*, vol. 26, no. 2, pp. 308–328.

Steele, L., Swaffer, K., Phillipson, L., & Fleming, R. (2019) 'Questioning Segregation of People Living with Dementia in Australia: An International Human Rights Approach to Care Homes', *Laws*, vol. 8, no. 3, pp. 1–26.

Swaffer, K. (2018) 'Human Rights, Disability and Dementia', *Australian Journal of Dementia Care*, vol. 7, no. 1, pp. 25–28.

Swaffer, K. (2019). 'Normal Human Responses: #Beyond BPSD', 29 November 2019. https://kateswaffer.com/2019/11/29/normal-human-responses-beyondbpsd/.

United Nations Committee on the Rights of Persons with Disabilities (2014) *General Comment No. 1 (2014). Article 12: Equal Recognition before the Law*, CRPD/C/GC/1.

United Nations Committee on the Rights of Persons with Disabilities (2015) *Guidelines on Article 14 of the Convention on the Rights of Persons with Disabilities: The Right to Liberty and Security of Persons with Disabilities.*

United Nations Committee on the Rights of Persons with Disabilities (2017) *General Comment No. 5 (2017) on Living Independently and Being Included in the Community*, CRPD/C/GC/5.

United Nations Committee on the Rights of Persons with Disabilities (2018) *General Comment No. 6 (2018) on Equality and Non-discrimination*, CRPD/C/GC/6.

Vatanabe, I.P., Manzine, P.R., & Cominetti, M.R. (2020) 'Historic Concepts of Dementia and Alzheimer's Disease: From Ancient Times to the Present', *Revue Neurologique*, vol. 176, no. 3, pp. 140–147.

Verbeek, H., Peisah, C., Lima, C.A.D.M., Rabheru, K., & Ayalon, L. (2021) 'Human Rights to Inclusive Living and Care for Older People with Mental Health Conditions,' *The American Journal of Geriatric Psychiatry*, vol. 29, no. 10, pp. 1015–1020.

Walrath, D., & Lawlor, B. (2019) 'Dementia: Towards a New Republic of Hope', *The Lancet (British Edition)*, vol. 394, no. 10203, pp. 1002–1003.

Werner, P., & Kim, S. (2021) 'A Cross-National Study of Dementia Stigma Among the General Public in Israel and Australia' *Journal of Alzheimer's Disease*, vol. 83, no. 1, pp. 103–110.

Young, J.A., Lind, C., Orange, J.B., & Savundranayagam, M.Y. (2019) 'Expanding Current Understandings of Epistemic Injustice and Dementia: Learning from Stigma Theory', *Journal of Ageing Studies*, vol. 48, pp. 76–84.

13 The carnival is not over

Cultural resistance in dementia care environments

Andrea Capstick and John Chatwin

Introduction

> To be means to communicate dialogically. When dialogue ends, everything ends. Thus dialogue, by its very essence, cannot and must not come to an end.
>
> (Bakhtin, 1984: 252)

Within the dominant biomedical model of dementia, disorders of language (such as dysphasia, aphasia and perseveration) feature prominently among diagnostic criteria. In this view, changes in ability to produce coherent speech or understand the speech of others are considered to be a direct and inevitable result of neuropathology. The alternative psychosocial account of communicative challenges in dementia places emphasis largely on problems with social positioning that arise in interpersonal communication between people with dementia and 'healthy others', as Sabat (2014) somewhat problematically terms them. Less emphasis has been placed on people with dementia as social actors who create meaning and draw on contextual clues in order to give shape to their interactions. In this chapter, we draw on Mikhail Bakhtin's concepts of the carnivalesque, heteroglossia, polyphony and dialogism to analyse a series of interactions involving people with dementia in day and residential care environments.

We spent significant amounts of time in each care environment discussed below, getting to know the people who lived or spent their time there. One of the main outputs from the first study described below as Care Environment 1 was a short film about the local city market, made with two women at the day centre in question. The second project involved a number of people from Care Environment 2 in the development of a short film to be used in practitioner education. In the final study (Care Environment 3), the participants co-produced individual short films about subjects of personal interest to them.

We will not describe the three studies in detail. Instead we want to discuss how spending time with people in such environments has increased our

DOI: 10.4324/9781003221982-17

understanding of the communicative challenges faced, and the strategies employed, by people with dementia in group care settings.

Discourses on communication and dementia

We might identify three specific discourses on language and communication in dementia. They can be described respectively as dominant, alternative and emergent. The dominant biomedical discourse attributes all actions and behaviour of the diagnosed person to the progression of neurological disease. The alternative, psychosocial discourse recognises that communication with others in a social environment is also part of the picture. A more recent and still-emergent socio-political discourse recognises that much of the verbal and non-verbal communication of people with dementia is agentic, either as a protest against their situation or as a way of keeping a sense of personal identity alive in unpropitious circumstances.

Biomedical discourse

Within the biomedical standard paradigm, problems with language are among the criteria required for a diagnosis of dementia (American Psychiatric Association, 2013). In biomedical texts, the utterances of people with dementia are often reported as symptomatic of their condition. In this view, also, there is a typology of language disorders, including dysphasia (word finding problems), aphasia (absence of speech) or perseveration (repetitive speech) which are considered to be solely the result of neuropathology in localised areas of the brain, independent of any environmental factors. Studies of dementia conducted within this deficit-focused paradigm have typically examined language elicited through standardised clinical tests or as a part of interviews or conversations with a researcher (see, for example, Shao et al., 2014; Weakley and Schmitter-Edgecombe, 2014). The focus of research is generally on the prevention or management of 'inappropriate' forms of communication on the part of the person with dementia, e.g. 'verbally disruptive' behaviours in nursing home residents (Randall and Clissett, 2016).

Psychosocial discourse

An alternative model of communication in dementia is grounded in humanistic psychology. Here, it is pointed out that the psychological needs of a person diagnosed with dementia remain unchanged, and that the responses and actions of others to that diagnosis can have a significant impact on the individual's well-being and sense of identity. From this psychosocial perspective – since the environments in which people with dementia find themselves are often less than ideal – word-finding problems are also recognised, at least in part, as the result of stress and frustration, absence of speech as the result of social disengagement and repetition as a result of others failing to respond to one's communication.

Much research within this psychosocial domain has focused on improving communication in dementia care settings. Different interactional contexts have been shown to result in differences in the language produced and comprehended by people with dementia. Ramanathan (1995), for example, identified conversational partners, and the relationship between them as an influential factor on the language formulations used by individuals with dementia. These studies have mainly employed observational and ethnographic approaches and have focused on aspects of daily living.

Although preferable to the biomedical model in many ways, these sources often imply a largely passive role for the person with dementia, who is positioned as the 'spoken to', 'spoken for' or 'spoken about'. He or she is constructed as somewhat dependent, needy and lacking in agency. Of concern here, for example, is the notion – central to all of Kitwood's work – that the status of 'personhood' can either be bestowed on or taken away from a person with dementia (Kitwood 1997). Sabat's (2014) designation of those able to carry out such bestowing or withholding as 'healthy others' further compounds the unequal status ascribed to 'bestower' and recipient. For all their attempts to alter the prevailing social milieu from a malignant to a benign one, then, such formulations perpetuate a climate in which, as Langdon et al. (2007) point out, people with dementia are rarely considered able to express their own views or contribute directly to social research.

Socio-political discourse

In our own research, what has impressed us more than the communicative difficulties faced by the participants is the persistence of their attempts to use every opportunity and means at their disposal to keep communication alive. The culture of care in the environments where our studies were carried out was relatively enlightened, but nevertheless we observed many instances of improvable communication on the part of professionals and direct care staff. We also witnessed a range of coping, sense-making and self-determining strategies, which can perhaps be summed up informally as 'answering back'. Rather than the 'challenging behaviour' viewed, from a biomedical perspective, as a symptom of dementia, it became increasingly clear over time that we were observing a form of *cultural resistance*.

This finding is consistent with the gradual emergence, over the last 20 years or so, of a more socio-political model of dementia which, as Bartlett and O'Connor (2010) suggest, has not yet been sufficiently theorised. Proctor (2001), for example, located her study on the power relationships between women with dementia and medical staff, in the context of feminism as well as disability studies. Baldwin and Capstick (2007) in their critical reading of Tom Kitwood's work on person-centred care suggested that dementia studies needed to learn once again that 'the personal is political'. Behuniak (2010: 237) pointed out that the politicisation of dementia 'enables us to question the use of power, the extent of authority to be exerted over people with dementia, and the responsibilities of the community', while Branelly (2016) notes, as an issue of social justice, that people living with dementia still face a fight to achieve rights and citizenship.

In this chapter, we therefore begin to identify new theoretical perspectives on the communication of people with dementia in formal care environments – ones which seem to us to do better justice to our research findings than the view from either biomedical science or humanistic psychology.

Why Bakhtin?

Since Bakhtin was a literary theorist working predominantly in the first half of the 20th century, it may seem on the face of things a far stretch to apply his work in the context of early 21st century dementia care. We have not, however, chosen to draw on Bakhtinian concepts at random, but because they have a good, mind-to-world fit with our observations of, and interactions with, people who have dementia. In the following sections, we explain how certain concepts of Bakhtin – the carnivalesque, polyphony, heteroglossia and dialogism – have fostered a different way of seeing action and interaction within the dementia care environments where our studies were carried out. For example, the polyphony or 'play of many voices' admired by Bakhtin in the work of Rabelais and Dostoevsky is a celebration of difference, of heterogeneity. What is radical about Bakhtin's thinking is precisely that it is drawn from real-world contexts and the day-to-day language of people who do not themselves produce literary texts, although they may be represented in them. So the methodological field which is a dementia care environment, as we view it through the lens of Bakhtin's theory, is a place of extreme differences, competing voices and multiple speaking positions. People with dementia, just like the unruly 'folk' attending Rabelais' feasts and fairs, cannot conveniently be bidden to the place set out for them by the official order. The various speakers who arrive here are not the ones imagined by either biomedical or psychosocial orthodoxy; they are prone to turning the world upside down.

The carnivalesque

Bakhtin uses the term 'carnivalesque' to describe popular humour, particularly when this is directed against officialdom. Historically, carnival was an expression of mockery against church and state, and folk humour of this kind is, in Bakhtin's view, a form of cultural resistance. *Rabelais and His world* (RHW), the text in which Bakhtin (1981a) advances his theory of the carnivalesque, demonstrates via the work of Rabelais (1494–1553) how carnival imagery was deeply embedded, and embodied, in the folk culture of the Middle Ages. This imagery is a form of robust, humorous and often ribald resistance to the attempts of church and state to organise society in their own image. Bakhtin's text is structured around five key themes, which are the subject of individual chapters: laughter; the marketplace and its language; popular-festive forms and images; banquet imagery; and the grotesque image of the human body, particularly what Bakhtin terms its 'lower stratum'. Bakhtin suggests that Rabelais 'so fully and clearly revealed the peculiar and difficult language of the laughing people, that his work sheds light on the folk culture of humour belonging to other ages' (RHW: 484). Carnival laughter 'builds its own world in opposition to the official world' and has 'an essential relation to freedom' (RHW: 88–89). Much of the humour we have observed is linked to a philosophy of laughing in the face of adversity. One woman who grew up in extreme poverty in the 1930s, for example, talks of herself as coming from '(Place name) – where they eat muck, but wash it first'.

We have found that the stories told to us by people with dementia, and their spontaneous speech with each other, often rich in vernacular detail, are neither dominated by official history nor compliant with it. Humour – sometimes scatological – is a frequent feature. Much of this humour is dismissed in biomedical discourse related to people with dementia, as, for example, 'verbal abusiveness' or 'sexual disinhibition'. Here it is the context which determines what is considered appropriate, so that an off-colour joke which would not be out of place in a bar-room or on a factory floor is classed as a symptom of dementia or form of challenging behaviour in the lounge of a voluntary sector care home.

The marketplace and its language

In Care Environment 1, footage recorded in the local market – a large, canopied, Victorian landmark building – was edited together with a soundtrack composed of the comments of two women in response to the images of various stalls. Although initially subdued, we found that the two women became increasingly animated as the film sequence went on; they seemed to regain a sense of ownership of the market and its contents, and to co-construct a dialogue related to their own roles as discerning shoppers (for a full discussion see Capstick 2011). Near the end of the film, for example, the two women comment, in relation to images of jars on a sweet stall:

P: We'll have *all* the top row….
C: …and we'll have *all* the bottom row; (to researcher) we'll give you one if you like!

An aspect of the film footage which no doubt made the market more real to the two women involved is the sound of various stall-holders shouting their wares in the background ('He's got lamb chops for sale', as one of them comments). This is very reminiscent of Bakhtin's discussion of the cries of the market place in Rabelais; these cries

> were an essential part of the marketplace and street, they merged with the general popular-festive and utopian world. Rabelais heard in them

the tones of a banquet for all the people, "for all the world". These uto-pian tones were immersed in the depths of concrete, practical life, a life that could be touched, that was filled with aroma and sound.

(Bakhtin 1984: 185)

We have found that participants in all three studies refer frequently to the buying and exchange of goods, shops and shopping, the challenges of find-ing and cooking food, and different kinds of traders and vendors of goods. One woman in Care Environment 3 often repeated a playground rhyme referring to 'tingalaries'. This word was not familiar to us, but we found that 'tingalary men' was a term used by the migrant Irish population in the area where she grew up to refer to street hawkers, barrel organ players and ice-cream vendors, who were predominantly Italian. We can trace a line of descent here from the 'peculiar culture of the marketplace' in the 16th cen-tury with its 'itinerant hawkers, gypsies, and ...popular argot' (RHW, 155) through to the street language (or 'billingsgate' as Bakhtin describes it) of the Northern UK in the 1930s.

Not having money to pay for things, or not having control over one's own money, is a frequent source of anxiety among people with dementia in for-mal care environments, particularly at mealtimes. After a morning spent talking about her life story in the garden at Care Environment 3, for exam-ple, one woman said, 'Thank you, I enjoyed that, and when I get some more money we'll have a *good* do'. This is simultaneously a rueful acknowledge-ment of not being able to return hospitality at the present moment, and an invitation to future gaiety. Another woman, visited in her own apartment at the same care environment, was worried that she didn't have 'anything in' to offer us to eat. On more than one occasion, she presented a plate of dry breakfast cereal rather than offer nothing to her guests.

Popular-festive forms

'Popular-festive forms', as described by Bakhtin, are 'deeply traditional and popular, bringing an atmosphere of freedom, frankness and familiar-ity' (RHW: 195). Within these popular-festive forms, singing is considered by Bakhtin to be a form of 'profane love'. In Care Environment 3, in par-ticular, self-initiated community singing is frequent, and the songs popular with participants tend to lie within the tradition of pub and piano sing-alongs, music hall and variety. Often these songs have humorously subver-sive themes such as the 'moonlight flit' (i.e. leaving rented accommodation under cover of night without paying off arrears) in 'My old man said follow the van'; the adulterous or bigamous relationship suggested by 'My wife won't let me'; and the veiled sexual allusions of 'Daddy wouldn't buy me a bow-wow'. Also popular were the more conventionally romantic love songs of the 1940s and 1950s. One woman had lived with her widowed mother and siblings in a public house owned by another family member for several years as a child. She knew a vast range of popular songs by heart and would often sing aloud, apparently as a way of preserving her own identity and personal relationships. One song of which she was particularly fond (*I don't care who knows it, I'm in love with you*) was always introduced with the words 'And my husband used to sing to me...'. Dance halls, cinemas, high days and holidays (the local 'feast', fair, sports day or races) were also frequent subjects in spontaneous reminiscence.

Banquet imagery

As already mentioned in the discussion of marketplace imagery above, discussions related to food, its sufficiency or inadequacy, the problems of cooking and 'having enough to go round' were frequent subjects of discussion. One fieldnote from Care Environment 3, for example, describes the following interaction between Residents 1 and 2:

RESIDENT 1: [singing] 'You're the cream in my coffee....' [Resident 1 can't get beyond this first line, which she repeats several times.]
RESIDENT 2: [emphatically] 'You're the SALT IN MY STEW!'
RESIDENT 2: [a few moments later] 'Stew and dumplings! Rice pudding! You never had any money, but you always got a proper dinner!'

'Not going hungry' in the face of poverty and wartime rationing was a repeated theme of several of the female participants in Care Environment 3 and was always associated with their mothers' or grandmothers' resourcefulness in baking their own bread, cakes and puddings, and being able to make meals out of anything. A woman who originated from Liverpool, which historically has had a large Irish-Catholic population, told us what seemed at first to be the unlikely story of a shop that sold nothing but potatoes (or 'spuds' as she described them) but this turned out to be true. One woman spoke in detail about her father buying eggs and other produce (presumably on the black market) from a work colleague who lived in the country, and how her mother's face 'lit up' when he brought them home. Another, who sadly did not live to see the end of the study, gave us the recipe for making a rabbit pie, down to detailed instructions for skinning the rabbit.

The bodily lower stratum

Discussions of marital relationships, childbirth and sex are more frequent among people living with dementia than might be expected on the basis of published research, which has traditionally indicated increasing sexual apathy among this population (e.g. Miller 1995). As Ward et al. (2005) pointed out, the almost constant surveillance in most long-term care facilities makes any overt sexual expression almost impossible. One woman in Care Environment 3 who worked in a maternity hospital was particularly interested in talking about how patients and their husbands often asked her for advice about intimate problems which she was able to help with. This same participant had an interesting double take on the seamier aspects of life, often telling us how her father did not allow bad language, and then regaling us with schoolyard jokes such as 'Have you got 'em; spots on yer bottom'. Another woman explained that she had a job 'sewing men's trouser flies', which was met with the laughing question from another 'Were the men in them at the time?' In one audio recording, three women are singing and laughing uproariously at a playground song about three old ladies locked in a lavatory.

The following sections present a more detailed analysis of some of the material from these transcribed audio recordings which we believe conform to Bakhtin's concepts of polyphony, dialogism and heteroglossia.

Polyphony: The play of many voices

Polyphony is a term Bakhtin (1981b) used to advance his belief that truth requires many voices and can neither be held within a single mind, nor spoken by a single mouth. According to Rudrum (2005: 34), Bakhtin views dialogue as 'a site where no single discourse absolutely triumphs over the rest'; each individual's voice is understood to shape the character of the others' speech. In the context of dementia, the concept of polyphony helps to remind us that people with dementia are not homogenised by their diagnosis but speak in many, and diverse, voices. The psychodynamics among groups of people living with dementia can, correspondingly, be very complex.

The following extract comes from an interaction recorded in Care Environment 3 between three female residents, all in their late 80s, who have relatively severe cognitive difficulties. A researcher is showing pictures (some of which have written captions) to one resident, Nora, while another resident, Olive, is sitting alongside them in the communal lounge. A third resident, Lily, is sitting on the opposite side of the room.

During our fieldwork, it had already become clear that Nora and Lily had a complex relationship with one another. Staff members told us that they had previously been close friends, and that Nora had often been called upon to placate Lily when she was upset about something. Over time, Nora had become less able to deal with these requests, and, while she was usually still warm towards Lily, she was now clearly trying to extricate herself from the emotional demands of the relationship. Nora frequently referred to Lily as 'my mother', so possibly aspects of this relationship were reminiscent of that with her own mother (the 'dear little mother' mentioned near the end of the extract below).

One of the pictures shows the Jarrow crusade of 1936, a historical event which Nora remembers from her childhood, and has spoken of before. The interaction proceeds as follows:

NORA: And I mean they would all, all be very poor. Well, I mean, we were all poor.

OLIVE: (Starts to count the people in the photograph) 'One, two, three...'
LILY: (Shouts loudly from her seat across the room) Nora!.. Nora!.. Nora!..
Where are we?
NORA: (To researcher) Would you do me a big favour; just tell my mother
where we are?
   She'll never rest.

(The researcher crosses the room and shows Lily a map of Leeds to indicate
where she is.)

OLIVE: I saw 'em on the telly
LILY: (To researcher) Well, aren't we staying here? Well, where are we going?
How long are we going to be here?
RES: We're going to be here until lunch time.
NORA: (Laughs nervously) Oh dear
OLIVE: And then we're having some lunch.
LILY: Where are we having it?
RES: Just down the corridor
LILY: What time?
RES: Er, at half past twelve
LILY: And what time is it now?
RES: Quarter to twelve
NORA: (To Olive) Does she know that, though? ...Oh look, the Jarrow
crusade!
OLIVE: (To Nora) Where's the – how's that then?
NORA: (Has turned to the next image and is reading a picture caption to
Olive) "But I had a lovely mother, a dear little mother..."
OLIVE: (Reading another picture caption) "But the money was tight." ...I
said they was there, cos the money was tight.

(Researcher returns to sit with Nora and Olive.)

NORA: (To researcher, indicating Lily) She's a bit clever, y'know!

Here at least three separate interactions are taking place: between Nora and
Olive about the images; between Nora and the researcher about reassuring
Lily; and finally between the researcher, Lily and Olive about lunchtime.
Nora delegates the researcher to respond to Lily, using the quite sophis-
ticated negotiating skill of requesting a favour. At no point in the extract
does Nora interact directly with Lily, yet her final remark to the returning
researcher, 'She's a bit clever, y'know!', is said in an almost conspiratorial
way, suggesting that Nora is well aware of the interactional ploys used by
Lily and admires them.

Dialogism: The struggle to be heard

Vice (1997: 45) suggests that three key characteristics of dialogism in Bakhtin's work are 'the mixing of intentions of speaker and listener...the creation of meaning out of past utterance, and the constant need for utterances to position themselves in relation to one another'. The next two extracts are taken from an interaction in Care Environment 2 initiated by Don, an 89-year-old man with dementia who was recovering from a recent hip operation. Here, we suggest, the simultaneously recorded dialogue of the care staff exemplifies several of the elements identified by Vice. In addition, it seems that the content of Don's narrative is itself a subliminal influence on the interaction of the staff members (Chatwin and Capstick, 2019).

Like many people with dementia, Don's long-term recall is good and he often recounts his experience of joining the RAF at the age of 17, and working on fuel supply in a variety of war zones during the Second World War. Our impression is that this story is often repeated as a form of cultural resistance. That is to say, Don does not believe himself to fit the place now ascribed to him, as an '89-year-old man with dementia', and he rejects this status by reiterating his exploits as a young man.

On the occasion when this next interaction took place, the day centre lounge was particularly noisy, making a clear sound recording of Don extremely difficult. Don was filmed talking to a researcher in a corner of the lounge often described as the 'Men's corner'. Across the room – 7 to 10 m away – several care workers (CW) in the kitchen area are carrying on a loud and animated discussion. It is unlikely that the staff group are in a position to hear what Don and the researcher are saying to each other. They will, however, have been aware that he liked to talk about his wartime experiences, and can probably anticipate what he is talking about now.

DON: I was there when the V bombs were coming over us. And the kites were chasing them. Before they got to London, they shot them down.
CW1: (on the other side of the room) Oh sorry!
CW2: Soldier!
DON: I was never still.
CW1: Bang! bang! bang! bang! –bang!!
DON: See I was in Transport and I was all over... (Tom talks about his experience of driving a field ambulance from Hamburg to Arnhem)...and Montgomery came back. I was with Montgomery in the Middle East.
CW1: Ahh, that's what that was.
CW2: When you carry a gun, you are fighting a war.
DON: It all seems like a dream to me now; you know what I mean?

This appears to be a striking example of the mixing of intentions of speaker and listener (Vice 1997). For example, Careworker 2 makes explicit reference to a 'soldier!', while Careworker 1 imitates gunfire. The fact that this is loud enough to be audible on the film footage means that Don will have been aware that he was competing with the interchange on the other side of the room. In this context his reference to 'never being still' – coming as it does between these two militaristic utterances – implies some resistance to his current situation. Possibly, it implies 'I was never still *like I am now*', referencing not only his immobility due to recent surgery, but also that he is confined to a corner of the room while the care staff's dialogue appears to exclude and dismiss him. Careworker 2 then delivers the line, 'When you carry a gun, you are fighting a war', at the same time that Don declares, 'It all seems like a dream to me now...'

The juxtaposition of military metaphors here is particularly fascinating. While we do not wish to impose any kind of interpretative closure on this material, it adds to our growing awareness of the complex and multifaceted nature of communication in dementia care environments. Whether or not the carers borrow, consciously or unconsciously, from what they already know of Don's story, the fact that such metaphors are chosen at all implies cultural resistance on their own part as well as Don's.

Heteroglossia: Subverting the other's word

Bakhtin's concept of heteroglossia suggests how the dominant or 'prestige' organisational language of the care environment extends its control, while the subordinated language of the residents tries, in White's words (1994: 137), 'to avoid, negotiate, or subvert that control'. Here, Olive, who featured earlier, draws on the presence of others to co-construct a form of dialogue which is more favourable to her own interests. This enables her to resist, at least momentarily, the prevailing regime of the care environment – one in which even the most basic physical functions are monitored and controlled by others. 'The word does not', as Bakhtin puts it, 'exist in a neutral and impersonal language... but rather it exists in other people's mouths, in other people's contexts, serving other people's intentions; it is from there that one must take the word, and make it one's own' (Bakhtin 1981b: 294).

As the recording begins, Olive is sitting in the main lounge area with a group of other residents. Two researchers are chatting informally with members of the group. There are various other activities going on around the room. The general atmosphere is lively and the audio recording from which this extract is taken has a background of jumbled noise including fragments of speech, singing and TV noise. We join the interaction as a care worker (CW) approaches to speak to Olive:

CW: Olive, it's your turn now; going to take you to the toilet and just check your pad
OLIVE: Whu-hh? I just had – I had one
CW: Just for five minutes...

OLIVE: Just for five minutes?

CW: Yes.

OLIVE: I've got somebody with me.

CW: Yea. I'll take you to the – I'll take you to the toilet.

OLIVE: To the where?

CW: To the *toilet*...

OLIVE: *Parlour*?

CW: To the *toilet*

OLIVE: I don't want to go to the toilet.

CW: I'll just check your *pad*.

OLIVE: No. I know when I want to go to the toilet.

CW: Yea...

OLIVE: And I always go...I've gone this morning

CW: (cajoling tone) Olive, sometimes it needs checking it needs checking, y'know?

    Sometimes it's soaking wet, 'cos it needs changing, needs changing, yea?

OLIVE: I really don't want to go.

CW: You don't want to go?

OLIVE: No.

OLIVE: (To the researcher) Do *you* want to go?

RES: No, I'm all right.

From the perspective of the biomedical model of dementia what is happening here might be described as 'non-compliance with personal care', and viewed as a behavioural or psychological symptom of dementia (BPSD). Interpreted from the psychosocial perspective, it would be viewed as multiple personal detractions (Kitwood 1997: 46) committed by the carer against Olive; for example, 'imposition' ('going to take you to the toilet and just check your pad'), 'stigmatisation' (referring to her need for continence aids in front of others) and 'invalidation' ('it needs checking/changing'). However, the care worker is clearly not responsible for the cultural regime of scheduled toileting but is put in the uncomfortable position of being required to implement it as a condition of her employment. The cajoling tone that the care worker adopts is evidence of a reluctance to persist with the 'organisationally scripted' interchange. In keeping with its generally apolitical stance, then, the psychosocial model is keener to point to the 'uncaring' and 'unhomely' nature of care environments, than it is to recognise that they are also workplaces where the rights of workers are frequently overlooked.

There is also evidence of cultural resistance on Olive's part; for example, she expresses autonomy, appeals to the researcher for solidarity and persists in the face of opposition.

While we need to be reflexive about the difference that factors such as our own presence might be making, over time our becoming familiar with staff led to a relaxation of any changes to their normal practice that might have been adopted for our benefit. We frequently noted, for example, that care staff came in already wearing rubber gloves and carrying packs of incontinence pads with them – something that falls well outside normal social behaviour. Olive seems to be resisting not only the suggested toilet visit but also a culture in which people can be subjected to this form of social embarrassment in front of visitors.

Conclusion

> Bakhtin's vision of carnival [...] is finally about freedom; the courage needed to establish it, the cunning needed to maintain it, and – above all – the horrific ease with which it can be lost.
>
> (Holquist 1984: xxi)

We have argued in this chapter that neither the dominant biomedical model of dementia nor its psychosocial alternative provides a sufficient account of the complexity of communication by, and between, people with dementia and those who care for them. In particular, such models tell us little about the resources drawn on by people with dementia as social actors in order to make sense of the situations in which they find themselves, or to resist the ways in which they are constructed by others.

The theory advanced in this chapter has emerged from in-depth encounters with people with dementia in a variety of contexts and over a number of years. As 'flies on the wall' we have no doubt been party to many interactions that would simply be missed by less immersive research methods. We have not, however, found the participants in these studies to be either the hapless victims of disease or the psychologically needy recipients of care who populate familiar accounts of dementia. On the contrary, we have found numerous examples of courage, persistence and humour on the part of people living with dementia, in their attempts to subvert prevailing institutional norms and regimes.

To date the emergent socio-political model of dementia has not drawn to any great extent on relevant inter- or trans-disciplinary fields. In this chapter, we have identified the work of Mikhail Bakhtin as having particular relevance. His concepts of the carnivalesque, dialogism, heteroglossia and polyphony seem to us to have much to offer this field. We do not, however, wish to impose closure on the analysis of this data, nor do we suggest that Bakhtin's work is the only source of theoretical value. Rather, we wish to see more theoretically informed debate on this subject. Studying the communicative strategies people with dementia adopt in order to keep dialogue alive – against odds which are often heavily stacked against them – is instructive. In this way, we may learn to reconstruct people with dementia as social actors, meaning-makers and partners in equal dialogue – the 'laughing people' described by Bakhtin who have always, collectively if not individually, prevailed in the face of adversity.

Acknowledgements

This chapter is an abridged version of an article previously published in the journal *Pragmatics and Society*.

Capstick, A. and Chatwin, J. (2016) The Carnival Is Not Over: Cultural Resistance in Dementia Care Environments. *Pragmatics and Society* 7(2): 169–195.

Published by John Benjamins Publishing Company, Amsterdam/Philadelphia https://benjamins.com/catalog/ps

References

American Psychiatric Association. (2013) *Diagnostic and Statistical Manual of Mental Disorders, Fifth Edition*. Arlington, VA: American Psychiatric Association. https://doi.org/10.1176/appi.books.9780890425787.

Bakhtin, M. (1981a) *Rabelais and His World*. Bloomington: Indiana University Press.

Bakhtin, M. (1981b) On Dialogism and Heteroglossia (the other(s)' word). In Bakhtin, M. (ed.), *The Dialogic Imagination: Four Essays*. Austin, TX: University of Texas Press.

Bakhtin, M. (1984) *Problems of Dostoevsky's Poetics*. Minneapolis: University of Minnesota Press.

Baldwin, C. and Capstick, A. (2007) *Tom Kitwood on Dementia: A Reader and Critical Commentary*. Maidenhead: Open University Press.

Bartlett, R. and O'Connor, D. (2010) *Broadening the Dementia Debate: Toward Social Citizenship*. Bristol: Policy Press.

Behuniak, S.M. (2010) Toward a Political Model of Dementia: Power as Compassionate Care. *Journal of Aging Studies*, 24: 231–240. https://doi.org/10.1016/j.jaging.2010.05.003.

Branelly, T. (2016) Citizenship and People Living with Dementia: A Case for the Ethics of Care. *Dementia*, 15(3): 304–315. https://doi.org/10.1177/1471301216639463.

Capstick, A. (2011) Travels with a Flipcam: Bringing the Community to People with Dementia through Visual Technology. *Visual Studies*, 26(2): 142–147. https://doi.org/10.1080/1472586X.2011.571890.

Chatwin, J. and Capstick, A. (2019) The Influence of Subliminal Crosstalk in Dementia Narratives. *Dementia: The International Journal of Social Research and Practice*, 18(5): 1740–1750 (first published online 6.9.17) https://doi.org/10.1177/1471301217724922.

Holquist, M. (1984) *Prologue to Rabelais and His World*. Bloomington: Indiana University Press, pp. xiii–xxiii.

Kitwood, T. (1997) *Dementia Reconsidered: The Person Comes First*. Buckingham: Open University Press.

Langdon, A., Eagle, A. and Warner, J. (2007) Making Sense of Dementia in the Social World: A Qualitative Study. *Social Science and Medicine*, 64: 989–1000. https://doi.org/10.1016/j.socscimed.2006.10.029.

Miller, B., Darby, A., Yener, G. and Mena, 1. (1995) Dietary Changes, Compulsions and Sexual Behaviour in Fronto-Temporal Degeneration. *Dementia*, 6: 195–199.

Proctor, G. (2001) Listening to Older Women with Dementia: Relationships, Voices and Power. *Disability and Society*, 16(3): 361–376.

Ramanathan, V. (1995) Narrative Well-Formedness in Alzheimer Discourse: An Interactional Examination across Settings. *Journal of Pragmatics*, 23: 395–419.

Randall, E.W. and Clissett, P.C. (2016) What Are the Relative Merits of Interventions Used to Reduce the Occurrences of Disruptive Vocalisation in Persons with Dementia? – A Systematic Review. *International Journal of Older People Nursing*, 11(1): 4–17. https://doi.org/10.1111/opn.12083.

Rudrum, D. (2005) Silent Dialogue: Philosophising with Jan Svankmajer. In Read, R. and Goodenough, J. (eds.), *Film as Philosophy: Essays on Cinema after Wittgenstein and Cavell*. London: Palgrave-Macmillan, pp. 114–132.

Sabat, S. (2014) A Bio-Psycho-Social Approach to Dementia. In Downs, M. and Bowers, B. (eds.) (2nd ed.), *Excellence in Dementia Care: Research into Practice*. Maidenhead: Open University Press. https://doi.org/10.1177/10.1177_14713012177 05483.

Shao, Z., Janse, E., Visser, K. and Meyer, A.S. (2014) What Do Verbal Fluency Tasks Measure? Predictors of Verbal Fluency Performance in Older Adults. *Frontiers in Psychology*, 5(772): 1–10. https://doi.org/10.3389/fpsyg.2014.00772.

Vice, S. (1997) *Introducing Bakhtin*. Manchester: Manchester University Press.

Ward, R., Vass, A.A., Aggarwal, N., Garfield, C. and Cybyk, B. (2005) A Kiss Is Still a Kiss?: The Construction of Sexuality in Dementia Care. *Dementia*, 4(1): 49–72.

Weakley, A., and Schmitter-Edgecombe, M. (2014) Analysis of verbal fluency in Alzheimer's Disease: The Role of Clustering, Switching, and Semantic Proximities. *Archives of Clinical Neuropsychology*, 29(3): 256–268. https://doi.org/10.1093/arclin/acu010.

White, A. (1994) Bakhtin, Sociolinguistics, Deconstruction. In J. Barrell, J. Rose, P. Stallybrass, J. White and S. Hall (eds.), *Carnival, Hysteria and Writing: Collected Essays and an Autobiography*. Oxford: Oxford University Press, pp. 135–159.

Part IV
Forging alliances

14 Convergences, collaborations, and co-conspirators

The radical potentiality of critical disability studies and critical dementia studies

Hailee M. Yoshizaki-Gibbons

Introduction

Dementia is an unstable and elusive concept. Medical, social, political, economic, and cultural views of dementia at times intertwine and at other times conflict. Dementia is deeply medicalised as a 'disease' and a sign of 'abnormal' or 'pathological' ageing while also being historically and culturally constructed as an expected, 'normal' outcome of ageing (Ballenger, 2006; Kelley-Moore, 2010). It has been positioned as the anti-thesis of 'successful ageing' and yet there is a growing focus on 'living well' with dementia (Daffner, 2010: Gibbons, 2016; Martyr et al., 2018). Dementia is often viewed as an illness 'without hope and beyond help' (Gilliard et al., 2005, p. 574) while also being the focus of billions of dollars each year in research funds (Alzheimer's Association, 2020). It is perhaps the most feared condition in modern society, but simultaneously it is an increasingly common human experience, a politicised identity, and a source of mobilisation and activism (Bartlett, 2012; Marist Institute for Public Opinion, 2014). The complexity of dementia has given rise to critical dementia studies, a field that seeks to 'think dementia differently' (Sandberg and Ward, 2019). In this chapter, I contend that to think dementia differently, it is important to engage in radical and disruptive collaborations with critical disability studies and other critical fields, recognise convergences between dementia and other social identities and locations, and co-conspire with feminist, anti-racist, postcolonial, queer-crip movements. Despite Alison Kafer's (2013) call for political, relational affinities and flexible alliances between disability and other social justice movements in her ground-breaking text *Feminist, Queer, Crip*, there has been little to no collusion or coalition-building between critical disability studies and critical dementia studies (Yoshizaki-Gibbons, 2018b, 2021). I argue that integrating critical disability studies and critical dementia studies is essential and has the radical potential to create crucial coalitions that can change the social, political, and economic landscape for people with dementia and other devalued 'bodyminds' (Price, 2015).

Building on Julie Avril Minich's(2016) and Sami Schalk and Jina B. Kim's (2020) work framing critical disability studies as a *methodology* rather than

DOI: 10.4324/9781003221982-19

a subject area devoted exclusively to the study of disabled people, I explore the radical potential of placing critical disability studies and critical dementia studies in conversation. Specifically, convergences between these critical fields traverse disciplinary boundaries, uncover new critical analyses of dementia, old age, disability, and care, and expand possibilities for radical coalition-building. To illustrate, I consider how critical disability studies theories, perspectives, and frameworks may be applied in new ways to dementia. Specifically, I focus on mental disability (Price, 2011), bodymind (Price, 2015; Schalk, 2018), debility (Puar, 2017), and crip-of-colour critique (Kim, 2017). In doing so, I elucidate how such an intersection furthers our understanding of the lived experiences of people with dementia, illuminates the structural and societal changes needed to work towards the collective liberation, and contributes to the emerging field of critical dementia studies.

Disability studies and dementia: An elusive connection

Broadly speaking, disability studies centres the study of disability from bodily, social, political, and economic perspectives, thereby countering individualised, medicalised approaches to disability. The field emerged in the 1980s, primarily in the Global North, in conjunction with disability rights activism. Disability studies is a highly interdisciplinary field, integrating disciplines such as history, literature, philosophy, cultural studies, anthropology, sociology, and psychology. While disability studies has grown extensively since its inception, there has been limited scholarly or activist engagement with dementia. As Baldwin (2008) lamented, 'The disability model of dementia is still relatively under-theorised' (p. 223). Although there are notable exceptions,[1] unfortunately, there has been insufficient progress in exploring dementia through disability studies. Shakespeare et al. (2019) observed, 'Dementia and disability seem like planets spinning on different axes, their inhabitants aware of each other's existence but apparently unable to communicate' (p. 1075). This lack of attention to dementia is unfortunate given the potential of disability studies as a transformative, liberatory field. As van Heuman (2012) argued, 'Disability studies can provide valuable insights and applications in reframing dementia because of its social explanations of disability, emancipatory nature, aim to interrogate and change elements of the disabling world, and interdisciplinary approaches' (p. 109). Disability studies could expand through explorations of dementia, yet this connection remains elusive.

From disability studies to critical disability studies

In recent years, disability studies has been critiqued as a discipline for privileging dominant perspectives and failing to acknowledge race, gender, class, sexuality, age, and nation as categories of analysis that intersect with disability (Bell, 2006; Erevelles, 2011; McRuer, 2006; Schalk and Kim, 2020; Yoshizaki-Gibbons, 2018b). Furthermore, as noted by Minich (2016) and

Schalk (2017), disability studies has been limited by reducing its scope to a specific subject of study—disabled people. Jennifer Eun-Jung Row (2022) explained:

> Until recently, scholarship in disability studies has emphasised that disability is an object—the object of inquiry, of social, medical, or legal studies of deformity or aberrance. These approaches endeavor to probe the origins of, correct, cure, or even eradicate disability. Although well-intentioned, these approaches can unknowingly perpetuate and reinforce hierarchies of ableism—the belief that abled bodyminds are superior to disabled ones.
>
> (p. 87)

This subject/object mode of inquiry has prevented disability studies from employing disability as an analytic or method to examine how particular bodyminds—including those not generally understood or labelled as 'disabled'—are pathologised, stigmatised, and devalued across intersecting axes of difference.

Such criticisms have led to the emergence of critical disability studies.[2] Critical disability studies is not seeking to merely replace or add to disability studies; rather, it seeks to expand and transform the field by emphasising critical perspectives, engaging in intersectional analyses, and working towards social justice (Goodley, 2013; Meekosha and Shuttleworth, 2009; Minich, 2016; Schalk and Kim, 2020; Yoshizaki-Gibbons, 2018a). As noted by Minich (2016), a critical disability studies methodology 'involves scrutinising not bodily or mental impairments but the social norms that define particular attributes as impairments, as well as the social conditions that concentrate stigmatised attributes in particular populations' (para 6). Whereas disability studies has predominately focused on disability and disabled people, critical disability studies seeks to examine how discourses, practices, and ideologies of ability and disability connect to broader, more expansive issues such as embodiment, self and identity, state and capitalistic violence, the environment, reproduction, healthcare, care and care work, and globalisation (Erevelles, 2011; Kafer, 2013; Minich, 2016; Schalk and Kim, 2020; Yoshizaki-Gibbons, 2020). Consequently, critical disability studies has produced important new insights into how disability is situated within overlapping and mutually constitutive systems of power, oppression, and resistance. Furthermore, critical disability studies has supported new approaches to and spaces for praxis, or the application of theory into activism and practice (Goodley, 2013; Minich, 2016).

An expansive, transformative approach

Examining dementia through the social model of disability illustrates how critical disability studies is expansive and transformative. The social model is useful as a case study because it is a foundational framework in disability studies and of the limited work that seeks to integrate disability studies and dementia, much of it focuses on the application of the social model of disability (e.g. Bartlett and O'Connor, 2010; Gilliard et al., 2005). The social model of disability contrasts the medical model of disability by locating the problem of disability in society (Oliver, 2009). Hence, the social model proposes that disability is socially constructed through prejudicial and discriminatory attitudinal, environmental, and structural barriers. In doing so, the social model distinguishes impairment—a functional limitation— from disability—a socially created system of oppression. This emphasis on disadvantages and restrictions caused by society has been used to organise for disability rights, including the rights for disabled people to live in the community, access public spaces and events, receive training and education, and work and earn a living wage (Llewellyn and Hogan, 2000; Wendell, 1996). The social model has the potential to demonstrate how attitudinal, environmental, and structural barriers marginalise and disable people with dementia. Hence, it can be used to address prejudice and discrimination, and adapt environments to fit the unique needs of individuals with dementia.

However, critical disability studies scholars have increasingly highlighted the limits of the social model and argued for a more expansive, inclusive approach to social and political change (Kafer, 2013; Meekosha and Shuttleworth, 2009; Puar, 2015). These constraints and opportunities become apparent when the social model is considered in the context of dementia. A major challenge is that the social model was developed primarily by white, cisheterosexual men with permanent, stable physical disabilities and excludes people with mental disabilities, chronic illnesses, and progressive or unpredictable disabilities (Price, 2011; Wendell, 2001). As noted by Shakespeare et al. (2019), 'Because the social model was developed to account for the experiences of people with static physical impairments, it fails adequately to contextualise impairments which are associated with pain; with limitation; with frailty; and with degeneration' (p. 1080). Furthermore, the social model distinguishes between impairment and disability, creating dichotomous, binary categories. As Kafer (2013) noted, 'Although I agree that we need to attend to the social, asserting a sharp divide between impairment and disability fails to recognise that both impairment and disability are social' (p. 7). In other words, impairment is also subject to socially constructed meanings and conditions related to difference, power, and oppression. For people with dementia, impairments such as memory loss and communication difficulties are interconnected with social understandings of the self and personhood. The impairment/disability distinction under the social model also often leads to overlooking or neglecting the significance of impairment in disabled people's lives, and the ways in which impairment may be disabling (Kafer, 2013). Impairments experienced by people with dementia, such as memory loss, disorientation, pain, and fatigue, cannot be alleviated or addressed solely through environmental manipulation and social change.

Additionally, the social model of disability is often used within disability rights movements in ways that support neoliberal capitalism. The social model reflects a generational system in disability studies, which focuses on youth and middle age and the roles associated with these life stages—specifically, education and employment (Priestley, 2003). These roles are deeply intertwined with neoliberal, capitalistic discourses of the normal, self-sustaining, successful citizen. The social model has been used to argue that the state must eliminate environmental and structural barriers for disabled people to engage in education and employment to become productive and thus valuable citizens (Puar, 2017). This tactic further marginalises people with dementia, who are viewed as 'too old' and 'too impaired' to contribute meaningfully to society. Consequently, despite the expansion of disability rights and protections, people with dementia continue to be largely excluded from society.

When dementia is centred, the limitations of the social model and rights frameworks become more apparent. Its inability to address issues of impairment and its entanglement with neoliberal capitalist ideologies constrain its usefulness when applied to dementia. To be clear, the field of critical disability studies does not advocate for entirely rejecting the social model and rights frameworks due to its potential usefulness for addressing the attitudinal, environmental, and structural barriers disabled people face. However, critical disability studies offers a way to move beyond the social model of disability to expansively theoretically engage with the complexity of dementia, leading to richer and more disruptive analyses of dementia.

Critical disability studies and dementia

Despite the bodily, social, political, economic, and structural entanglements of disability and dementia, there remains a dearth of critical disability studies scholarship on dementia (Yoshizaki-Gibbons, 2018b). The lack of engagement with dementia in critical disability studies has several significant consequences. First, it limits intersectional analyses of dementia that are grounded in feminist, anti-racist, queercrip politics. Second, it deprioritises and makes invisible people with dementia who are further marginalised by race, class, gender, sexuality, and age (for further discussion of these intersections see Chapters 15 and 16). Third, it maintains existing power structures and systems of oppression rather than achieve critical disability studies' goal of 'producing knowledge in support of justice for people with stigmatised bodies and minds' (Minich, 2016, para 6). Additionally, dementia can develop, complicate, and transform critical disability studies due to its implications for theorising issues such as memory (Price, 2017; Yoshizaki-Gibbons, 2020), temporality (Kafer, 2013; Yoshizaki-Gibbons, in press), cognition (Dowse et al., 2009), selfhood and citizenship (Minich, 2014). Relatedly, centring people with dementia pushes critical disability studies to consider who is included and excluded from disability scholarship and political movements.

Thus, it is essential that scholars and activists apply critical disability studies theories and frameworks to dementia. Doing so will also do the crucial work of placing critical disability studies and critical dementia studies in conversation with each other, serving as a foundation to coalition-building for 'more accessible futures' (Kafer, 2013, p. 169). In what follows, I examine dementia through four critical disability studies theories and frameworks: mental disability (Price, 2011), bodymind (Price, 2015; Schalk, 2018), debility (Puar, 2018), and crip-of-colour critique (J. B. Kim, 2017).[3]

Mental disability and 'demented' bodyminds

In recent years, debate has emerged over whether dementia should be categorised as a disability (All-Party Parliamentary Group on Dementia, 2019; Shakespeare et al., 2019). While these debates have focused on semantic, functional, and legal definitions, critical disability studies urges examinations of language that do not only centre on meaning but also explore 'what our current articulations of disability are saying in the here and now' (Titchkosky, 2001, p. 138) and moreover, how these articulations are grounded in social, cultural, and material realities.

Dementia is predominately understood, medically and culturally, as an impairment of the mind. The very origins of the word dementia reflect this reality, as dementia is derived from the Latin 'de mentis' which means 'out of one's mind.' In this regard, dementia is a 'mental disability,' defined broadly by Margaret Price as a disability located in one's mind (2011, 2013). This classification is important, as Price deployed mental disability as a category of analysis, or a way of examining how certain minds are pathologised as 'unwell,' 'mentally ill,' 'demented,' or 'cognitively deficient,' and how these constructions are rooted in categorisations of racialised, gendered, classed, aged, and nationalised difference (Price, 2011, 2015). Cultural constructions of women as 'hysterical' support patriarchal ideologies of gender and disability that position women as weaker and mentally incapable without the support of a strong, rational male figure (Yoshizaki-Gibbons and O'Leary, 2018). Shifting criteria for schizophrenia in the *Diagnostic and Statistical Manual II* emphasised hostility, aggression, and violence which led to Black men being over-diagnosed and placed in institutions for the 'criminally insane' (Metzl, 2010). In the context of dementia, ageist ideas that old people should be 'nice,' 'docile,' and 'cooperative' merge with ableist notions of people with dementia as 'agitated,' 'unmanageable,' and 'combative' to justify the overuse of anti-psychotics in dementia units of nursing homes (Mason, 2018). Similarly, a loss of cognitive control has been connected to a failure to normatively perform gender, at times resulting in an aggressive and dehumanising reinforcement of gender norms for people with dementia (Baril and Silverman, 2022; Sandberg, 2018). Such examples emphasise the mutually constitutive nature of mental disability across axes of difference and highlight its relevance to dementia.

In addition to serving as an analytic, mental disability is a collective category. It is intentionally broad in scope, challenging rigid systems of diagnosis and categorisation that produce exclusions and limit alliances (Kafer, 2013). Hence, mental disability has coalitional potential, uniting people with diverse bodyminds who are constructed as disabled, including Autistic people, people with psychiatric diagnoses, people who do not follow norms in terms of attention or learning processes, and, I would add, people with dementia (Lewiecki-Wilson, 2003; Price, 2011). Such a coalition unites people with different mental disabilities who have been segregated into silos based on diagnosis, medical treatment, and cultural discourses and ideologies, yet who share experiences as people with stigmatised and devalued minds (see also Chapter 18, which strikes a note of caution about potential coalitions along these lines).

Yet, dementia and other mental disabilities do not exist within disembodied minds. Whereas dementia is often associated with cognitive experiences such as memory loss, disorientation, confusion of time and place, disorganisation, and aphasia, various bodily experiences may also co-exist, including pain, mobility impairments, incontinence, and difficulty performing rote tasks such as chewing and swallowing. These mental and physical manifestations intertwine and cannot be examined singularly. Dementia is not unique in this regard, as many mental disabilities involve a complex overlapping of the body and mind.

Given this, Price (2011, 2015) highlights the usefulness of examining mental disability through the term 'bodymind'—a term Price adopted to communicate the importance of mental disability as an analytic while also grappling with the complexity that the mind cannot be easily separated from the body. Under the Cartesian dualism of Western philosophy, the body and mind are considered distinct entities—a view that has been widely embraced in the Global North (Price, 2015). Indeed, mainstream disability studies has reflected this dualism by historically focusing on and privileging the perspectives of those with physical disabilities while disregarding mental disabilities, including dementia. As a critical disability studies concept, bodymind seeks to challenge the differentiation between mind and body. As observed by Schalk (2018), the term 'bodymind' emphasises 'the inextricability of mind and body and highlights how processes within our being impact one another in such a way that the notion of a physical versus mental process is difficult, if not impossible to clearly discern' (p. 5). As a material feminist disability studies concept, bodymind has applications far beyond more traditional understandings of disability. For instance, Schalk (2018) considers how bodymind is a useful framework for examining the toll racism and white supremacy have on Black, Indigenous, and other People of Colour—a toll that manifests physically, mentally, and even at a cellular level. Patsavas (2014) draws on the framework of bodymind to uncover how pain is not easily located within the body or the mind, but instead is a slippery concept that is simultaneously imbricated in the bodymind and leaking, or occurring between, bodyminds. Thus, the theory of bodymind supports critical analyses of oppression, pain, trauma, and other human experiences.

Applying the concept of bodymind to dementia reveals the ways in which certain aged and disabled bodyminds are constructed as 'demented'—as bodies with minds that are so deeply impaired, one is unable to function or care for oneself, mentally and physically. The 'demented' bodymind is viewed as an empty body, a body without a working, logical, and productive mind, a body in which one is 'trapped' (Aquilina and Hughes, 2006). This classification of course applies to older people with dementia but it is also relevant to those of us labelled as insane, crazy, irrational, and psychotic. The very word 'demented' conjures images of older people staring at nothing as they sit in wheelchairs in nursing homes or patients in psychiatric wards shuffling around under the haze of intense psychiatric medications (Zeilig, 2013). While these cultural stories are troubling, such depictions also illustrate the structures to which those of us with 'demented' bodyminds are subjected, such as pathologisation, overmedicalisation, and institutionalisation.

Dementia as debility and crip-of-colour critique

The concept of bodymind is also useful when considering the ways in which dementia and dementia care are debilitating. Debility has emerged in recent years as a category that connects to and convolutes disability (Livingston, 2005; Puar, 2017). Within Western medicine and American culture, debility is widely associated with weakness, frailty, or infirmity. Consequently, the employment of debility as a theoretical lens in disability studies may initially appear to pathologise or re-medicalise impaired, injured, or aged bodyminds (Price, 2015). However, debility offers an opportunity to contextualise impairment. As Livingston (2005) noted, 'Debility...has a history, in the sense that impairment and disfigurement arise out of particular junctures...and thus gives us insights into people's historical experiences and changing assumptions about personhood and self' (p. 2). Similarly, Puar (2017) theorised debility as bodily injury and exclusion related to cultural, economic, and political factors. This conceptualisation seeks to disrupt the disabled/non-disabled binary by arguing that marginalised populations, such as Black, Indigenous, People of Colour, those in the Global South, and poor people, are often subjected to ongoing violence and trauma through state violence, colonisation, and imperialism. The impairments that arise out of these junctures are often not viewed as disability, as defined by Western, white neoliberal rights frameworks. These groups 'may well be debilitated, in part by being foreclosed access to legibility and resources as disabled' (Puar, 2017, p. xv). Thus, while the social model has been criticised for disregarding impairment, debility centres impairment. It allows us to consider the ways in which impairment is created by and subject to economic, political, cultural, and social forces. In this regard, debility follows

Kafer's (2013) assertion that impairment, like disability, is subject to social meanings and assemblages but it is distinct due to its examination of how impairment via debilitation occurs over time and thus exists outside of ability and disability categorisations and systems.

Focusing on debility also uncovers the myriad ways that marginalised and vulnerable people are targeted for debilitation. Puar (2017) connects debility to Lauren Berlant's (2007) concept of 'slow death,' or the wearing out of populations experiencing structural inequality under neoliberal capitalism. Schalk and Kim (2020) illustrate debilitation through the Flint Water Crisis. In Flint, Michigan, a predominately working-class, Black, post-industrial city, those in power elected to shift the residents' water source from the treated Detroit Water and Sewage Department to the toxic and corrosive Flint River as an austerity measure. This water contamination debilitated children and adults through lead poisoning and exposure to harmful bacteria, which over time led to numerous physical and mental health issues, including neurological damage, cognitive decline, increased anxiety and depression, hypertension, and kidney and cardiovascular disease. Thus, rather than presenting disablement as a one-time, traumatic event, debility highlights the ways marginalised people are vulnerable to ongoing violence and oppression (Morrison and Casper, 2012; Puar, 2017). Viewing debilitation as a process occurring over the life course complicates the disabled/non-disabled binary and creates new possibilities for explorations of people marginalised by gender, race, class, and age with a wide range of impairments who may not identify as disabled or be recognised as disabled by others or the state (Kafer, 2013; Puar, 2017).

Relatedly, as highlighted by Puar (2017), debility provides a way to disrupt disability rights discourses grounded in the social model that further the power of the state, privilege dominant groups, and reify oppressive notions of productivity, value, and personhood. Critical disability studies has increasingly critiqued identity-based, rights-based frameworks as an avenue for social change (Schalk and Kim, 2020). Puar (2017) stated:

> Debility is…a crucial complication of the neoliberal transit of disability rights. Debility addresses injury and bodily exclusion that are endemic rather than epidemic or exceptional and reflects a need for rethinking overarching structures of working, schooling, and living rather than relying on rights frames to provide accommodationist solutions.
>
> (p. xvii)

Neoliberal disability rights platforms reinforce the power of the state by allowing the state to define and determine the boundaries of the category of 'disability' and allocate rights, protections, and services accordingly (Puar, 2017). The state also has the power to decide the parameters of disability rights laws and policies, and if, when, and how such laws and policies are enforced. Moreover, rights do not equally benefit all members of a marginalised group or protected class. According to Schalk and Kim (2020), rights-based frameworks 'tend to primarily benefit the most elite occupants of any given identity category while prioritising assimilation into dominant institutions' (p. 43). Additionally, as Dean Spade (2015) observed, rights-based frameworks position the state as benevolent and protective. Hence, marginalised groups subject to state violence are excluded and invisibilised, and critical analyses of state violence are limited. Although disability rights have had a significant impact on disabled people in Western countries, particularly those who are white, male, well-educated, and physically disabled, debility refocuses our attention on people and groups who have been ignored by or ostracised from disability rights movements and are subject to ongoing suffering under neoliberal capitalism.

In the context of dementia, rights-based frameworks would primarily benefit and support those who are able to access a diagnosis of Alzheimer's disease or related dementias, those who are considered to be in the 'early stages' of dementia and retain normative abilities such as verbal communication skills, and those in privileged categories of race, gender, and class. Such rights-based approaches fail to acknowledge those with dementia who are controlled, confined, brutalised, and debilitated by the state through slow violence and slow death, such as the rapidly increasing population of people with dementia in prison and other carceral systems or those in poverty and undocumented people with dementia unable to access welfare and similar supports.

In addition to the limits of the neoliberal rights framework sponsored by the state, it is also essential to understand how dementia and dementia care are connected to state and capitalistic violence. Jina B. Kim (2017) forwards a 'crip-of-colour critique,' which is 'a mode of analysis that urges us to hold racism, illness, and disability together, to see them as antagonists in a shared struggle, and to generate a poetics of survival from that nexus' (para 2). J.B. Kim (2017) further elaborates that a crip-of-colour critique centres precarious populations. In doing so, it understands the state not as a site of protection but rather a site of control, violence, and disablement and capitalism as a debilitating, deadly imperative.

Furthermore, employing a crip-of-colour critique in the context of debility allows critical disability studies and critical dementia studies to grapple with the complex ways in which dementia is intertwined with gender, racialisation, class, disablement, and deep old age, and how these matrices of oppression operate within neoliberal capitalism and state power. Dementia is often portrayed as a public health epidemic from which no one is 'immune' or 'safe' (Thompson, 2017). However, Puar (2017) argued that debilitation is 'a practice of rendering populations available for statistically likely injury' (p. xviii) and examining the demographics of people with dementia reveals that dementia is in fact unexceptional and endemic for marginalised groups. Approximately, two-thirds of people with dementia are women (Alzheimer's Association, 2022). Additionally, older Black people are about two times as likely and older Latinx people are about one and one-half times as likely to have Alzheimer's disease or related dementias than older white people (Alzheimer's Association, 2021). Recent research has connected dementia to stress, poverty, racism, pollution, and deprived living conditions (Kunkle, 2017; Wong, 2017), revealing the ways in which marginalised and vulnerable groups are subject to ongoing debilitation under state and capitalistic violence that places them at risk for dementia in old age.

For multiply marginalised elders, dementia may be the final form of debilitation, which marks them as the 'living dead,' and subjects them to institutionalisation—creating an opportunity for the medical industrial complex to profit (Behuniak, 2011; Yoshizaki-Gibbons, 2020). As a crip-of-colour critique highlights, institutionalisation is one way that the state and capitalism intersect to simultaneously provide older people with dementia and care workers with a means of survival while also subjecting them to debilitation, isolation, exploitation, and violence. As Puar asked, 'What debilitated bodies can be reinvigorated for capitalism, and which cannot?' (p. 153). Older women, particularly older women of colour, are increasingly confined in nursing homes, the majority of which are private companies, as their middle- and upper-class white peers opt for community-based care (Feng et al., 2011). Consequently, the gendered, racialised, and classed demented subject is transformed into a consumer of care, on local and transnational levels (Kolářová, 2015). This transformation is key in the process of debilitation and central to what Puar (2017) referred to as 'the right to maim,' or the right of sovereign power to impair or debilitate (compare to Robertson and Travaglia's argument on necropolitics, Chapter 11). Puar (2017) further contextualised the right to maim, explaining, 'Maiming is a source of value extraction from populations that would otherwise be disposable' (pp. xviii–xix). Although dementia is classified as a terminal disease, people may live anywhere from 1 to 20 years after diagnosis. In this liminal place between life and death, 'useless' and 'unproductive' old and demented bodyminds—the 'living dead'—are converted into lucrative bodies that benefit the nursing home industry and medical industrial complex.

Once people with dementia are incarcerated in nursing homes, they are excluded from society and subject to further maiming through placement in locked wards, physical or pharmacological restraints, neglect, abuse, and other forms of violence (further discussed in Chapter 12). Consequently, people marginalised by gender, race, and class with dementia experience an old age that is not the time of leisure, health, or opportunity society imagines—but rather one marked by shifting and intensifying forms of surveillance, discipline, and control.

Furthermore, a crip-of-colour critique reveals how those who care for people with dementia are also often subject to debilitation and state violence. Approximately two-thirds of dementia caregivers are women (Alzheimer's Association 2022; Bartlett and O'Connor, 2010), and in institutional settings, many of these women are further marginalised by race, class, and immigrant status (Allen and Cherry, 2006; Khatutsky et al., 2011). As noted by Puar (2017), 'Caretakers of people with disabilities often come from chronically disenfranchised populations that endure debilities themselves' (p. xvi). These multiply marginalised women often experience difficult working conditions with increasing levels of bureaucracy and control due to state regulations. They frequently work for minimum wage, and without access to benefits such as paid leave, health insurance, disability insurance, or retirement packages. Consequently, neoliberal capitalism and the state exploit both sides of the care dialectic in dementia care—simultaneously contributing to the debilitation of people with dementia and their caregivers.

Conclusion

Although the social model of disability and other forms of mainstream disability studies scholarship are useful for examining the attitudinal, environmental, and social barriers older people with dementia face, critical disability studies theories, perspectives, and frameworks offer new, expansive, and transformative ways to think about dementia. As noted by Ward and Sandberg (2019), 'Ultimately, a move toward critical dementia studies is a chance to ask afresh what dementia means, what it does and the outcomes it has for people' (para 5). In this chapter, I have sought to make a case for scholar-activists in critical disability studies and critical dementia studies to co-conspire and engage in liberatory, coalitional politics in order to think dementia differently. Placing critical disability studies and critical dementia studies in conversation is important for several reasons. First, it will further unsettle dominant cultural discourses and ideologies of devalued bodyminds by drawing from diverse critical feminist, anti-racist, postcolonial, and queercrip critiques. Second, it will open possibilities for racialised, gendered, classed, and nationalised analyses of dementia, which are currently missing in mainstream disability and dementia studies. Third, it will challenge disabling social structures and systems of oppression, thereby creating 'more accessible futures' for older people with dementia, particularly for those with advanced dementia who are excluded by identity-based, rights-based, and citizenship frameworks (Kafer, 2013). Lastly, it will integrate disability and dementia political movements in important ways, such as creating structures of care that foreground the social and material conditions of those giving and receiving care, working towards collective access in our communities (Hamraie, 2013), and seeking abolition of carceral systems, including nursing homes and other institutions (Ben-Moshe, 2020). The radical potentiality of critical disability studies and critical dementia studies is infinite and can lead to new forms of scholarship and activism that uses intersectional politics to centre diverse older and disabled bodyminds as we work towards social justice.

Notes

1 See Bartlett and O'Connor (2010); Gilliard et al. (2005); Shakespeare et al. (2019)·
2 It is essential to note that critical disability studies is intertwined with other critiques and expansions of disability studies, including feminist disability studies (Kafer, 2013), feminist-of-colour disability studies (Schalk and Kim, 2020), materialist feminist disability studies (Price, 2015), black feminist disability studies (Bailey and Mobley, 2018), and transnational feminist disability studies (Erevelles, 2011).
3 I selected theories and frameworks that I viewed as particularly relevant to dementia, but there are many others that may be useful for analysing dementia that I was unable to cover due to space constraints, such as crip theory (McRuer, 2006), curative time and curative violence (Kafer, 2013; E. Kim, 2017), compulsory able-bodiedness/able-mindedness (Kafer, 2013; McRuer, 2006), compulsory youthfulness (Gibbons, 2016), and collective access (Hamraie, 2013).

References

Allen, P.D., and Cherry, K. (2006). Race Relations in the Nursing Home Setting. *Race, Gender & Class*, 13(1/2), pp. 36–45. JSTOR. https://www.jstor.org/stable/41675219.

All-Party Parliamentary Group on Dementia. (2019). Hidden No More: Dementia and Disability. https://www.alzheimers.org.uk/sites/default/files/2019-06/APPG_on_Dementia_2019_report_Hidden_no_more_dementia_and_disability_media.pdf.

Alzheimer's Association. (2022). 2022 Alzheimer's Disease Facts and Figures. https://www.alz.org/media/documents/alzheimers-facts-and-figures.pdf

Alzheimer's Association. (2021) Special report Race, ethnicity and Alzheimer's in America https://www.alz.org/media/Documents/alzheimers-facts-and-figures-special-report-2021.pdf

Alzheimer's Association. (2020). *Fiscal Year 2021 Alzheimer's Research Funding.* https://act.alz.org/site/DocServer/2015_Appropriations_Fact_Sheet__FY16_.pdf?docID=3641.

Aquilina, C. and Hughes, J.C. (2006). The Return of the Living Dead: Agency Lost and Found? In J.C. Hughes, S.J. Louw, and S.R. Sabat (Eds.), *Dementia: Mind, Meaning, and the Person* (pp. 143–162). Oxford University Press.

Bailey, M. and Mobley, I.A. (2018). Work in the Intersections: A Black Feminist Disability Framework. *Gender & Society*, 33(1), pp. 19–40. https://doi.org/10.1177/0891243218801523.

Baldwin, C. (2008). Narrative(,) Citizenship and Dementia: The Personal and the Political. *Journal of Aging Studies*, 22(3), pp. 222–228. https://doi.org/10.1016/j.jaging.2007.04.002.

Ballenger, J.F. (2006). *Self, Senility, and Alzheimer's Disease in Modern America: A History.* John Hopkins University Press.

Baril, A. and Silverman, M. (2022). Forgotten Lives: Trans Older Adults Living with Dementia at the Intersection of Cisgenderism, Ableism/Cogniticism and Ageism. *Sexualities*, 25(1–2), pp. 117–131. https://doi.org/10.1177/1363460719876835.

Bartlett, R. (2012). The Emergent Modes of Dementia Activism. *Ageing and Society*, 34(4), pp. 623–644.

Bartlett, R. and O'Connor, D. (2010). *Broadening the Dementia Debate: Towards Social Citizenship*. The Policy Press.

Behuniak, S.M. (2010). The Living Dead? The Construction of People with Alzheimer's Disease as Zombies. *Ageing and Society*, 31(1), pp. 70–92. https://doi.org/10.1017/s0144686x10000693.

Bell, C. (2006). Introducing White Disability Studies: A Modest Proposal. In Davis, L. (Ed.), *The Disability Studies Reader* (pp. 275–282). Routledge.

Ben-Moshe, L. (2020). *Decarcerating Disability: Deinstitutionalization and Prison Abolition*. University of Minnesota Press.

Berlant, L. (2007). Slow Death (Sovereignty, Obesity, Lateral Agency). *Critical Inquiry*, 33, pp. 754–780. https://www.jstor.org/stable/10.1086/521568?seq=1.

Daffner, K.R. (2010). Promoting Successful Cognitive Aging: A Comprehensive Review. *Journal of Alzheimer's Disease*, 19(4), pp. 1101–1122. https://doi.org/10.3233/JAD-2010-1306.

Dowse, L., Baldry, E. and Snoyman, P. (2009). Disabling Criminology: Conceptualising the Intersections of Critical Disability Studies and Critical Criminology for People with Mental Health and Cognitive Disabilities in the Criminal Justice System. *Australian Journal of Human Rights*, 15(1), pp. 29–46. https://doi.org/10.1080/1323238x.2009.11910860.

Erevelles, N. (2011). *Disability and Difference in Global Contexts: Enabling a Transformative Body Politic*. Palgrave Macmillan.

Feng, Z., Fennell, M.L., Tyler, D.A., Clark, M., and Mor, V. (2011). Growth of Racial and Ethnic Minorities in US Nursing Homes Drive by Demographics and Possible Disparities in Options. *Health Affairs*, 30(7), pp. 1358–1365. https://doi.org/10.1377/hlthaff.2011.0126.

Gibbons, H.M. (2016). Compulsory Youthfulness: Intersections of Ableism and Ageism in "Successful Aging" Discourses. *Review of Disability Studies*, 12(2 & 3), pp. 70–88.

Gilliard, J., Means, R., Beattie, A., and Daker-White, G. (2005). Dementia Care in England and the Social Model of Disability: Lessons and Issues. *Dementia*, 4(4), pp. 571–586. https://doi.org/10.1177/1471301205058312.

Goodley, D. (2013). Dis/entangling Critical Disability Studies. *Disability & Society*, 28(5), pp. 631–644.

Hamraie, A. (2013). Designing Collective Access: A Feminist Disability Theory of Universal Design. *Disability Studies Quarterly*, 33(4). https://dsq-sds.org/article/view/3871/3411.

Kafer, A. (2013). *Feminist Queer Crip*. Indiana University Press.

Kelley-Moore, J.A. (2010). Disability and Ageing: The Social Construction of Causality. In D. Dannefer and C. Phillipson (Eds.), *The SAGE Handbook of Social Gerontology* (pp. 96–110). SAGE.

Khatutsky, G., Wiener, J., Anderson, W., Akhmerova, V. and Jessuprti, E.A. (2011). *Understanding Direct Care Workers: A Snapshot of Two of America's Most Important Jobs: Certified Nursing Assistants and Home Health Aides*. U.S. Department of Health and Human Services. https://aspe.hhs.gov/system/files/pdf/76186/CNAchart.pdf.

Kim, E. (2017). *Curative Violence: Rehabilitating Disability, Gender, and Sexuality in Modern Korea*. Duke University Press.

Kim, J.B. (2017). Toward a Crip-of-Color Critique: Thinking with Minich's "Enabling Whom?" *Lateral*, 6(1). https://doi.org/https://doi.org/10.25158/L6.1.14

Kolářová, K. (2015). 'Grandpa Lives in Paradise Now': Biological Precarity and the Global Economy of Debility. *Feminist Review*, 111, pp. 75–87.

Kunkle, F. (2017). Stress of Poverty, Racism Raise Risk of Alzheimer's for African Americans, New Research Suggests. *Washington Post*. https://www.washingtonpost.com/local/social-issues/stress-of-poverty-and-racism-raise-risk-of-alzheimers-for-african-americans-new-research-suggests/2017/07/15/4a16e918-68c9-11e7-a1d7-9a32c91c6f40_story.html?utm_term=.b099963f5f50.

Lewiecki-Wilson, C. (2003). Rethinking Rhetoric through Mental Disabilities. *Rhetoric Review*, 22(2), pp. 156–167. https://www.jstor.org/stable/3093036.

Livingston, J. (2005). *Debility and Moral Imagination in Botswana*. Indiana University Press.

Llewellyn, A. and Hogan, K. (2000). The Use and Abuse of Models of Disability. *Disability & Society*, 15(1), pp. 157–165. https://doi.org/10.1080/09687590025829.

Marist Institute for Public Opinion. (2014). "Alzheimer's Most Feared Disease." *Marist Poll*.

Martyr, A., Nelis, S.M., Quinn, C., Wu, Y.-T., Lamont, R.A., Henderson, C., Clarke, R., Hindle, J.V., Thom, J.M., Jones, I.R., Morris, R.G., Rusted, J.M., Victor, C.R. and Clare, L. (2018). Living Well with Dementia: A Systematic Review and Correlational Meta-Analysis of Factors Associated with Quality of Life, Well-being and Life Satisfaction in People with Dementia. *Psychological Medicine*. Cambridge University Press, 48(13), pp. 2130–2139. https://doi.org/10.1017/S0033291718000405.

Mason, B. (2018). *Mitigating the Impact of Structural Discrimination for People with Dementia Residing in Long-Term Care Facilities*. Master's Thesis. St. Johns: Memorial University of Newfoundland.

McRuer, R. (2006). *Crip Theory: Cultural Signs of Queerness and Disability*. New York University Press.

Meekosha, H., & Shuttleworth, R. (2009). What's So 'Critical' about Critical Disability Studies? *Australian Journal of Human Rights*, 15(1), pp. 47–75. https://doi.org/10.1080/1323238X.2009.11910861.

Metzl, J. (2010). *The Protest Psychosis: How Schizophrenia Became a Black Disease*. Beacon.

Minich, J.A. (2014). *Accessible Citizenships: Disability, Nation, and the Cultural Politics of Greater Mexico*. Temple University Press.

Minich, J.A. (2016). Enabling Whom? Critical Disability Studies Now. *Lateral*, [online] 5(1). https://csalateral.org/issue/5-1/forum-alt-humanities-critical-disability-studies-now-minich/.

Morrison, D.R. and Casper, M.J. (2012). Intersections of Disability Studies and Critical Trauma Studies: A Provocation. *Disability Studies Quarterly*, 32(2). https://doi.org/10.18061/dsq.v32i2.3189

Oliver, M. (2009). *Understanding Disability: From Theory to Practice*. Palgrave.

Patsavas, A. (2014). Recovering a Cripistemology of Pain. *Journal of Literary & Cultural Disability Studies*, 8(2), pp. 203–218. https://doi.org/10.3828/jlcds.2014.16.

Price, M. (2011). *Mad at School: Rhetorics of Mental Disability and Academic Life*. University of Michigan Press.

Price, M. (2015). The Bodymind Problem and the Possibilities of Pain. *Hypatia*, 30(1), pp. 268–284. https://doi.org/10.1111/hypa.12127.

Price, M. (2017). Are They Still in There? Memory Loss and the in/human. Conference on College Composition and Communication. Portland, OR.

Priestley, M. (2003). Disability and Old Age. In M. Priestley (Ed.), *Disability: A Life Course Approach* (pp. 143–165). Polity Press.

Puar, J. (2015). Bodies with New Organs: Becoming Trans, Becoming Disabled. *Social Text,* 33(3), pp. 45–73.

Puar, J. (2017). *The Right to Maim: Debility, Capacity, Disability.* Duke University Press.

Row, J.E. (2022). Marvelous Monstrosity and Disability's Delights: New Directions in Premodern Critical Disability Studies. *Exemplaria,* 34(1), pp. 87–101. https://doi.org/10.1080/10412573.2021.2021003.

Sandberg, L. (2018). Dementia and the Gender Trouble?: theorising Dementia, Gendered Subjectivity and Embodiment. *Journal of Aging Studies.* 45(June), pp. 25–31.

Schalk, S.D. (2017). Critical Disability Studies as Methodology. *Lateral,* [online] 6(1). https://csalateral.org/issue/6-1/forum-alt-humanities-critical-disability-studies-methodology-schalk/.

Schalk, S.D. (2018). *Bodyminds Reimagined: (Dis)ability, Race, and Gender in Black Women's Speculative Fiction.* Duke University Press.

Schalk, S.D. and Kim, J.B. (2020). Integrating Race, Transforming Feminist Disability Studies. *Signs: Journal of Women in Culture and Society,* 46(1), pp. 31–55. https://doi.org/10.1086/709213.

Shakespeare, T., Zeilig, H. and Mittler, P. (2019). Rights in Mind: Thinking Differently about Dementia and Disability. *Dementia,* 18(3), pp. 1075–1088. https://doi.org/10.1177/1471301217701506.

Spade, D. (2015). *Normal Life: Administrative Violence, Critical Trans Politics, and the Limits of Law.* Duke University Press.

Thompson, B. (2017). No One Immune to Alzheimer's Touch. *Chronicle.* http://www.chronicleonline.com/news/local/no-one-immune-to-alzheimer-s-touch/article_8d70f5ee-b20e-11e7-a8a5-9349ef650f59.html.

Titchkosky, T. (2001). Disability: A Rose by Any Other Name? "People-first" Language in Canadian Society. *Canadian Review of Sociology/Revue Canadienne de Sociologie,* 38(2), pp. 125–140. https://doi.org/10.1111/j.1755-618X.2001.tb00967.x.

van Heuman, L. (2012). Challenging the Way We Think about Dementia. In J. Jansen and T. Dobbelaar (Eds.), *Zie meer Kijk anders. Tien jonge wetenschappers over disability studies (See More by Looking in a Different Way. Ten Young Scientists on Disability Studies)* (pp. 101–114). ZonMw.

Ward, R. and Sandberg, L. (2019, August 30). Calling for (a more) Critical Dementia Studies - Critical Dementia Network. *International Network for Critical Gerontology.* https://criticalgerontology.com/calling-for-a-more-critical-dementia-studies-critical-dementia-network/.

Wendell, S. (1996). *The Rejected Body: Feminist Philosophical Reflection on Disability.* Routledge.

Wendell, S. (2001). Unhealthy Disabled: Treating Chronic Illnesses as Disabilities. *Hypatia,* 16(4), pp. 17–33. https://doi.org/10.1111/j.1527-2001.2001.tb00751.x.

Wong, E. (2017). Pollution Leads to Greater Risk of Dementia among Older Women, Study Says. *The New York Times.* https://www.nytimes.com/2017/02/04/world/asia/pollution-dementia-women.html.

Yoshizaki-Gibbons, H.M. (2018a). Critical Disability Studies. In T. Heller, S. Parker Harris, C. Gill, and R. P. Gould (Eds.), *Disability in American Life: An Encyclopedia of Concepts, Policies, and Controversies* (pp. 149–152). ABC-CLIO.

Yoshizaki-Gibbons, H.M. (2018b). Engaging with Ageing: A Call for the Greying of Critical Disability Studies. In K. Ellis, R. Garland-Thomson, M. Kent, and R. Robertson (Eds.), *Manifestos for the Future of Critical Disability Studies* (pp. 179–188). Routledge.

Yoshizaki-Gibbons, H.M. (2020). Time and again: Old Women and Care Workers Navigating Time, Relationality, and Power in Dementia Units [Doctoral dissertation, University of Illinois at Chicago]. Proquest Dissertations Publishing.

Yoshizaki-Gibbons, H.M. (2021). Integrating Critical Disability Studies and Critical Gerontology to Explore the Complexities of Ageing with Disabilities. In M. Putnam and C. Bigby (Eds.), *Handbook of Aging with Disability*. Routledge. London: Routlege, pp. 32–43.

Yoshizaki-Gibbons, H. M. (In Press.) "She's going to forget everything": Entanglements of disability and aging in films centered on dementia. In S. Falcus, H. Hartung and R. Medina (eds.) *The Bloomsbury Handbook to Ageing in Contemporary Literature and Film*. London: Bloomsbury.

Yoshizaki-Gibbons, H.M., and O'Leary, M.E. (2018). Deviant Sexuality: The Hypersexualization of Women with Bipolar Disorder in Film and Television. In J. Leeson-Schatz and A. George (Eds.), *The Image of Disability: Essays on Media Representations* (pp. 93–106). McFarland.pp.93-106

Zeilig, H. (2013). Dementia as a Cultural Metaphor. *The Gerontologist*, 54(2), pp. 258–267. https://doi.org/10.1093/geront/gns203.

15 Thinking dementia differently

Dialogues between feminist scholarship and dementia studies

Linn J. Sandberg

What does feminist scholarship have to offer dementia studies? Over several decades, feminist researchers have provided a wealth of knowledge on men and women's lives and the workings of gendered power asymmetries and other forms of oppression, both how they are sustained and challenged. A lot of this research has been and will continue to be of great value for studying things such as the organisation of formal and informal dementia care and the citizenship and everyday lives of people with dementia, of which a vast majority are older women (for some notable work on gender and dementia, see, for example, Boyle, 2019; Hulko, 2009; Proctor, 2001). Beyond this, feminist scholarship also provides a range of critical 'tools' for rethinking knowledge production, including the ways we may understand dementia as an Othered position and people with dementia as a marginalised or oppressed group. These 'tools' will provide the focus for this chapter. The overall aim is to engage in a critical dialogue between dementia studies and feminist scholarship.

Some of the most perceptive analyses of illnesses and disabilities as social and political conditions have emerged from prominent feminist scholars, such as Patti Lather's (Lather & Smithies1997) work on HIV/AIDS and Audre Lorde's (1997) and Eve Kosofsky Sedgwick's (1999) work on cancer to name but a few. Surprisingly, however, dementia has rarely been the centre of feminist attention. Thus, it is my ambition to show some of the ways feminist work can be engaged with to critically think and rethink dementia.

Needless to say, feminist studies is a broad terrain of concepts and theories and in this brief chapter I have been forced to limit my discussion to some sections of this terrain. Specifically, I focus on how feminist scholarship invites us to think dementia through the lens of *difference* and of thinking dementia as a fundamentally political category and condition. I approach dementia and difference through two different feminist theoretical genealogies. The first part of my argument draws on the work of feminist difference theorists to argue for *dementia as difference*. The second part of my argument draws on feminist standpoint theory and discusses *differences between people with dementia* and how people with dementia may be understood as holding 'epistemic privilege', a unique positioning from

DOI: 10.4324/9781003221982-20

which to understand cognitive ableism. The first part of my argument is situated in a post-structuralist and post-materialist realm, focusing on ways of rethinking the cultural imaginaries of dementia. The second is to a greater extent emerging from materialist roots, inspired by Marxism and radical feminism. The focus of feminist standpoint theory is consequently on the different material conditions and lived experiences of people with dementia, including their experiences of oppression both from cognitive ableism and other forms of power asymmetries.

My motivation for exploring these theoretical genealogies stems from the influential work of feminist philosopher Sandra Harding (1986) who maps out three different feminist epistemologies: feminist empiricism, feminist standpoint theory and post-modern feminist epistemology. Feminist empiricism primarily seeks to remove gender bias and include women further in scientific research, and in terms of dementia this could, for example, involve including women in medical studies and women's possibilities for a timely diagnosis. The latter two, in comparison, aim at more radical revisioning of knowledge production, something I find imperative for critical dementia studies. Consequently, although the two approaches discussed in this chapter are different in epistemological terms, they both allow dementia scholars to go beyond both the bio-medical realm and a liberal humanist realm that focuses on personhood, citizenship and human rights, and move towards a more critical knowledge production in dementia studies.

Thinking dementia as difference: Beyond loss or 'living well'

Are women *different*? Are people with dementia *different*? As suggested by feminist theorist Rosi Braidotti (1994, p. 148), 'difference' within feminist thinking is a site of intense conceptual tension'. For many feminists, from Simone de Beauvoir onwards, overcoming the devaluation and othering of women/femininity and achieving equality has been linked to the rejection of a purported difference/otherness of women. Difference has often been dismissed by feminists as 'a hopelessly "essentialistic" notion', as formulated by Braidotti (1994, p. 148). Moreover, the rejection of difference, in the work of many feminists but also more broadly in liberal-humanist scholarship, could also be linked to the tarnished history of difference. In European fascism and colonialist projects historically, as well as in present-day populist right-wing discourse, the purported difference of racialised, indigenous and other minority populations has been used as the legitimation for subjugation and even extinction of Others (for more applied discussions on otherness and difference, see, for example, Chapters 7, 17 and 18 in this volume).

However, for Braidotti and other feminist difference theorists such as Elisabeth Grosz (1994) and Luce Irigaray (1985), the problem is not difference itself, but rather how difference is always constituted in negative and pejorative terms, as loss and lack. For feminists, these discussions have primarily centred on sexual difference and how the female body and subjectivity have been equated with lack, loss and castration. But this is equally relevant in terms of other differences, such as ageing and/or disabled bodyminds (Roets & Braidotti, 2012; Sandberg, 2013; Shildrick, 2009; for a discussion of the concept of bodymind, see Chapter 14 in this volume). In their chapter on cognitive disabilities, Roets and Braidotti (2012) argue:

> Ever since modernity, a vision of the subject as a unitary and rational self is pursued in knowledge production and the aim has been to control, govern and discipline the individual according to this norm. In this universalistic frame of reference, a binary logic of self-other reduces differences to a pejorative and disqualified phenomenon.
>
> (p. 164)

However, instead of trying to do away with difference, feminist difference theorists have proposed an affirmation of difference. In these versions, difference is not used as negation but as a proliferative and productive force – a way of thinking bodies and subjectivities as being set in constant processes of becoming. In the case of Braidotti, she is inspired specifically by a Deleuzian approach to difference. As I will go on to argue, this kind of approach is also useful for theorising the bodyminds of people living with dementia as it provides ways of acknowledging the embodied specificities and the different subjectivities that may emerge when living with dementia illnesses, without being trapped within a framework in which these differences are either pathologised or assimilated into a cognitive ableist world.

There is a long history of equating dementia with decline and loss and it is thus very visible the way in which dementia is constituted in terms of negative difference and otherness. As discussed in several chapters in this volume, biomedicine and its focus on the degeneration of cognitive capacities have played a significant role in positioning dementia as primarily a matter of deterioration. But narratives of negativity and loss have also been perpetuated in cultural and media discourses, where the person with dementia has commonly been portrayed as abject or monstrous (Behuniak, 2011; Peel, 2014, also Chapter 9 in this volume). Altogether this has fuelled what McParland and colleagues (2017) refer to as a 'tragedy discourse' on dementia.

While discourses on ageing and later life have increasingly focused on successful/positive/active/healthy ageing, dementia has come to function as the unsuccessful underbelly of ageing (Gilleard & Higgs, 2013). Dementia is thus continuously portrayed as the most fearful state of ageing (Lock, 2013) and the ultimate example of 'growing old "badly"' (Latimer, 2018). This has resulted in an increasing emphasis on managing and taking responsibility to prevent cognitive illness. Thus, the 'ageing brain can be managed' through brain exercises and life style choices, and the slide into the othered position of dementia can supposedly be avoided (Latimer, 2018). However, in a contemporary 'neuroculture of healthy aging', this also entails that those who experience memory loss and cognitive impairments are continuously positioned as 'failed' and remain in a position as Other (Williams et al., 2011, p. 242).

To challenge the pervasive discourses centred on negativity, loss and tragedy, a new discourse of 'living well with dementia' has, over the years, emerged within academia, policy-making and civil society (McParland et al., 2017). This discourse seeks to underscore the remaining capacities of persons with dementia and how personhood may be sustained. Clearly a living well discourse is more positive, seeks to invoke hope and to shift the perspectives on dementia from a terminal to a chronic illness, and to underline the normality of people with dementia. As argued by Kate Swaffer (2015, p. 4) who is living with dementia, to 're-invest in life' poses a significant challenge to the pervasive approach that prescribes disengagement after a dementia diagnosis. Clearly, the emergence of a 'living well with dementia' discourse in many ways mimics developments within policies on ageing, chronic illness and disabilities more broadly. However, the surfacing of a living well discourse also carries with it a similar set of problems that has engaged critical gerontologists and disability scholars for some time. Simply that an emphasis on normality and the good life when living with illness/disability/old age continues to rest on an obscuring and othering of those with the most severe conditions. As McParland and colleagues astutely point out, the living well with dementia discourse by and large focuses on a relatively agentic group of people with dementia, but still tends to exclude the most vulnerable and frail, including those residing in formal care:

> While the newly visible group of people living well with dementia strive to convince society that they are part of its normality, the more vulnerable group of people living with advanced dementia continue to epitomise deviance, differentness or 'otherness'.
>
> (McParland et al., 2017, p. 265)

As McParland and colleagues go on to argue, the current dichotomising of dementia, as either tragedy or living well, does not rightfully reflect the complex experiences of people living with dementia and risks creating dividing lines between people with dementia who are understood as living successfully and those who remain in the position of the failed Others, due to more severe forms of impairment. I suggest that what is essentially 'the elephant in the room' is *difference*. While it may seem as if a living well discourse provides a greater acceptance of difference, one may also argue that it is still largely invested in Western modernist and humanist ideals of relatively active, agentic, autonomous, and contained subjects. As such this discourse could not be considered a fundamental challenge to hegemonic subjectivity and cognitive ableism. Living well discourses are thus primarily assimilationist discourses that seek to underscore normality and sameness – 'Look, they/we are just like us/you!'.

Moreover, one may argue that the living well discourse by and large imitates successful ageing discourses and their rejection of negative affects, including pain and suffering and abject embodiment (Bülow & Holm, 2016; Sandberg, 2015). Just as the production of successful ageing implies the potential of failure, the emphasis on living well clearly indicates 'living badly' with dementia. The turn to positivity may as such become an imperative for happiness and the good life. Still, living with dementia also involves considerable suffering (Bartlett et al., 2017) and a 'living well' discourse may as such become a form of 'cruel optimism' to use a term coined by cultural theorist Lauren Berlant (2011). In Berlant's words, 'cruel optimism exists when something you desire is actually an obstacle to your flourishing' (Berlant, 2011, p. 1). In the case of dementia, the struggle to 'live well' with dementia may then essentially lead to additional suffering when one cannot achieve this idealised state and overcome difference.

So, what would it mean to turn to another version of difference, an affirmative version as proposed by feminist difference theorists? First, this would enable ways of thinking dementia neither from the perspective of biomedicine as a pathological difference nor through an assimilationist lens which risks effacing the embodied and lived specificities of the experience of dementia. This would allow for radically new ways of imagining dementia beyond dichotomised approaches of decline/loss/tragedy or living well.

Second, thinking dementia as affirmative difference would enable ways of thinking subjectivity in new and more radical ways. Historically, subjectivity in dementia has predominantly been defined in terms of loss or unbecoming (see discussion in Chapter 6). There has since the end of the last century been significant work done to challenge these definitions, primarily by underscoring how subjectivity in dementia may be sustained in social interactions and by others supporting or 'holding' the person with dementia in their identities (Hydén et al., 2014; Kitwood, 1997). Still these alternative versions of subjectivity, beyond loss, do not fundamentally challenge the premise of Western hegemonic subjectivity as singular, stable (enduring) and primarily built on cognitive capacities. Turning to feminist difference theorist such as Braidotti would, in contrast, promote ways of thinking 'the subject as a multiple, open-ended and interconnected identity that occupies a variety of possible subject positions, at different places (spatially) and at different times (temporally), across a multiplicity of constructions of self (relationality)' (Braidotti, 1994, p. 158). This kind of construction of subjectivity is not bound to reinforcing continuity with an assumed stable self from the past, but instead allows bodyminds in dementia to go in new and unforeseen directions, to become different from what they were, without being 'lost'. This kind of approach to dementia as difference resonates with the argument of Ward and Price (2016, p. 167) who suggest that experiences of dementia sometimes involve 'loosening of the customary ties to social convention' which may in turn open up to the possibilities of exploring 'hidden, forgotten, or quite new aspects of self and identity'. In more concrete terms, dementia could, for example, entail 'forgetting' heteronormativity and enable new and different gendered and sexual subjectivities to emerge (Baril & Silverman, 2022; Capstick & Clegg, 2013; see also Chapter 17 in this volume).

Third, turning to feminist difference theorists to think dementia is also a way to further explore and emphasise dementia as embodied. For feminists, embodiment has surely been a site of potential trouble and concern. Since women have often been reduced to their bodies and biological determinist and essentialist arguments have been frequently used to legitimise the subordination of women, many feminists, including feminist scholars, have been prone to evade the material specificities of gendered and sexed bodies (Lykke, 2010). This in many ways parallels developments within disability studies as well as social and cultural gerontology and dementia studies. Almost two decades ago, feminist gerontologist Julia Twigg (2004, p. 59) argued that the attempts of social and cultural gerontologists to challenge the dominance of the bio-medical paradigm and its focus on physiological and pathological aspects of old age had effectively resulted in the avoidance of the 'topic of the body'. A parallel tendency can be seen in the history of dementia studies where person-centred approaches have tended to focus on social interaction in ways which have often overlooked embodiment (Kontos & Martin, 2013). Although things have changed in the last decades in feminist studies as well as gerontology, disability and dementia studies, the fear of biological determinism when turning to questions of embodiment still seems to linger in many instances. However, turning to feminist difference theorists offers non-deterministic and non-essentialist ways of understanding embodiment and corporeality in dementia. This implies regarding dementia as a site for the production of embodied difference, not as *being* different but constantly in a process of *becoming* different from itself. This includes attending to the materiality and the plasticity of brains with dementia, but also how technological assemblages such as robot care protheses might enable embodied becomings in dementia (DeFalco, 2018; Jenkins, 2017). Moreover, disorientation and 'getting lost' as very concrete embodied manifestation of dementia position people on a different slant, in a different positioning, from which the world can be approached and knowledge produced (Ward et al., 2022). This leads me to my next discussion on difference, where I argue that the different standpoints that people with dementia inhabit need to be put at the centre of knowledge production in dementia studies.

The different positionalities of dementia: Thinking through feminist standpoint theory

So far I have discussed feminist difference theorists and how their attempts to formulate affirmative versions of difference may be useful to dementia studies. But difference has also figured in other ways in feminist research, as differences between women (and other subjugated groups) and how intersections of various power asymmetries affect and shape women's lives differently. In the discussion that follows, where I discuss differences between people with dementia, I will particularly draw on the theoretical genealogies of feminist standpoint theory to argue for these different experiences of oppression to form the basis of knowledge production in dementia studies.

Among those living with dementia, does it matter whose voice is amplified? A central question for feminist studies has been whose voices get heard and listened to and who are understood as legitimate subjects of knowledge. This question is of great relevance also to dementia research where historically people with dementia were not included and heard in their own voice. Since people with dementia were not historically (and often still are not) understood as capable of accounting for their own lives and experiences, instead the accounts of scientists, professionals, families and carers have repeatedly been those which are heard and prioritised (see Chapter 4). Indeed, understandings of people with dementia as not lucid or coherent enough to be involved and questioned about their views reflect a longer history of disregarding the voices of disempowered groups. As suggested by Proctor (2001), the reasons for not including the perspectives of people with dementia in research have been the very same as those used to exclude people with mental health problems, children, people with learning difficulties and women: 'In fact almost every oppressed and disempowered group in society' (p. 362).

However, a growing emphasis on citizenship, agency and self-determination in the last decade has meant that people with dementia are increasingly involved in research, policy-making and advocacy. Still, as noted in the introduction to this volume, the use of the category 'people with dementia' tends to overlook how this collective is not one and the same but located differently in relation to power and privilege depending on social location (Hulko, 2009). This raises further questions about *who* among the vast group of people with dementia gets to have a voice – who is heard and represented not only in research but also in policy and advocacy. (See for example discussion on whiteness and race in Chapter 8.) Moreover, from a critical perspective, one may also question to what extent bringing people with dementia into research in its current forms alters existing 'regimes of truth' as Foucault (1993) terms the discursive production of some knowledges as truths. Does the involvement of people with dementia as participants and co-producers effectively challenge the dominance of biomedicine or do these voices merely become supplemental at best or tokenistic at worst?

However, turning to feminist standpoint theory goes beyond the mere involvement of people with dementia and offers a more radical epistemological shift in dementia studies. This entails an understanding of people with dementia as a subjugated group who due to their specific positionality hold an 'epistemic privilege'. This 'epistemic privilege' is particularly held by those living with dementia who are also experiencing other forms of oppression and systemic injustices, including but not limited to sexism, homophobia, racism, poverty and precarity. This notion of epistemic privilege refers to the central idea in feminist standpoint theory: that the standpoint of the oppressed is a privileged vantage point from which to theorise, an idea which originated from Marxist theory (Hartsock, 2004; Smith, 1974). This implies that women, either in general terms or in more specific terms such as black women, third-world women or women workers, are understood as carrying specific knowledge and insight into the workings of gendered power asymmetries (Collins, 1986; hooks, 2000; Lykke, 2010). As argued by Sandra Harding (1993, p. 54), although those in a dominant position in a society may have the best of intentions, 'the activities at the top both organise and set limits on what persons who perform such activities can understand about themselves and the world around them' (Harding, 1993, p. 54). Standpoint theory thus advocates a radical shift where 'the activities of those at the bottom of such social hierarchies can provide starting points for thought – for everyone's research and scholarship – from which human relations with each other and the natural world can become visible' (p. 54). This epistemological approach has subsequently been the foundation to emancipatory feminist methodologies such as institutional ethnography (Devault, 2006; Smith, 2005), memory work (Haug, 1987) and feminist autoethnography (Stanley, 1992).

Bringing the standpoint approach into dementia studies would entail a radical shift in terms of knowledge and truth in relation to dementia. If currently the perspectives of people with dementia are often dismissed or at best understood as supplemental to the hegemonic knowledge regimes of medicine and the health sciences, a *'demented' standpoint* would turn the existing order on its head. I am very aware of the problems of the term 'demented' and how it functions to stigmatise and dehumanise people living with dementia (Sabat et al., 2011). Still I am using the term 'demented', rather than for example standpoint of the person with dementia, as a conscious provocation to underscore how some people considered 'out of their minds' are systematically positioned as Other, too different, to have their perspectives positioned at the centre of knowledge production. A 'demented' standpoint is a way to recast dementia from a medical category to a political one, and to prioritise the perspectives of people with dementia before those of professionals, the health sciences and medicine in ways which have hitherto been regarded as unthinkable. While few today would dispute women in general terms as rational and capable of knowledge, people with dementia, in particular women and others on the margins living with dementia, are in society dominated by cognitive ableism still not understood as legitimate producers of knowledge. As such, the 'demented' standpoint is a necessary and long overdue intervention in research on dementia, which parallels the emergence of terminologies such as queer, crip and mad in other critical fields. However, the term 'demented' standpoint should be seen as provisional, reflecting the current absence of a critical term coming from within dementia activism, and should preferably in the future be substituted with a terminology of critical activists themselves.

Notably, my proposal to further introduce standpoint theory into dementia studies is not only parallel to feminist scholarship but also to developments within the field of mad studies, which has emerged and solidified in the last decade (see, for example, LeFrançois et al., 2013). Mad studies, in a similar vein as critical dementia studies, takes its inspiration from other critical fields such as disability studies, feminist, queer studies, decolonial and postcolonial studies and challenges the dominance of bio-medical psychiatry for understanding mental illness. As argued by Faulkner (2017), experiential knowledges by survivors and mental health users are key to this transformative research agenda and are closely linked to peer support and collective knowledge building as political acts:

> Telling our stories and listening to each other's stories is the cornerstone of peer support, empowerment and recovery. But it is also a political act and begins the process of creating and building our experiential knowledge.
>
> (Faulkner, 2017, p. 13)

In disability studies more broadly disabled people have themselves been conducting research and the phrase 'nothing about us without us' has been a guiding principle for many decades (Charlton, 1997). Although people with dementia are now increasingly employing this term, particularly in contexts with strong self-advocacy movements such as in the UK, the role and significance of experiential knowledge have been much more marginal in dementia studies in other parts of the world. Moreover, voices of people with dementia are often emerging from the most articulate within dementia communities and on established platforms such as Alzheimer's Disease International, often aligned with discourses of agentic citizenship. A 'demented' standpoint would, in contrast, seek to centre the multiply marginalised and start from other modes of knowing than verbal articulations and recalling, points I will develop in the following section.

Limits and challenges to a 'demented' standpoint: Towards situated knowledge and imagination in dementia studies

While a 'demented' standpoint could be a significant critical intervention in dementia studies, there are some evident challenges and unresolved issues coming with this position.

First, it is worth noting that feminist scholarship, similarly to many other critical fields, has emerged and been based in the needs and interests of the oppressed group. A 'demented' standpoint should thus be the outcome of people with dementia as an epistemic community, not that of researchers as suggested above. It is also worth noting how feminist standpoint theorists differentiate between a feminist standpoint and a women's viewpoint. Nancy Hartsock (2004) does, for example, underline that a feminist standpoint is something achieved through political consciousness-raising and cannot simply be understood as women's everyday experiences.

This is an evident challenge when it comes to critical dementia studies. In the last decade, there has been a rise in dementia advocacy movements in places like the UK, Australia and Canada, driven by people with dementia themselves. Although these movements have also made impressions on the research agenda, they are still marginal and very unevenly distributed across the globe. One may also ask whether these movements by definition contribute to transformative knowledge. As Örulv discusses in Chapter 18 of this volume, for the self-advocates participating in her research obtaining a medical diagnosis has been of the utmost importance and they do not refute a cure for dementia (in contrast to for example the existing movement of activists or self-advocates with autism or other neurodiversities). Consequently, the formation of an epistemic community of people with dementia, which aligns with other disability movements (Shakespeare et al., 2019) and focuses on dementia in terms of oppression, is still missing in most places. Is it thus possible to move towards a 'demented' standpoint, when the collective critical mobilising of people with dementia and the formation of a critical epistemic community are largely absent?

Moreover, my call for a 'demented' standpoint needs to be referred back to the questions and concerns I raised earlier in this chapter: who within current dementia advocacy and within dementia research is heard and listened to? And is a term such as 'people with dementia' useful or is it too homogenising and risks overshadowing the different positionalities within the group? Early feminist standpoint theorists' unreflexive use of the notion of women has been critiqued for overlooking the diversity and difference among women and over the years the feminist standpoint has increasingly been revised to encompass intersectionality and difference. Similar questions also need to be posed to the 'demented' standpoint – what constitutes the standpoint: the diagnosis, the community, a political position or something else? And what is the shared positionality of dementia across differences such as gender, race, class and age? The evident limits of standpoint theory, in particular the risks of homogenising and essentialising the oppressed subject and obscuring differences within the oppressed group, in turn also reflect the potential limits of a 'demented' standpoint.

An alternative to the 'demented' standpoint could be Donna Haraway's (1988) concept of 'situated knowledge'. This could provide a way of avoiding standpoint theory's totalising gestures and instead point to the fragmented and contradictory experiences of people with dementia across different social locations. Haraway's concept has emerged in close dialogue with standpoint epistemologies including Sandra Harding's concept of 'strong objectivity' and shares assumptions of standpoint theory that claims for truth are always partial. As Haraway argues, knowledge production is always dependent on the embodied 'sites' and 'sights' of the researcher and research participants – and as such there is no neutral point from which truth can be observed. However, situated knowledge draws to a greater extent than classical standpoint theory on a post-structuralist epistemology and its focus on multiple co-existing narratives of the world. This should not be understood as a recourse to relativism. Instead, the concept proposes a form of strong objectivity through the combination of multiple heterogenous narratives. From this, it is not one singular 'demented' standpoint which is holding epistemic privilege, but the multifarious standpoints of subjects with dementia of different social locations. In the words of Mark Stoetzler and Nira Yuval Davis (2002, p. 315), this kind of approach to knowledge 'views the process of approximating the truth as part of a dialogical relationship among subjects who are differentially situated'. This perspective is concomitant with a more intersectional turn in dementia studies and would also further acknowledge how people living with dementia may be situated at the intersections of both privilege and marginalisation (Hulko, 2009). Situated knowledges thus draw on the strengths of standpoint theory's 'bottom-up approach' and its challenge to universal and decontextualised knowledge, but they also open up to multifarious, local, contextual, unstable and fragmented 'demented' standpoints.

Another limitation of standpoint theory, as well as the sister theory of situated knowledge, is how they do not really go beyond rational faculties and to a great extent prioritise rational agentic subjects who may produce coherent narratives of their lives and experiences. One may thus argue that feminist standpoint theory, for example, is a largely cognonormative epistemological approach and as such of limited use to research involving people with cognitive illness. I thus propose that a more feminist dementia studies is not only about knowing differently but also about the uses of imagination. Dementia studies is not only in need of thinking through situated knowledges but also 'situated imagination', as introduced by Mark Stoetzler and Nira Yuval-Davis (2002). Situated imagination, emerging in close dialogue with standpoint theory, is a concept that attempts to position imagination 'at the heart of the construction of all kinds of knowledge' (p. 321). Any kind of knowledge is ultimately tied to our potential for imagining, and imagination is both something that transgresses and creates boundaries. In the words of Stoetzler and Yuval-Davis (2002, p. 324), the creative force of imagination is thus both 'the source of freedom, change and emancipation as much as a source of the borders and boundaries that emancipation wants to challenge'. While imagination is often primarily thought of in individual terms, situated imagination should, similarly to the concept of situated knowledge, be understood as both individual, based on a corporeal and affective reality, and social and collective, based on a wider political landscape. Notably, the significance of imagination is increasingly recognised in dementia studies, in particular studies that draw on arts-based methodologies (Ward et al., 2021; Zeilig et al., 2014). However, this research rarely acknowledges the social and political dimensions of imagination and how imagination is shaped and conditioned by social positioning. Situated imagination is, in contrast, a more critical position that allows for what Hulko refers to as 'alternative worldmaking' on dementia (see Chapter 16 in this volume). This kind of endeavour is a way of imagining dementia differently, centring the voices and imaginings of people with dementia most on the margins, beyond ageist, ableist, colonialist and sexist knowledge regimes on dementia.

Thinking from the epistemological positions of situated knowledges and situated imagination also leads to questions of critical methodologies in dementia studies (which we discuss further in Chapter 19). A lot of emancipatory feminist research as well as qualitative research in dementia studies has been based on methods that rely on the capacities to remember, retell and produce coherent narratives. To incorporate different voices and to centre imagination further would also require further exploration of creative methodologies, including methods where the researchers are willing to challenge the control and authority in the research process further.

Moving towards more situated knowledges in dementia also requires careful consideration of how those with dementia being most on the margins become increasingly involved. As argued by Capstick and Njoki (2020), recruitment of people with dementia for research is often very difficult, in particular when recruiting from marginalised groups. In the process of recruitment, time is thus crucial in order to build relationships and rapport and for researchers to become accomplices, as formulated by Hulko in Chapter 16. Another crucial aspect is the situatedness of researchers in dementia studies. To what extent are people's own experiences of ableism, heteronormativity and racism for example made present in the field of dementia studies? Having more researchers with experiences of neurodiversity or who are part of various queer, disabled or ethnic minority communities may both enable recruitment and impact on the knowledge produced. The situatedness of researchers also inevitably impacts, as clearly illustrated in Chapters 8 and 18 in this volume.

Finally, more creative and critical methodological discussions are also vital to enable critical epistemic communities to emerge. Researchers in dementia studies may for example support the formation of feminist groups for women with dementia or decolonial dementia spaces where indigenous understandings and knowledges on ageing and memory loss are centred and 'welcomed in' (Changfoot et al., 2021). It is also notable how perspectives from Western countries predominate in dementia studies (which is also reflected in this volume). To resist dementia as a decontextualised and ahistorical phenomenon, there is a need to strengthen the perspectives from a wider non-Western context and to foster 'transversal conversations' (Lykke, 2020) between differently situated people with dementia from different parts of the world, perhaps facilitated by researchers as accomplices in these conversations.

Final remarks: Imagining dementia differently

In this chapter, I have introduced two feminist theoretical genealogies and how they may offer critical dementia studies ways of thinking and rethinking dementia and difference. The aim has been to show how feminist scholarship is useful, not only to study gender and dementia, but how it also provides critical tools for dementia researchers in a broader sense, to analyse dementia as a political category, linked to wider questions of Othering and oppression. As argued in several chapters in this volume, existing research on dementia remains to a great extent apolitical, does not challenge the basic premises of mainstream academic and policy discourses, and often reinforces whiteness, coloniality and heteronormativity (see, for example, Chapters 7, 8, 16 and 17). Feminist scholarship (together with other critical scholarship) is useful as it urges us to ask more critical questions in dementia studies, including: who is understood as a legitimate producer of knowledge, what kinds of knowledges matter and how may we reimagine the dominant cultural imaginaries of dementia? Dialogues with feminist scholarship thus invite us to conceptualise dementia differently, which opens up other ways of doing research.

I have chosen to focus specifically on difference in this chapter because it is such a contentious issue in both feminist scholarship and dementia studies. I see some evident parallels in how some feminists have sought to evade the otherness of women by emphasising sameness and how person-centred dementia scholars and campaigners have fought hard to normalise and advocate for the sameness of people with dementia. But what is then the standing or status of those with more severe cognitive impairments, who are too dependent, too frail, *too different* to be fully incorporated into a Western liberal-humanist framework with its hegemonic subject characterised by autonomy, rationality and control? But, as I have argued, feminist scholarship, in the versions of both difference theorists and standpoint theorists, also points us in other directions where social, material and embodied difference is understood in political terms and where difference is not ultimately tied to otherness. I also see some evident parallels between homogenising notions 'women' and 'people with dementia' which have overshadowed different positionalities. Feminist dementia studies thus needs to find ways of doing research that further involve the most marginalised within dementia communities.

Although the aim of this chapter has primarily been to outline possible theoretical directions, this has also led me to raise questions on methodology. In the future, I hope to see more exploration of how feminist emancipatory methodologies, which challenge objectifying, uniform and detached knowledge production in favour of subjective, diverse and situated knowledges, have been or can be used in studies of dementia. But as a lot of feminist work is based on a cognonormative framework, I also see how feminist dementia scholars will invigorate methodological discussions and point to new and different ways of doing research, where situated knowledge as well as situated imagination is explored.

References

Baril, A., & Silverman, M. (2022). Forgotten Lives: Trans Older Adults Living with Dementia at the Intersection of Cisgenderism, Ableism/Cogniticism and Ageism. *Sexualities*, 25(1–2), 117–131.

Bartlett, R., Windemuth-Wolfson, L., Oliver, K., & Dening, T. (2017). Suffering with Dementia: The Other Side of "Living Well". *International Psychogeriatrics*, 29(2), 177–179.

Behuniak, S.M. (2011). The Living Dead? The Construction of People with Alzheimer's Disease as Zombies. *Ageing and Society*, 31(1), 70–92.

Berlant, L. (2011). *Cruel Optimism*. Durham: Duke University Press.

Boyle, G. (2019). Beyond Lipstick and Woodwork: Why Gender Matters When Living with Dementia. In S. Pickard and J. Robinson (Eds.), *Ageing, the Body and the Gender Regime: Health, Illness and Disease across the Life Course*. Abingdon: Routledge, pp. 113–127.

Braidotti, R. (1994). *Nomadic Subjects: Embodiment and Sexual Difference in Contemporary Feminist Theory*. New York: Columbia University Press.

Bülow, M.H., & Holm, M.-L. (2016). Queering 'Successful Ageing', Dementia and Alzheimer's Research. *Body & Society*, 22(3), 77–102.

Capstick, A., & Clegg, D. (2013). Behind the Stiff Upper Lip: War Narratives of Older Men with Dementia. *Journal of War & Culture Studies*, 6(3), 239–254.

Capstick, A., & Njoki, M. (2020). Recruiting People with Dementia to Research: Why Is It Still So Difficult? https://memoryfriendly.org.uk/programmes/critical-dementia-network/blog/recruiting-people-with-dementia-to-research-why-is-it-still-so-difficult/ (Accessed 2022-10-15).

Changfoot, N., Rice, C., Chivers, S., Williams, A.O., Connors, A., Barrett, A., Gordon, M., & Lalonde, G. (2021 ahead of print). Revisioning Aging: Indigenous, Crip and Queer Renderings. *Journal of Aging Studies*, 100930. https://doi.org/10.1016/j.jaging.2021.100930.

Charlton, J. (1997). *Nothing About Us Without Us: Disability Oppression and Empowerment*. Berkeley: University of California Press.

Collins, P.H. (1986). Learning from the Outsider Within: The Sociological Significance of Black Feminist Thought. *Social Problems*, 33(6), S14–S32.

DeFalco, A. (2018). Beyond Prosthetic Memory: Posthumanism, Embodiment, and Caregiving Robots. *Age, Culture, Humanities: An Interdisciplinary Journal*, 3, 1–31.

Devault, M.L. (2006). Introduction: What Is Institutional Ethnography? *Social Problems*, 53(3), 294–298.

Faulkner, A. (2017). Survivor Research and Mad Studies: The Role and Value of Experiential Knowledge in Mental Health Research. *Disability & Society*, 32(4), 500–520.

Foucault, M. (1993). *Diskursens Ordning: Installationsföreläsning vid College de France den 2 december 1970*. Stockholm: Brutus Östlings förlag.

Gilleard, C., & Higgs, P. (2013). The Fourth Age and the Concept of a 'Social Imaginary': A Theoretical Excursus. *Journal of Aging Studies*, 27(4), 368–376.

Grosz, E.A. (1994). *Volatile Bodies: Toward a Corporeal Feminism*. Bloomington: Indiana University Press.

Haraway, D. (1988). Situated Knowledges: The Science Question in Feminism and the Privilege of Partial Perspective. *Feminist Studies*, 14(3), 575–599.

Harding, S. (1993). Rethinking Standpoint Epistemology: What Is "Strong Objectivity. In L. Alcoff & E. Potter (Eds.), *Feminist Epistemologies*. London: Routledge, pp. 49–82.

Harding, S.G. (1986). *The Science Question in Feminism*. Ithaca: Cornell University Press.

Hartsock, N. (2004). The Feminist Standpoint: Developing the Ground for a Specifically Historical materialism. In S. Harding (Ed.), *The Feminist Standpoint Theory Reader: Intellectual and Political Controversies*. London: Routledge, pp. 35–53.

Haug, F. (1987). *Female Sexualization: A Collective Work of Memory*. London: Verso.

Hooks, B. (2000). *Feminist Theory: From Margin to Center*. London: Pluto Press.

Hulko, W. (2009). From 'Not a Big Deal' to 'Hellish': Experiences of Older People with Dementia. *Journal of Aging Studies*, 23(3), 131–144.

Hydén, L.-C., Lindemann, H., & Brockmeier, J. (2014). *Beyond Loss: Dementia, Identity, Personhood*. Oxford: Oxford University Press.

Irigaray, L. (1985). *This Sex Which Is Not One*. Ithaca: Cornell University Press.

Jenkins, N. (2017). No Substitute for Human Touch? Towards a Critically Posthumanist Approach to Dementia Care. *Ageing and Society*, 37(7), 1484–1498.

Kitwood, T.M. (1997). *Dementia Reconsidered: The Person Comes First*. Buckingham: Open University Press.

Kontos, P., & Martin, W. (2013). Embodiment and Dementia: Exploring Critical Narratives of Selfhood, Surveillance, and Dementia Care. *Dementia*, 12(3), 288–302.

Lather, P., & Smithies, C. (1997). *Troubling the Angels: Women Living with HIV/AIDS*. Boulder: Westview Press.

Latimer, J. (2018). Repelling Neoliberal World-Making? How the Ageing–Dementia Relation is Reassembling the Social. *The Sociological Review*, 66(4), 832–856.

LeFrançois, B.A., Menzies, R., & Raume, G. (Eds.). (2013). *Mad Matters: A Critical Reader in Canadian Mad Studies*. Toronto: Canadian Scholars' Press.

Lock, M.M. (2013). *The Alzheimer Conundrum: Entanglements of Dementia and Aging*. Princeton, NJ: Princeton University Press.

Lorde, A. (1997). *The Cancer Journals*. San Francisco: Aunt Lute Books.

Lykke, N. (2010). *Feminist Studies: A Guide to Intersectional Theory, Methodology and Writing*. New York: Routledge.

Lykke, N. (2020). Transversal Dialogues on Intersectionality, Socialist Feminism and Epistemologies of Ignorance. *NORA - Nordic Journal of Feminist and Gender Research*, 28(3), 197–210. https://doi.org/10.1080/08038740.2019.1708786.

McParland, P., Kelly, F., & Innes, A. (2017). Dichotomising Dementia: Is There Another Way? *Sociology of Health & Illness*, 39(2), 258–269.

Peel, E. (2014). 'The Living Death of Alzheimer's' Versus 'Take a Walk to Keep Dementia at Bay': Representations of Dementia in Print Media and Carer Discourse. *Sociology of Health & Illness*, 36(6), 885–901.

Proctor, G. (2001). Listening to Older Women with Dementia: Relationships, Voices and Power. *Disability & Society*, 16(3), 361–376.

Roets, G., & Braidotti, R. (2012). Nomadology and Subjectivity: Deleuze, Guattari and Critical Disability Studies. In D. Goodley, B. Hughes, & L. Davis (Eds.), *Disability and Social Theory*. Basingstoke: Palgrave Macmillan, pp. 161–178.

Sabat, S.R., Johnson, A., Swarbrick, C., & Keady, J. (2011). The 'Demented Other' or Simply 'a Person'? Extending the Philosophical Discourse of Naue and Kroll through the Situated self. *Nursing Philosophy*, 12(4), 282–292.

Sandberg, L. (2013). Affirmative Old Age—The Ageing Body and Feminist Theories on Difference. *International Journal of Ageing and Later Life*, 8(1), 11–40.

Sandberg, L. (2015). Towards a Happy Ending? Positive Ageing, Heteronormativity and Un/happy Intimacies. *Lambda Nordica*, 20(4), 19–44.

Sedgwick, E.K. (1999). *A Dialogue on Love*. New York: Beacon Press.

Shakespeare, T., Zeilig, H., & Mittler, P. (2019). Rights in Mind: Thinking Differently About Dementia and Disability. *Dementia*, 18(3), 1075–1088.

Shildrick, M. (2009). *Dangerous Discourses of Disability, Subjectivity and Sexuality.* Basingstoke: Palgrave Macmillan.

Smith, D.E. (1974). Women's Perspective as a Radical Critique of Sociology. *Sociological Inquiry*, 44(1), 7–13.

Smith, D.E. (2005). *Institutional Ethnography: A Sociology for People*. Walnut Creek, CA: AltaMira.

Stanley, L. (1992). *The Auto/biographical I: The Theory and Practice of Feminist Auto/Biography*. Manchester: Manchester University Press.

Stoetzler, M., & Yuval-Davis, N. (2002). Standpoint Theory, Situated Knowledge and the Situated Imagination. *Feminist Theory*, 3(3), 315–333.

Swaffer, K. (2015). Dementia and Prescribed Disengagement™. *Dementia*, 14(1), 3–6.

Twigg, J. (2004). The Body, Gender, and Age: Feminist Insights in Social Gerontology. *Journal of Aging Studies*, 18(1), 59–73.

Ward, M.C., Milligan, C., Rose, E., Elliott, M., & Wainwright, B.R. (2021). The Benefits of Community-based Participatory Arts Activities for People Living with Dementia: A Thematic Scoping Review. *Arts & Health*, 13(3), 213–239.

Ward, R., & Price, E. (2016). Reconceptualising Dementia towards a Politics of Senility. In Westwood, S. & Price, E. (Eds.) *Lesbian, Gay, Bisexual and Trans* Individuals Living with Dementia: Concepts, Practice and Rights*. London: Routledge, pp. 65–78.

Ward, R., Rummery, K., Odzakovic, E., Manji, K., Kullberg, A., Clark, A., & Campbell, S. (2022). Getting Lost: Encounters with the Time-Space of Not Knowing. *Health and Place*. 78 (November), 102940.

Williams, S.J., Katz, S., & Martin, P. (2011). Neuroscience and Medicalisation: Sociological Reflections on Memory, Medicine and the Brain. In M. Pickersgill & I. Van Keulen (Eds.) *Sociological reflections on the Neurosciences*. Bingley: Emerald Group Publishing Limited, pp. 231–254.

Zeilig, H., Killick, J., & Fox, C. (2014). The Participative Arts for People Living with a Dementia: A Critical Review. *International Journal of Ageing and Later Life*, 9(1), 7–34.

16 Revolutionising dementia policy and practice

Guidance from 'the memory girl', an accomplice

Wendy Hulko

Accomplice: One who aligns with equity-seeking groups and minoritised peoples, takes direction from the members and/or leaders of said groups, *and* actively assists in their social, economic, and climate justice efforts without undue regard for personal risks and/or benefits. While allies often self-identify, this is insufficient for accomplices. See also consensual ally (Hunt & Holmes, 2015) and co-conspirator (Garza, 2016).

Revolutionise: Bring about a new social order that is radically different from the preceding one.

> The Memory Girl:
> After the others had said hello [to Nancy at her 87th birthday party], I came over and said hello and she greeted me warmly by name and then exclaimed "you're the memory girl". I reminded her of why I was there – to observe and take pictures and at mention of the pictures, she said with a grin "and I'll say I don't remember."
>
> (Hulko, 2004, p. 165)

The aim of this chapter is to demonstrate how critical perspectives can be integrated into dementia policy and practice and revolutionise the way we work with persons living with dementia, their families, and communities. Drawing on insights from anti-colonial, intersectional feminist, queer, critical race, and disabilities scholars working alongside or at the margins of dementia care, as well as my own research, practice, and teaching experience in Canada, this chapter offers concrete guidance for students, practitioners, and policymakers wanting to change the current social order with respect to dementia policy and practice. Readers will be guided towards becoming accomplices in efforts to change the systems, structures, and discourses that limit the possibilities of sur-thrivance (McNeil-Seymour, 2017) for persons with dementia and their families. These concepts will be discussed in more depth below.

This chapter is a 'worldmaking' endeavour, informed by Duong's (2012) conceptualisation of queer worldmaking: 'the making of a commons, itself realisable only through claims for a common world that does not yet exist,

DOI: 10.4324/9781003221982-21

which is technically unimaginable but nevertheless retained as a possibility' (p. 379). The world that the contributors to this book and others are engaged in making is one in which persons living with dementia are seen and heard – in all their diversity and complexity – and their contributions to those in their midst and the world at large are acknowledged/celebrated. In this world, dementia is 'welcomed in' (Changfoot et al., 2021). This requires seeing agency 'along different registers and temporalities…[and] orienting and attuning to others "altered subjectivities"', which Changfoot et al. (2021, pp. 5–6) frame as a means of cripping and queering ageing and dementia. At the same time, it is helpful to view dementia as a bio-psycho-social phenomenon rather than a neurocognitive disorder and persons living with dementia as a heterogenous group of people, who have a number of identities and affinities.

Building on previous chapters identifying the limitations of historical and contemporary approaches to dementia, and proposing instead the adoption/integration of critical gerontology, critical disability studies, anti-racism, feminist theory, and posthumanism, this chapter proposes a critically informed/engaged praxis. It starts with a note on terminology and a brief introduction to anti-oppression gerontology, including the key concepts of agency, equity, resilience, and resistance, as well as the use of counter-storytelling methodology (Hulko et al., 2020). The counter-story[1] of Harpreet and Olive is woven throughout this chapter so that readers see Harpreet's growing appreciation of Olive, first as a person and then as a citizen, and her gradual adoption of a more critical/radical approach to dementia that prepares her to serve as an accomplice. Along with presenting 'facts about dementia' and highlighting counter-hegemonic knowledges, I demonstrate how anti-oppression gerontology (AOG) – which is informed by anti-colonialism, critical race, queer theory, critical disabilities, and intersectional feminism – can be applied to practice. This shows how critical dementia studies has the potential not only to revolutionise dementia policy and practice but also to destabilise the dementia subject.

A note on terminology

Secwepemc two-spirit scholar and activist McNeil-Seymour uses sur-thrivance to signal the possibility that survivors of trauma may *thrive*, as well as *survive*. This includes Indigenous people for whom the cognate term 'sur-vivance' was conceptualised in an effort to reject or destabilise the 'victimry' poured onto Indigenous people; however, sur-thrivance has been adopted by trans folk too (McNeil-Seymour, 2017). Perhaps, then, this concept can be applied to persons with dementia – whether they be Indigenous and/or trans or two-spirit or not – as they too continue to be positioned as victims – of a ravaging disease – with no hope of further growth and development.

An accomplice would necessarily reject such framing and instead align with persons with dementia to eradicate the 'malignant social psychology'

(Kitwood, 1997) surrounding them and the ageism and ableism and other systems of oppression at its core. Accomplice and related terms like co-conspirator and comrade have been adopted by critical scholars moving away from the idea of allyship. Claiming the identity of an ally is often 'nonperformative' (Ahmed, 2021) in that it does not bring about the action, but rather it *is* the action. Powell and Kelly (2017) see the concept of 'risk' as distinguishing between white allies and white accomplices; their critique of allyship is motivated by the 'proliferating number of people identifying as allies who are not working toward disrupting the heteropatriarchy but are rather cycling through and maintaining systems of privilege and oppression' (p. 45). Indigenous Action Media (2014) suggests that accomplices 'seek ways to leverage resources and material support and/or betray their institution to further liberation struggles [and should] strategise with, not for and not be afraid to pick up a hammer' (p. 5). Accomplice, co-conspirator, and comrade may be used interchangeably; the important distinction is between those identifying or being identified in this way and those claiming 'allyship' without actually performing it.

Being more than critical, i.e. walking the talk

Concerned with the inattention to ageing and older adults within anti-oppressive social work and the lack of meaningful engagement with diversity and difference in gerontology, Hulko et al. (2020) proposed eight anti-oppression gerontology (AOG) principles that challenge normative understandings of ageing and foreground agency, equity, resilience, and resistance. The actions they recommend fall at the personal, cultural-relational, and structural levels and start with being 'critically self-reflexive and humble' and end at 'working towards a more socially just and equitable world' (Hulko et al., 2020, p. 5). The method they use to enact these principles is counter-storytelling, developed by critical race theorist Richard Delgado (1989) as a means of documenting and/or amplifying the stories of minoritised people to challenge dominant or master narratives about the social world. Stories may be created by members of equity-seeking groups or those working as accomplices to said groups. This includes older adults and persons with disabilities like dementia. Hulko et al. (2017) demonstrate this in their chapter on anti-oppressive social work with older adults, which includes seven counter-stories written by the authors based on their research and practice with older adults from equity-seeking groups. Counter-storytelling such as this challenges dominant or mainstream narratives of ageing and disability and destabilises interlocking systems of oppression such as ageism and ableism. Through analysing counter-narratives of dementia, Bitenc (2018) argues that 'positioning and performance are more critical than referentiality and factuality'; that is, what the person with dementia conveys to their interlocuter is more relevant than what has objectively occurred between the two. This underscores the power held by the listener/observer to grasp the intent/meaning of the person with dementia's utterances, i.e. position them as 'sensical'.

> Harpreet is a social worker in a care home in Quesnel (small city in the Cariboo region of British Columbia, Canada) where the majority of the residents have a diagnosis of dementia[2], often alongside other complex chronic diseases (CCD). Many of these older adults living with dementia were known to the staff from long before they started having memory problems and/or moved to the care home as they lived in Quesnel and nearby rural towns where the staff live. Harpreet herself is from Vancouver and only moved to this much smaller city when her partner got a full-time teaching position at a local high school. While she misses her family and the much larger Sikh community in Vancouver, this move was not unwelcome, as it meant leaving child protection work which Harpreet had done for the past five years. It also gave her the chance to spend more time with her grandparents who have lived in Quesnel for over 40 years, having chosen to stay there after her grandfather's retirement from the mill. While Harpreet had never worked with older adults, she had taken a class on aging during her Bachelor of Social Work (BSW) degree and has always enjoyed spending time with her grandparents.
>
> The second week at her new job, Harpreet is tasked with organising a family meeting as a resident named Olive has been climbing into her roommate's bed at night. Staff are concerned about how Olive's husband – who still lives at home and visits her daily – will react to this. They also worry about the safety of the other resident who has no family that they know of. Harpreet decides to meet with Olive's two daughters first to gain their support and then speak with the husband; she does not consider involving Olive as the head nurse has told her that while Olive is a lovely woman, she doesn't understand anything that's going on.

Dementia: What is it and whose knowledge counts?

Dementia refers to 'a range of memory loss inducing, disorienting, and judgement impairing conditions that most often occur in later life and are usually permanent (chronic)' (Hulko et al., 2020, p. 134) and was reclassified as a neurocognitive disorder in the fifth edition of the *Diagnostic and Statistical Manual* (Sachdev et al., 2014). Canada's national dementia strategy states that the symptoms 'are caused by neurodegenerative and vascular diseases or injuries' (Public Health Agency of Canada [PHAC], 2019, p. 82) and indicates that 6.9% of those aged 65 or older are living with diagnosed dementia, 63% of whom are women (PHAC, 2019). This figure is actually 1.1% lower than the 2007 estimate (Canadian Institutes of Health Research, 2007), consistent with global evidence that rates for high-income countries are decreasing, while rates for low- and middle-income countries are increasing (Patterson, 2018). In spite of this, there continues to be an over-concentration on dementia and dementia care in the Global North and a concomitant lack of engagement with or outright dismissal of non-white and minority ethnic understandings of dementia (Fletcher, 2020; see Zubair, this volume). Fletcher (2020) tells the story of Dr Carter Solomon Fuller, an African-American physician and pathologist who discovered in the early 1900s that 'senile dementia' was no different than 'presenile dementia', and explains how the overlooking or silencing of Fuller's research allowed this false distinction to hold sway until the 1970s. This serves as testament to the 'systemic silencing of black voices and promotion of white culture as absolute truth' (Fletcher, 2020, p. 3) in dementia research.

The predominance of the biomedical model and/or the 'neuro-psychiatric biopolitics of dementia' (Fletcher et al., 2021) and the suppressing of minoritised knowledge are significant not only on a global scale but also within nation states. Rates of dementia do vary within high-income countries, with Indigenous people in Canada and other countries experiencing an increase in dementia prevalence (Hulko et al., 2019; Walker & Jacklin, 2019; Warren et al., 2015), and 'more socially disadvantaged groups' such as Black, Asian, and ethnic minority people consistently identified as being more at risk (Livingston et al., 2020). The onset of dementia tends to be earlier for Indigenous people as well as people with Down Syndrome, though for different reasons; these two groups are at higher risk, as are women, older adults, and those with previous health conditions like hypertension (PHAC, 2019).

> As Harpreet learns more about dementia through her work at the care home, she begins to recognise the signs of disorientation. For example, Jimmy will get restless at the end of the day and search for his hat, coat, and briefcase. He believes that it is time for him to leave work and go home for dinner and Harpreet understands this to mean that he is disoriented to time and place. This occurs a few hours after Clara begins to ask when her mother is picking her up from school. Harpreet witnesses the staff reorienting both of these residents to the present and wonders if this is the best approach as Clara is distressed to learn that her mother has died and Jimmy worries that he has lost or will lose his job given that is not the place he has spent the day. Harpreet starts to think it might be better to 'jump into their realities' (Vittoria, 1998) rather than reorient them to her time and place.

In addition to the silencing of Black and minority ethnic knowledges, the impact of gender on dementia has received little attention beyond the recognition that the majority of those living with dementia are women, as are those providing both informal and formal care (Alzheimer Society of Canada, 2018; Patterson, 2018). Further, much of the limited research on women and dementia concentrates on caregiving (Bartlett et al., 2018; Errol et al., 2015). Intersectional feminist studies of dementia are distinct from the nascent literature on gender and dementia in that these researchers do not isolate gender from other categories of difference such as racialisation, ethnicity, sexual orientation, class, and Indigenous status (Hulko, 2002, 2009, 2016; O'Connor et al., 2010; Westwood, 2014) and make use of other difference-centred theories such as queer theory (Sandberg, 2018; Sandberg & Marshall, 2017; Ward & Price, 2016). These researchers have shown that gender makes a difference, yet their more critical and difference-centred work tends to be overlooked or marginalised within dementia studies, much like Black and minority ethnic knowledges, whether intersectionality is addressed or not.

> Before the family meeting, Harpreet learns more about Olive from reading the chart notes which depict Olive as frequently disoriented, unable to form complete sentences, and restless. The notes also query whether climbing into her neighbor's bed is a sign of sexual disinhibition. Harpreet asks the head nurse whether the previous social worker had completed a social history with Olive and/or her family and wonders if this might help the team better understand Olive's current behavior and provide more person-centred care. Learning that the previous social worker felt Olive was too cognitively impaired to be a reliable informant, Harpreet feels reassured that her plan to meet with the daughters makes sense.
>
> When she meets with the daughters and apprises them of Olive's nocturnal activities, they do not seem concerned about this and report that their mother has always been an adventurous person. They ask if the neighbor and/or her family are upset at all and Harpreet says the team's concern has been Olive's husband, rather than the neighbor as the latter appears comfortable with this arrangement. The daughters suggest they allow this to continue though ask that Harpreet continue to withhold this information from their father so as not to upset him.

Approaching the dementia subject

I was taught as a social worker to 'start where the client is at', thus I have always tried to approach a person with dementia before their care partner(s) and to privilege the stories and opinions of those disabled by society on the basis of their declining cognitive abilities. Harpreet did not start this way with Olive; rather, she took at face value both the official and family accounts of Olive and her (Harpreet's) efforts to learn about 'the person behind the disease' came much later. The story of Olive and Harpreet is indicative of the gendered nature of dementia noted above. Harpreet's reliance on the dominant (biomedical) discourse about Olive could result in Olive's 'de-gendering' (e.g. 'too cognitively impaired') while adopting person-centred care could serve to 're-gender' her (e.g. 'lovely woman'); as Sandberg (2018) argues, the options are limited in terms of diverse expressions of gender identity (and their affirmation) as long as we employ binary notions of gender, i.e. stay within the confines of the sex/gender system.

In dementia studies, we have largely moved on from a time (1940s–1950s England) when 'the dements' was a label applied to persons with dementia and the focus was primarily on supporting families (Manthorpe, 2016). The introduction of personhood and person-centred care (Kitwood, 1997) initiated this shift and eventually led to the emergence of self-advocacy and other forms of dementia activism (Bartlett, 2014; Shakespeare et al., 2017). Since Kitwood first defined personhood as 'a standing or status bestowed on one human being, by others, in the context of relationship and social well-being' (1997, p. 8), a range of theories have been put forward to describe or explain a person with dementia in their environment (see Chapters 6 and 7 in this volume). This expansion of dementia theorising has added or emphasised consideration of the body of the person with dementia as communicative and/or expressive of self (Kontos, 2003). It has also incorporated relationships with family members and other care partners as facilitating or inhibiting identity maintenance and experiences of care (Adams & Gardiner, 2005; Kontos et al., 2017) – as well as highlighting the social-cultural context as impacting the rights and responsibilities of persons living with dementia (Bartlett & O'Connor, 2010; Cahill, 2020; Hulko, 2009). Kitwood (1997) framed personhood as both personal and relational which is echoed in Hennelly and O'Shea's (2021) identification of key elements of personhood as interests and preferences, life course experiences, social interaction, family, and place. The structural level is neglected in all but those theories addressing the socio-cultural context of dementia, yet this is the third component of an AOG perspective.

A few days after meeting with Olive's daughters, Harpreet happens upon Olive's husband Milton in the dining room and introduces herself as the new social worker. Milton seems keen to talk with her and tells her of how the couple met at university when they were both graduate students and student activists who crossed paths frequently at protests and demonstrations, as well as social gatherings. Harpreet enjoys listening to his tales of being on the frontlines of civil rights and anti-war protests as it reminds her of why she wanted to be a social worker in the first place and also why she left child protection work. Milton describes Olive as a 'real firecracker' who always made life interesting, smiling in fondness at his wife's antics in their younger years. He talks of Olive's involvement in the women's movement and her anger over the ousting of lesbian women – 'the lavender menace' in the 1970s – and the couple's support of gay rights. Milton then leans towards her and says quietly, "Olive was in a relationship with a woman before we met and she still likes women, you know". Harpreet thanks Milton for sharing this with her and invites him to stop by her office and chat the next time he comes to visit Olive. As she walks away, she smiles to herself, thinking about

Olive and her roommate and wondering if Olive is 'in the closet' or if her daughters have put her in there. Harpreet is intrigued by this image of Olive that Milton conjures for her and wonders if she might get to know this person. She decides the starting point has to be seeing Olive as a person living with dementia – as she was taught in her BSW program – rather than suffering from it – as the media and so many health professionals depict it. She decides to try and speak directly with Olive and brings along some images of older adults so that she can try photo elicitation and third-party questioning, a technique she recalls reading about in the BCASW newsletter and her AOP social work textbook.

(Baines, 2017)

The story of Olive in this chapter is sadly rather typical in that persons with dementia are often excluded from discussions and decisions about their care. Women (and trans, two-spirit, and non-binary people) are probably excluded more often than cisgender men. The reasons for this exclusion – assumptions of incapacity, family member preference, communication difficulties, time constraints, no/few opportunities, and delegation of decision-making to others (Donnelly et al., 2018) – may vary by gender. Researchers have yet to address this, however. What is rare – though increasing – is the approach that Harpreet adopts after learning more about Olive as a person, an approach more aligned with the strengths perspective (McGovern, 2015; Saleebey, 1996) or the capabilities approach (Robeyns, 2005). The strengths perspective in social work, as articulated by Saleebey (1996), focuses on the strengths, resources, and possibilities of service users rather than their perceived deficits, barriers, and limitations. Similar to applying a social model of disability to dementia (Marshall, 1998), the capabilities approach is concerned with what older adults with disabilities are able 'to do and to be' and incorporates the core values of 'care, dependence and dignity'. Importantly, this approach considers structural factors as impacting care providers and causing unmet needs of care recipients (Berridge, 2012) in line with the compelling argument from residential care researchers that 'the conditions of work are the conditions of care' (Baines & Armstrong, 2018).

Having begun to consider how not only ageism but also ableism and hetero-sexism apply to Olive and the other persons with dementia with whom she is working, Harpreet now wonders how other aspects of the residents' social locations including ethnicity, racialisation, Indigenous ancestry, and class are impacting their lives and care.

Considering culture…and sharing power

While there is widespread acknowledgement that culture significantly impacts dementia and dementia care, the distinctions between different culture-based approaches is often omitted (Hulko et al., 2021). The difference between cultural safety and related approaches (e.g. cultural sensitivity, cultural competence, and cultural appropriateness) is that the former asks us to consider power in our interactions with service users and stresses the need to transfer (more) power to the service user so that the outcome of our intervention is one they consider to be culturally safe. Based on her critical ethnography of intercultural care in a Jewish long-term care facility, Stern (2012) calls for a culturally safe approach to dementia care, recognising that:

> Current models of cultural competency tend to focus on education that examines the relationships between static and defined cultural groups that do not take into account the wide range of cultural identities that individuals can construct. It fails to make the next step that recognises the diversity of both the people receiving care and those providing it (p. 9, see similar argument by Zubair in this volume).

Seeing cultures as fluid and recognising diversity within cultural groups is an important aspect of a culturally safe approach. For Indigenous Elders, this means avoiding pan-Indigenising, i.e., treating all Indigenous people the same, whether they are Métis, Inuit, or First Nations, and regardless of their specific nation. One way culturally safe dementia care can be achieved is through

> consulting with Elders or other community members to learn cultural and health status information [as this] can shift the power differential from one in which the health care provider is the "expert" to one in which the Elder teaches or guides the provider about the cultural aspects of their memory loss and care needs.
>
> (Hulko et al., 2010, p. 375)

As cultural safety is applicable to cultural groups other than those based on ethnicity or racialisation, a culturally safe approach to Olive would include acknowledging the fluidity of her sexual identity, for example. Engaging in dialogue with Olive will allow Harpreet to explore the range of her cultural identities, including Olive's ethno-cultural and class background, the intersections of these identities, and how these relate to the conditions of her care. Harpreet will need to reflect on her own positionality and how that mediates her role and influence in the care home (the conditions of her work), and consider ways to balance what she learns directly from residents with any collateral information provided by family members and the care team. These are considerations for Harpreet as she continues to work with Olive and also begins to interact with other residents.

> *As Harpreet gains more experience being a member of the inter-professional health care team, gets to know Olive as a person, and meets other residents in the care home, she wonders if social histories might be of benefit. After listening to Olive talk about both her past and present,*

Harpreet is particularly interested in applying an intersectional life course approach to make evident the diversity of the residents' lives and the ways in which they have shown resilience and resistance in the face of inter-locking oppressions, much like her own grandparents. She decides to try constructing a social history for a newly admitted First Nation man who has dementia as there are no other Indigenous residents in the home and staff have not yet taken the provincial Indigenous Cultural Safety (ICS) training[3]. Below is the first social history Harpreet writes:

Michael is a 76-year old Dene man who has lived away from his home community in the Northwest Territories since he was 6. He and his siblings were taken away to a residential school down South where Michael spent eight painful years before he ran away from it with his older brother Stan. They made their way to the Prince George, B.C. area where they found work in a mill and relied on one another for sup-port as they had in the residential school. Stan returned to their home community in the North five years later, seeking reconnection with his culture, family, and community, and healing from his residential school experiences. Michael stayed as he had met and fallen for a local white woman named June who he married the following year after which they moved to a small town outside Prince George. June's family never fully accepted him and that was one of the reasons the couple decided not to have children. Michael had good friends at the mill with whom he enjoyed fishing and hunting on the weekends. He was forced to retire eight years ago when he was diagnosed with dementia and three years later June died suddenly, leaving him on his own to take care of himself and their small house. For a long time, Michael managed on his own, but with his increasing cognitive and physical challenges and having few supports due to Stan and the rest of his Dene family and commu-nity being far away and his friends still working full-time, it became unsafe for him to live alone. As a result, he has been 'placed' in this care home in Prince George. It is an hour's drive from the small town where Michael lived for over 60 years and he is the only Indigenous resident. Michael was sent to residential school at the age of 6. During that time, he lost both of his parents. Not all of his siblings survived residential school and Michael has tried to forget the abuse they all suffered there, yet the memories remain.

After spending time with Michael to write his social history, Har-preet speaks to the Head Nurse about making both trauma-informed practice (TIP) and the San'yas ICS training a priority for all staff. She offers to facilitate a discussion at the next staff meeting and/or host an in-service on ways they can all make the care home more culturally safe, not only for Michael, but also for the staff. This includes the two Car-rier (a First Nation in Northern BC) nurses and the Métis cook with whom she has spoken about their interactions with the white residents, as well as the few racialised staff, including herself and two South Asian care aides who are casual employees. Knowing that dementia rates are increasing for Indigenous people and having seen how the first available bed policy[4] plays out, Harpreet expects there to be more Indigenous residents in the future, as well as more Sikh residents until her community is able to build its own care home. She has invited a few of her colleagues to the Gurdwara (Sikh temple) which she visits every weekend with her grandparents to enjoy a meal with the community and attend the service. Harpreet believes that if more people understand that her religion is a peaceful and loving one and that the Gurdwara is open to all, then they will be better able to provide culturally appropriate or safe care to the Sikh residents. Harpreet would like to have a dialogue about racism in the workplace as well; however, she thinks it might be safer to start with the residents and is hopeful that her white colleagues who claim to be allies will broaden the discussion to include racism experienced by both residents and staff. In constructing Michael's social history, she has enjoyed the opportunity to expand her knowledge and skills beyond strengths and person-centred approaches and looks forward to learning more about cultural safety and other approaches more aligned with AOP social work.

A social history such as the one Harpreet constructed has the potential to sensitise care staff to the losses and trauma that residents have endured throughout their life course as well as their resilience in the face of settler colonialism and other forms of structural violence. Shifting to a more critical approach to dementia, such as citizenship as practice, de-centres dementia as an 'individual experience' and focuses instead on how people with dementia are shaped by socio-cultural practices and discourses. For example, Olive may not be the only resident who was a feminist and civil rights activist and has been in a relationship with a woman, as the majority of those living in residential care are women and many of them are baby boomers like herself. Also, Michael may not be the only Indigenous person in the home; there may be Métis residents or others with Indigenous ancestry who are perceived to be white by the staff or are passing as white like they did when they were younger and it was not as safe to identify as Indigenous as it is perceived to be now. While there may be increased sensitivity towards and tolerance of Indigenous people than in the past, white supremacy and settler colonialism remain significant ideologies impacting all Black, Asian, minority ethnic, and Indigenous people.

Welcoming in dementia

The principles and tactics introduced in this chapter through the counterstory of Harpreet, a newly hired health care professional working in a care home, and Olive, an older woman with dementia living in the same care home, demonstrate some of the ways we can engage in AOG and alternative worldmaking, in creating a world where dementia is welcomed in. Yet if we don't ask about culture (broadly defined), create space and time for people to talk about their multiple and complex identities, and affirm their marginalised social statuses when they disclose them to us, then we miss the opportunity to see how socio-cultural practices and discourses have shaped their lives and hence be able to engage in critically informed/engaged praxis. If persons with dementia run into communication problems during assessments, for example, then we can employ some of the techniques Österholm and Hydén (2016) have observed social workers use: allow time for the person with dementia to 'self-repair' rather than jumping in to help or correct, acknowledge that communication is a challenge and express appreciation for their contributions, and make use of forced response (yes/no) questions when input cannot be elicited otherwise. Similarly, validation therapy techniques such as mirroring (the actions of the person with dementia), touching, and maintaining genuine, close eye contact (Feil, 2002), and the use of photo elicitation and third-party questioning (Hulko, 2004; Hulko et al., 2010) can be part of our repertoire. We can assist persons with dementia to express their needs and desires by being creative and adaptive with our *own* communication strategies and following the lead of persons with dementia – as accomplices – to build inclusive and accessible communities that welcome in dementia and other forms of difference. This includes promoting a sense of community and encouraging peer support and self-advocacy in care homes and considering how to support persons living with dementia to create more inclusive communities in rural towns, small cities, and large urban areas or take a neighbourhood-centred approach (Ward et al., 2021). We should envision how to shift our practice and that of others to reflect the belief that persons with dementia are still citizens with rights and responsibilities and that their social locations not only vary, but mediate their experiences of dementia (Hulko, 2009).

> While preparing a rationale for ICS Sanyas and TIP training for the Head Nurse and researching federal policies related to family sponsorship for a resident originally from Vietnam, Harpreet learned about GBA+ (Gender-Based Policy + intersectionality). The plus indicates an expanded focus beyond gender to include other categories of difference that also impact on lived experiences and the provision of health and social care. Harpreet began to consider how she might apply GBA+ analysis to the care home's organisational policies on features of daily life like rooms, meals, and furnishings, as well as provincial policies governing the location and funding of care homes and staffing ratios.

Although GBA+ is mandated for the development and analysis of federal policies in Canada, i.e., public servants must complete the training and demonstrate that they have considered gender alongside other categories of difference such as age, disability, nationality, race, and class, GBA+ does not appear to have been applied to the federal dementia strategy released in 2019 (Wyndham-West, 2020). This is unsurprising, given that person-centred care is still promoted as best practice and culture is barely mentioned (PHAC, 2019). There is much scope to do better and to do differently with respect to both practice and policy in dementia studies.

Conclusion – Whose side are we on?

People living with dementia are increasing in influence, if not in numbers. There has been a gradual shift from viewing persons with dementia as incapable and sub-human to recognising them as citizens with lives left to be lived and contributions to be made. This is occurring as persons with dementia author their own stories, engage in self-advocacy on Twitter, create and exhibit art, speak at conferences, and advise on policy and practice (see the section 'Reclaiming and Recasting' in this volume). The experiences of persons with dementia are as varied as those who live with cognitive impairment in later life. There is no master narrative about dementia nor are persons with dementia a homogenous group; rather, their views on and experiences of dementia are profoundly shaped by socio-cultural and political-economic contexts, as are ours as health and social care providers, researchers, and educators.

I conclude by posing a series of questions for researchers, practitioners, students, and activists.

- If being an accomplice requires one to take risks, then what risks are we willing to take to ensure persons with dementia are able to sur-thrive?
- Are we willing to take the lead from persons with dementia about the best ways to support or care for them?
- Are we willing to challenge our co-workers on their disabling practices?
- Are we willing to accept and promote all knowledges about dementia, including Black, Indigenous, minority ethnic, and/or queer ones that may challenge our own and/or dominant understandings of dementia and dementia care?
- Are we willing to advocate for culturally safe and queer-affirmative care?
- Are we willing to engage in job action to ensure adequate levels and appropriate types of care?

These are questions that arise for critical dementia studies, particularly if we have decided that being a 'dementia friend' is insufficient or problematic, that allyship is performative and self-serving, and that being an accomplice – like the memory girl – will get us closer to bringing to fruition the world we envision, one in which dementia is welcomed in – in a destabilised form.

Notes

1 This is an expanded version of the counter-story in Hulko et al.'s (2020) chapter on dementia, personhood, and citizenship as practice. The fictional characters are based on a variety of persons with dementia, practitioners, and students with whom the author has worked during her career and serve to illustrate key concepts and principles.
2 Sixty-seven percent of older adults in residential care have dementia (Canadian Institute of Health Information, 2017, p. 16)·
3 San'yas ICS is an online training programme for health care providers in BC developed by the Provincial Health Services Authority to educate health care practitioners on the impacts of colonisation and residential schools on Indigenous peoples and prepare them to work in a more respectful (culturally safe) way. It takes 8–12 hours to complete the programme and is mandatory for staff working in publicly funded health care (Browne et al., 2019).
4 This policy dictates that those awaiting transition to a care home, most of whom are older adults, must accept the first bed that becomes available in any of the homes they have selected.

References

Adams, T., & Gardiner. P. (2005). Communication and Interaction within Dementia Care Triads: Developing a Theory for Relationship-Centred Care. *Dementia: International Journal of Social Research and Practice, 4*(2), 185–205.

Ahmed, S. (2021). *Complaint!* Duke University Press.

Alzheimer Society of Canada (ASC). (2018, January 2). *Alzheimer Awareness Month. SPREADING awareness about the 72%.* Retrieved from http://www.alzheimer.ca/en/the72percent.

Baines, D. (2017). *Doing Anti-oppressive Practice: Social Justice Social Work* (3rd ed.). Halifax, NS: Fernwood Publishing.

Baines, D., & Armstrong, P. (2018). Promising Practices in Long Term Care: Can Work Organisation Treat Both Residents and Providers with Dignity and Respect? *Social Work & Policy Studies: Social Justice, Practice and Theory,* 1(1), 1–26.

Bartlett, R. (2014). The Emergent Modes of Dementia Activism. *Ageing & Society, 34*(4), 623–644. doi:10.1017/S0144686X12001158.

Bartlett, R., Gjernes, T., Lotherington, T.A., & Obstefelder, A. (2018). Gender, Citizenship and Dementia Care: A Scoping Review of Studies to Inform Policy and Future Research. *Health and Social Care in the Community, 26*(1), 14–26. doi: 10.1111/hsc.12340.

Bartlett, R., & O'Connor, D. (2010). *Broadening the Dementia Debate: Toward Social Citizenship.* Bristol, UK: Policy Press.

Berridge, C. (2012). Envisioning a Gerontology-Enriched Theory of Care. *Affilia: Journal of Women and Social Work, 27*(1), 8–21. doi:10.1177/0886109912437498.

Bitenc, R. (2018). "No Narrative, No Self?": Reconsidering Dementia Counter-Narratives in Tell Mrs. Mill Her Husband Is Still Dead. *Subjectivity, 11*, 128–143.

Cahill, S. (2020). New Analytical Tools and Frameworks to Understand Dementia: What Can a Human Rights Lens Offer? *Ageing & Society,* 1–10. doi:10.1017/S0144686X20001506.

Canadian Institute for Health Information. (2017). *Seniors in Transition: Exploring Pathways Across the Care Continuum.* https://www.cihi.ca/en/seniors-in-transition-exploring-pathways-across-the-care-continuum.

Canadian Institutes of Health Research. (2007). *The Future Is Aging: The CIHR Institute of Aging Strategic Plan 2007–2012.* http://www.cihr-irsc.gc.ca/cgi-bin/print-imprimer.pl.

Changfoot, N., Rice, C., Chivers, S., Williams, A.O., Connors, A., Barrett, A., Gordon, M., & Lalonde, G. (2021). Revisioning Aging: Indigenous, Crip and Queer Renderings. *Journal of Aging Studies.* doi:10.1016/j.jaging.2021.100930.

Delgado, R. (1989). Storytelling for Oppositionists and Others: A Plea for Narrative. *Michigan Law Review, 87*(8), 2411–2441.

Donnelly, S., Begley, E., & O'Brien, M. (2018). How Are People with Dementia Involved in Care-Planning and Decision-Making? An Irish Social Work Perspective. *Dementia, 18*(7–8), 1–19. doi:10.1177/1471301218763180.

Duong, K. (2012). What Does Queer Theory Teach Us about Intersectionality. *Politics & Gender, 8*(3), 370–386.

Errol, R., Brooker, D., & Peel, E. (2015, June). *Women and Dementia: A Global Research Review.* London: Alzheimer Disease International.

Feil, N. (2002). *The Validation Breakthrough: Simple Techniques for Communicating with People with "Alzheimer's-type Dementia"* (2nd ed). Baltimore, MD: Health Professions Press.

Fletcher, J.R. (2020). Black Knowledges Matter: How the Suppression of Non-white Understandings of Dementia Harms us All and How We Can Combat It. *Sociology of Health & Illness, 43*, 1–8. doi:10.1111/1467–9566.13280.

Fletcher, J.R., Zubair, M., & Roche, M. (2021). The Neuropsychiatric Biopolitics of Dementia and Its Ethnicity Problem. *The Sociological Review, 70*(5), 1–20. doi:10.1177/00380261211059920.

Garza, A. (2016, June). *Ally or Co-conspirator? A Conversation with Jesenia Santana and Alicia Garza.* https://movetoendviolence.org/blog/ally-co-conspirator-means-act-insolidarity/.

Hennelly, N., & O'Shea, E. (2021). A Multiple Perspective View of Personhood in Dementia. *Ageing & Society, 1*–19. doi:10.1017/S0144686X20002007.

Hulko, W. (2002). Making the Links: Social Theories, Experiences of People with Dementia, and intersectionality. In A. Leibing & L. Scheinkman (Eds.), *The Diversity of Alzheimer's Disease: Different Approaches and Contexts* (pp. 231–264). Rio de Janeiro: CUCA-IPUB.

Hulko, W. (2004). *Dementia and Intersectionality: Exploring the Experiences of People with Dementia and their Significant Others.* Stirling: University of Stirling.

Hulko, W. (2009). From 'Not a Big Deal' to 'Hellish': Experiences of Older People with Dementia. *Journal of Aging Studies, 23*(3), 131–144. Doi:10.1016/j.jaging.2007.11.002.

Hulko, W. (2016). LGBT* Individuals and Dementia: An Intersectional Approach. In S. Westwood & L. Price (Eds.), *Lesbian, Gay, Bisexual and Trans* Individuals Living with Dementia: Concepts, Practice, and Rights* (pp. 35–50). Abingdon: Routledge.

Hulko, W., Brotman, S., & Ferrer, I. (2017). Counter-Storytelling: Anti-Oppressive Social Work with Older Adults. In D. Baines (Ed.), *Doing Anti-Oppressive Practice: Social Justice Social Work* (3rd ed., pp. 193–211). Halifax: Fernwood Publishing.

Hulko, W., Brotman, S., Stern, L., & Ferrer, I. (2020). *Gerontological Social Work in Action: Anti-Oppressive Practice with Older Adults, their Families, and Communities.* Milton Park: Routledge Press.

Hulko, W., Camille, E., Antifeau, E., Arnouse, M., Bachynksi, N., & Taylor, D. (2010). Views of First Nation Elders on Memory Loss and Memory Care in Later Life. *Journal of Cross Cultural Gerontology, 25*(4), 317–342. doi:10.1007/s10823-010-9123-9.

Hulko, W., Mahara, S., Wilson, D., & Campbell-McArthur, G. (2021). Culturally Safe Dementia Care: Building Nursing Capacity to Care for First Nation Elders with Memory Loss. *International Journal of Older People Nursing, 16*, e12395. doi:10.1111/opn.12395.

Hulko, W., Wilson, D., & Balestrery, J. (Eds.). (2019). *Indigenous Peoples and Dementia: New Understandings of Memory Loss and Memory Care.* Vancouver, BC: UBC Press.

Hunt, S., & Holmes, C. (2015). Everyday Decolonization: Living a Decolonizing Queer Politics. *Journal of Lesbian Studies, 19*(2), 154–172.

Indigenous Action Media. (2014). *Accomplices, Not Allies: Abolishing the Ally Industrial Complex. An Indigenous Perspective and Provocation* (Ver. 2). https://www.indigenousaction.org/wp-content/uploads/Accomplices-Not-Allies-print.pdf.

Kitwood, T. (1997). *Dementia Reconsidered: The Person Comes First.* Buckingham, UK: Open University Press.

Kontos, P. (2003). 'The Painterly Hand': Embodied Consciousness and Alzheimer's Disease. *Journal of Aging Studies, 17,* 151–170.

Kontos, P., Miller, K.-L., & Kontos, A. (2017). Relational Citizenship: Supporting Embodied Selfhood and Relationality in Dementia Care. *Sociology of Health and Illness, 39*(2), 182–198. doi:10.1111/1467-9566.12453.

Livingston, G., Huntley, J., Summerlad, A., Ames, D., Ballard, C., Banerjee, S., … Mukadam, N. (2020). Dementia Prevention, Intervention, and Care: 2020 Report of the Lancet Commission. *The Lancet, 396,* 413–446. doi.org/10.1016/S0140-6736(20)30367-6.

Manthorpe, J. (2016). The Dement in the Community: Social Work Practice with People with Dementia Revisited. *Dementia, 15*(5), 1100–1111. doi:10.1177/1471301214554810.

Marshall, M. (1998). Environment: How It Helps to See Dementia as a Disability. *Journal of Dementia Care, 6*(1), 15–17.

McGovern, J. (2015). Living Better with Dementia: Strengths-Based Social Work Practice and Dementia Care. *Social Work in Health Care, 54*(5), 408–421. doi:10.1080/00981389.2015.1029661.

McNeil-Seymour, J. (2017). *Two-Spirit Sur-Thrivance and the Art of Interrupting Narratives.* https://www.neverapart.com/features/two-spirit-sur-thrivance-and-the-art-of-interrupting-narratives-panel-discussion-qa/.

O'Connor, D., Phinney, A., & Hulko, W. (2010). Dementia at the Intersections: A Unique Case Study Exploring Social Location. *Journal of Aging Studies, 24,* 30–39. doi:10.1016/j.jaging.2008.08.001.

Österholm, J.H., & Hydén, L.-C. (2016). Citizenship as Practice: Handling Communication Problems in Encounters between Persons with Dementia and Social Workers. *Dementia, 15*(6), 1457–1473. doi:10.1177/1471301214563959.

Patterson, C. (2018). *World Alzheimer Report 2018. The State of the Art of Dementia Research: New Frontiers*. London: Alzheimer Disease International. https://www.alz.co.uk/research/world-report-2018.

Powell, P., & Kelly, A. (2017). Accomplices in the Academy in the Age of Black Lives Matter. *Journal of Critical Thought and Praxis, 6*(2), 42–65.

Public Health Agency of Canada. (2019). *A Dementia Strategy for Canada: Together We Aspire*. Ottawa: Public Health Agency of Canada. https://www.canada.ca/en/public-health/serices/publications/dieases-conditions/dementia-strategy.html.

Robeyns, I. (2005). The Capabilities Approach: A Theoretical Survey. *Journal of Human Development, 6*(1), 93–117.

Sachdev, P.S., Blacker, D., Blazer, D.G., Ganguli, M., Jeste, D.V., Paulsen, J.S., & Petersen, R.C. (2014). Classifying Neurocognitive Disorders: The DSM-5 Approach. *Nature Reviews Neurology, 10*, 643–642. doi:10.1038/nrneurol.2014.181.

Saleebey, D. (1996). The Strengths Perspective in Social Work: An Extension and a Caution. *Social Work, 41*(3), 297–305.

Sandberg, L. (2018). Dementia and the Gender Trouble?: Theorising Dementia, Gendered Subjectivity and Embodiment. *Journal of Aging Studies, 45*, 25–31. doi:10.1016/j.jaging.2018.01.004.

Sandberg, L., & Marshall, B. (2017). Queering Aging Futures. *Societies, 7*(21), 1–11. doi:10.3390/soc7030021.

Stern, L.A. (2012). *The Cultural Whisper in Our Ear: Intercultural Dementia Care in a Jewish Long-term Care Facility*. Vancouver, BC: University of British Columbia (doctoral thesis).

Vittoria, A. (1998). Preserving Selves: Identity Work and Dementia. *Research in Aging, 20*(1), 91–136. doi:10.1177/0164027598201006.

Walker, J., & Jacklin, K. (2019). Dementia Prevalence. In W. Hulko, D. Wilson & J. Balestrery (Eds.), *Indigenous Peoples and Dementia: New Understandings of Memory Loss and Memory Care* (pp. 24–40). Vancouver, BC: UBC Press.

Ward, R., & Price, E. (2016). Reconceptualising Dementia: Towards a Politics of Senility. In S. Westwood, & E. Price (Eds.), *Lesbian, Gay, Bisexual and Trans* Individuals Living with Dementia: Concepts, Practice and Rights* (pp. 65–78). London: Routledge Press.

Ward, R., Rummery, K., Odzakovic, E., Manji, K., Kullberg, A., Keady, J., Clark, A., & Campbell, S. (2021). Beyond the Shrinking World: Dementia, Localization and Neighbourhood. *Ageing & Society*, 1–22. doi:10.1017/S0144686X21000350.

Warren, L.A., Shi, Q., Young, K., Borenstein, A., & Martinuik, A. (2015). Prevalence and Incidence of Dementia among Indigenous Populations: A Systematic Review. *International Psychogeriatrics, 27*(12), 1959–1970. doi:10.1017/S1041610215000861.

Westwood, S. (2014). Dementia, Women and Sexuality: How the Intersection of Ageing, Gender and Sexuality Magnify Dementia Concerns among Lesbian and Bisexual Women. *Dementia, 0*(0), 1–21. doi:10.1177/1471301214564446.

Wyndham-West, M. (2020). Gender and Dementia National Strategy Policymaking: Working toward Health Equity in Canada through Gender-Based Analysis Plus. *Dementia, 0*(0), 1–24.

17 Taking a queer turn – The significance of queer theory for critical dementia studies

Andrew King

Introduction

As this edited collection attests, there has been a move in recent years to explore the ways that dementia is a socially and culturally constructed phenomenon and to challenge biomedical understandings that locate it in purely pathological and reductive terms. The aim of my chapter is to contribute further to that exegesis and to consider the significance of queer theory in that endeavour. I contend that queer theory has much to offer for critical dementia studies and ways of understanding dementia that move beyond the pathological, the normative and the disciplinary. To achieve this, the chapter begins with a summary of dementia as a social construction. Following this, queer theory is introduced, together with a discussion of three queer turns, or themes within and across queer theory and what those could imply for how we understand dementia. Subsequently, I consider some queer troubles, or ways in which queer theory can be regarded as limited in relation to studies of dementia, before offering a short conclusion.

Dementia, a social construction

Readers of this collection know that dementia is considered a significant health issue among ageing populations worldwide. The World Health Organization (WHO) notes that

> Dementia is currently the seventh leading cause of death among all diseases and one of the major causes of disability and dependency among older people worldwide. Dementia has physical, psychological, social and economic impacts, not only for people living with dementia, but also for their carers, families and society at large.
>
> (World Health Organization, 2021)

This not only indicates the extent that dementia is a global phenomenon, with significant effects on people's well-being, their experiences and understanding of ageing, but that it has social (and economic) impacts; in short,

DOI: 10.4324/9781003221982-22

although the WHO subscribes to the view that dementia is primarily a phys-iological phenomenon, brought about by disease and/or bodily processes, it has global social consequences.

Nonetheless, in regarding dementia in this way, as pre-social, the WHO ignores issues that have been highlighted within the humanities and social sciences, by a diverse and multi-disciplinary group of writers. These com-mentators have not only explored the framing of dementia but questioned the biomedical narrative that positions it in pathological and biologically reductive terms. This has included, but is not limited to: questioning whether diagnoses of dementia using CT scanning are actually pre-social (Harding and Palfrey, 1997); the need for person-centred approaches to understand and reconsider neuropathology (Kitwood, 1997); and the need to de-pathol-ogise dementia, focusing instead on cognitive differences rather than abnor-malities (Baldwin and Capstick, 2007).

More recently critical studies of dementia have further challenged the pre-social, biomedical view of dementia, opening up a whole series of ques-tions about the place of structural inequalities (Hulko, 2004; Sandberg, 2018), the complexity of temporality and the imposition of normative ideas of time on self and identity (Gjødsbøl and Svendsen, 2019; Haeusermann, 2019) and the ways in which space and place form important and complex contexts for people living with dementia (Odzakovic et al., 2021; Ward et al., 2018).

Critical dementia studies have also drawn on a rich and varied theoret-ical corpus, especially post-structuralism, phenomenology, intersection-ality, crip, trans and, to an extent, queer theory (Baldwin and Capstick, 2007; Baril and Silverman, 2022; Davis, 2004; King, 2021; Sandberg, 2018). Despite differences in vocabulary and emphasis, all these perspectives ques-tion the decline/pathological/abnormal narrative that underlies the bio-medical framing of dementia and demonstrate the symbolic (and actual) violence that can be done when this epistemological and ontological fram-ing is not deconstructed (see also Chapters 14 and 18 in this volume). Sil-verman and Baril (2021) have drawn on crip and trans theories to highlight how new understandings of the self and its fluidity need to be developed in order that critical studies of dementia do not re-inscribe normative notions of self, time and embodiedness that, albeit unwittingly, reimpose the 'cis-cognonormative terror related to the loss of self in dementia... [and that it] can be reduced by reconceptualizing what it means to live with cognitive disability'.

I have argued elsewhere that queer theory offers a rich conceptual frame-work for unpicking and deconstructing understandings of dementia – par-ticularly in how it offers alternative ways of thinking through issues of time and forgetfulness (King, 2016, 2021). However, in the remainder of this chapter I want to critically revisit and extend some of these ideas with a more nuanced and comprehensive examination of the value of queer theory, particularly aspects that speak to three queer turns that have taken place since its emergence in the late 1980s, together with an assessment of what they imply for critical ways of understanding dementia.

Queer theory and three queer turns

Queer theory is not a unified theoretical perspective. In a recent publication assessing its contemporary significance, McCann and Monaghan (2020, p. 1) suggest that 'queer theory finds its radical potential as a term to challenge, interrogate, destabilise and subvert, but it also means there is difficulty in pinpointing queer theory's meaning'. My preferred definitions of queer theory come from Sullivan (2003, p. vi) who argues that *to queer* is 'to make strange, to frustrate, to counteract, to delegitimise, to camp up – (heteronormative) knowledge and institutions', whilst Edelman (2004, p. 17) suggests that queer 'can never define an identity; it can only ever disturb one'. Indeed, it is the radical potential of queer theory to disrupt, to make strange and to disturb that I find most useful in relation to the argument I am putting forward in this chapter: that queer theory, through a series of queer turns, provides critical dementia studies with a valuable conceptual armoury to challenge the pathological and reductive construction of dementia.

Interestingly, the development of queer theory itself was provoked by an emergent and growing health crisis, as well as more academic debates about the nature of knowledge and being. During the late 1980s and early 1990s, activists grappling with the AIDS pandemic began to radically question the validity of the existing, assimilationist Lesbian and Gay Movement to deal with this crisis and particularly state responses to it, especially in the United States of America and, to a lesser extent, the United Kingdom, as well as the perceived profiteering of drug companies (Green, 2007; McCann and Monaghan, 2020). This was coupled with academic debates influenced by post-structuralism and post-modernism that deconstructed notions of foundation, origin and authorship. These two emergent currents in queer theory, activism and radical deconstruction, were often interchangeable – with activism having a direct relationship with scholars who were writing critically about mainstream lesbian and gay politics.

Over the past 30 years, there has been what I will call a series of queer turns, which others have identified as a process wherein queer writers and scholars have come to focus on specific aspects of epistemology and ontology, i.e. knowledge and being related to self, identity, time, difference and pathologisation, and opened them up to critical (re)interpretation (McCann and Monaghan, 2020). These queer turns are not necessarily linear – as the focus of writing shifts around topics, with some apparently discarded, returned to and reconsidered.

As queer theorists adopt an anti-foundational perspective towards questions of knowledge, being, self and identity, which calls into question the very idea of original foundations, they centre instead on the social, political

and, above all, discursive construction of diversity, difference and norma-
tivities. However, it is important to note that queer theory, although primarily speaking to LGBTQI+ lives and experiences, can be applied more
widely to questions including ageing, agency and repression (Sandberg and
King, 2019), to critically question what makes 'successful ageing' (Sandberg
and Marshall, 2017) and indeed how dementia is constructed as an Other,
without a future (King, 2021). I therefore want to outline why these queer
turns make it a useful theoretical and conceptual framework to critically
engage with the social construction of dementia. The following sub-sections
therefore draw out three queer turns which trouble aspects of knowledge
and being and consider their implications for critical dementia studies.

Troubling identity, subjectivity and normativities

A critical issue within studies of dementia is the notion of personhood
(Bartlett and O'Connor, 2007; Gjødsbøl and Svendsen, 2019; Kitwood,
1997), although as others have noted (Baril and Silverman, 2019; Silverman
and Baril, 2021), personhood, identity and self are often used interchangeably within the literature. A questioning of identity and subjectivity and how
norms related to the nature of being are encapsulated in these debates is also
central to the early work of a number of queer theorists.

   Judith Butler's (1990) ground-breaking book *Gender Trouble* is often
regarded as crucial to the emergence of a queer theoretical canon, introducing ideas about the performativity of identity and subjectivity, i.e. that there
is no original doer behind a deed and that identity is simply the repeated
stylisation of acts that give the appearance of substance. In effect, we are
what we do, within highly prescribed discursive limits. However, it is in her
book *Bodies That Matter* that Butler (1993) provides a very useful and critical reappraisal of what embodied identity and subjectivity can mean in this
sense:

> [gender] is thus not the product of choice, but the forcible citation of a
> norm, one whose complex historicity is indissociable from relations of
> discipline, regulation, punishment. Indeed, there is no 'one' who takes
> on a gender norm. On the contrary, this citation of the gender norm
> is necessary in order to qualify as a 'one', to become viable as a 'one',
> where subject-formation is dependent on the prior operation of legiti-
> mating gender norms.
>
> (1993, p. 232)

Here, to be a subject, an identifiable person, a self, one must be recognised
as a viable subject; one must have an identity and self that align with normative expectations. To step outside of these norms is, as Butler (2004, 2010)
has argued, to become a non-person, to be abnormal and to have a life that
is precarious. Although Butler's work primarily relates this to norms of

gender and, to an extent, citizenship more broadly, as I have argued else-where, cognonormativity (King, 2016), the forcible citation of norms about cognition and cognitive capacity is central to being recognised as a person with or without dementia. Indeed, cognonormativity can be considered a discursive and systemic framing that manifests such a binary separation, in ways similar to those associated with heteronormativity. And as with the case of norms related to gender and sexuality, such norms are constituted both biomedically and behaviourally. If we extend Butler's ideas here with additional writings from other queer theorists, we can see another aspect to this process that I think gets to the very root of ways that dementia is socially constructed as Other-ness. This is through the troubling of differ-ence and the demarcating of those with identities and subjectivities deemed to be abnormal, pathological, precarious, troubled. Again, influenced by post-structuralist and post-modernist notions of challenging and decentring meta-narratives and binary logics, queer theory can shed light on a system-atic epistemological and ontological philosophy of normative cognition that permeates Western society and arguably now does so globally.

In Diana Fuss' work on the dichotomy between heterosexuality and homosexuality, which queer theorists see as important to explain the inter-nal logic of a normative heterosexuality, or heteronormativity, Fuss states:

> [t]he language and law that regulates the establishment of heterosexu-ality as both an identity and an institution, both a practice and a sys-tem, is the language and law of defence and protection: heterosexuality secures its self-identity and shores up its ontological boundaries *by pro-tecting itself from what it sees as the continual predatory encroachments of its contaminated other*, homosexuality.
>
> (Fuss, 1991, p. 2, my emphasis)

Whilst dementia and sexuality are different, if we now substitute hetero-sexuality in this quote with cognonormativity and homosexuality with dementia, we can see how Fuss's queer ideas have value for critical dementia studies. It is through the creation of a binary system around cognition and rationality and their associated practices (one can think of biomedical and clinical practices here) and behaviours deemed to be odd, strange, different and markers of cognitive decline that the cultural fear of a 'contaminated other' – a non-rational cognition – a de-cognition – illustrates how what is called dementia is constructed as an-other. To be normal, cognitively speak-ing, is not to be identified or subjectified as having dementia. Putting it very starkly and for hyperbolic effect, normal people may be older but they are not 'demented'.

This is not to deny the dis/stress that such a process and behaviours incul-cate in those living with dementia. Having personal experience of caring for my father who was diagnosed with vascular dementia three years before he suffered a fatal cerebral haemorrhage, I have come to look at how deeply ingrained ideas of cognonormativity are in my own thinking and responses to cognitive difference, and how difficult it is to shed them. Over time, I have struggled with not becoming irritated or wanting to correct when being addressed as a dead relative, for the umpteenth time, or when cleaning up another kitchen sink full of urine because it was regarded as the bathroom toilet. Indeed, this echoes Butler's point, quoted earlier, about the forcible citation of a norm; we are, mostly unwittingly, required to cite these norms as they are at the basis of understanding our own cognition, understanding and sense making. To question such normativity is to attempt to extricate oneself from the very disciplinary and regulatory bio-power (Foucault, 1978) that as individuals we are all caught within. Moreover, it is a form of bio-power that has its own temporal logics and I will now take another queer turn by discussing the usefulness of queer theory to question notions of time and temporality, particularly a normative life course and ideas about futurity and forgetting.

Troubling times

Several queer theorists have grappled with ideas of temporality and the highly normative idea that life has a linear logic within which cognition is binary. Three in particular are Lee Edelman (2004) in the book *No Future: Queer Theory and the Death Drive*, Elizabeth Freeman (2010) in *Time Binds: Queer Temporalities, Queer Histories* and J.J. Halberstam (2011) in *The Queer Art of Failure*, which itself builds on arguments made in *In a Queer Time and Place* (Halberstam, 2005).

Edelman's (2004) work addresses the way in which heterosexuality is associated with a life force, or jouissance, that relies on the negation of an-other, the queer, which in psychoanalytic terms comes to be associated with a death drive. For Edelman, this happens through a social and cultural trope of futurity. Moreover, the markers of a normative life course – birth, marriage, reproduction, death to name but a few – are reliant on a casting out, an expulsion of those deemed other, queer, abject. Edelman gives a whole range of examples, drawn from popular culture, to illustrate this thesis, but what I believe is relevant for critical studies of dementia is how (again) this provides a whole conceptual framework for exploring how dementia is deemed abject, death-driven with no future. Elsewhere, I have illustrated the usefulness of this approach with a close textual reading of normative family imagery in an Alzheimer's Society advertisement (King, 2021) – the way that dementia is represented as disruptive of normal family relationships and a normative family time but can be recuperated and re-framed into a story of hope and futurity largely by erasing issues of loss and death. Dementia, as something queer, can be put back in its place, as it were.

In addition to Edelman's queer(y)ing of futurity, Freeman's work underscores the neo-liberal imperative for time to be (re)productive and to follow a chrononormative logic. By this, Freeman means: 'the use of time to organize individual human bodies toward maximum productivity'

(2010, p. 3). This has the effect of creating a certain temporal patterning to the life course that is symbolically embedded within capitalism and heterosexual family life. Hence, to be queer is to be outside of this temporal and indeed spatial framing, or to be positioned as antithetical to it. Whilst Freeman's work is primarily about how LGBT+ people are positioned as non-productive according to this logic, it is also possible to apply it to people living with dementia. To have dementia is often regarded as non-productive, or to be deemed as a burden on family caregivers (Lindeza et al., 2020). Again, I am not trying to downplay the effects that caring for someone with dementia can have on others; but I think the point to remember is that this is usually framed and investigated from a social scientific view in negative, familial and normative ways.

One of the so-called burdens of caring for people with dementia relates to dealing with loss of memories, of forgetting and cognitive difference. Within cultures that are subject to the discourse of cognitive decline within a biomedical framing, there seems to be no way of conceptualising forgetting other than negatively. Although Edelman and Freeman's queer writings can highlight the way in which time and temporality are circumscribed to produce a (hetero)normalising of chronology and thereby creating chronological temporal cognitions in normative ways, the work of Halberstam (2011) has much to add to this in their writings.

In *The Queer Art of Failure*, Halberstam (2011) emphasises the radical potential of forgetting, stupidity and the absence of memory through a close reading of a number of films and novels that suggests these can be transformative without framing them (necessarily) as pathological by recourse to entering the lifeworld of those said to be displaying these characteristics on their own terms. As Halberstam notes:

> To say that we may want to think about memory and forgetting differently is in fact to ask that *we may start seeing alternatives to the inevitable and seemingly organic models we use for marking progress and achievement*
>
> (Halberstam, 2011, p. 70, my emphasis)

I believe this can be read as a further call to trouble notions of cognonormativity and chrononormativity and to add to studies of dementia what Halberstam (2011) calls 'jamming the smooth operations of the normal and the ordinary' (p. 70).

Indeed, Halberstam's point that failure should be embraced rather than erased or pathologised does appear to offer critical studies of dementia with a different route, a queer turn, through debates about rationality and cognition and how these are normalised and measured. However, as I will discuss shortly, there are counter-critiques to this view and indeed to the possibility that queer theory may be somewhat less radically deconstructionist in this respect, than it may first appear. Before that, I want to focus on another queer turn, one that in many ways begins to highlight the limits of queer theory and why, sometimes, queer theory needs to be aligned with, brought into dialogue with, other theoretical perspectives.

Troubling intersections

Since its inception, there have been numerous criticisms of queer theory, largely that its radically deconstructionist imperative can become an apologist for neo-liberalism, and hence it is actually both reactionary and regressive (Hennessy, 2000; Kirsch, 2000). Furthermore, the deconstruction of identities has the potential to overlook important structural inequalities, related to class, race, ethnicity and ableism, among others (McCann and Monaghan, 2020). To this end, other writers have sought to challenge and realign queering with other theoretical frameworks, including intersectionality, critical race studies and disability studies (ibid.). I cannot discuss all these in detail in this chapter, but I want to highlight ones that I think have added to queer theory in ways that make its usefulness to critical dementia studies particularly apposite.

Emerging from black feminism and critiques of the occlusion of race in feminism, intersectionality refers to the way that multiple structural marginalities co-construct each other to create disempowerment and privilege (Choo and Ferree, 2010). Intersectionality has been used effectively in studies of ageing to highlight the ways that age is always racialised, gendered, sexualised and classed (Hulko, 2009; Warner and Brown, 2011; Westwood, 2016). It highlights the ways that ageing is not only diverse but happens at the complex intersection between a range of identities and sources of social division; one is never 'just' an older person, but an older, gendered, racialised, dis/abled, sexualised, classed person, etc. However, in these writings, the significance of identities is not deconstructed as in queer theory, but it is decentred in the sense that age and ageing are social processes not decoupled from others. In this respect, whereas queer theory could be said to reify difference, turning difference into a form of pride and empowerment, intersectionality retains a focus on the practices and processes of marginalisation and how the intersection of different but co-constructing identities work to disempower along multiple axes of self.

Some writers have incorporated intersectionality into queer theory, particularly to redress the erasure of ethnic and racial difference. For instance, José Esteban Muñoz (1999, p. 4) discussed the processes of disidentification practised by drag performers of colour as:

> The survival strategies the minority subject practices in order to negotiate a phobic majoritarian public sphere that continuously elides or punishes the existence of *subjects who do not conform to the phantasm of normative citizenship.*

(my emphasis added)

Muñoz indicates that disidentification occurs for these drag performers of colour because of the intersection of gender, sexuality and race, and it is a way in which all aspects of their identities are transformed. Muñoz suggests that disidentification practices occur in counterpublics: locales where minoritised subjects are gathered and in which they can engage in actions which counter the dominant ideology, or 'survival strategies'.

Ferguson (2019) also argues that queers of colour are further marginalised in any queer theory that focuses on a single – one-dimensional – issue without a full assessment of historical and political complexity: that queer liberation cannot be disengaged from the racialised projects of neo-liberal capitalism. Meanwhile, Moussawi and Vidal-Ortiz (2020) argue that decentring whiteness in queer theory is important if it is to avoid replicating existing power structures and marginalities.

The points raised regarding the importance of decentring whiteness in queer theory are emphasised specifically in relation to dementia by Kontos et al. (2021) who argue that it is time to reimagine dementia in ways that recognises multiple marginalities, particularly how dementia care can repeat practices of segregation and social control experienced by people of colour. If a queer of colour critique is incorporated into such studies of dementia, then the intersections of dementia, race, sexuality, gender identity and further sources of social division within a historical and political context are clearly needed (see also Chapter 8). It is not simply that a queer approach to dementia needs to challenge issues of chrononormativity, cognonormativity and issues around time and space, but that this project will be incomplete as one of challenging inequality and privilege and creating empowerment unless it recognises intersectionality, especially the systemic and systematic practices of ethnic and racial exclusion.

Queer troubles

In a critique of an implicit ableism contained within queer theory, Johnson (2015) argues that in seeking to de-pathologise conditions that are normatively constructed as pathological, or illnesses or disabilities, ideas about queer failure in the work of Halberstam inadvertently romanticise or fetishise these conditions. Arguably, the notion I have put forth in this chapter, that a series of queer turns within queer theory provides useful ideas and concepts that can be applied within critical dementia studies, could be said to be problematic because, to a greater extent, queer theory has not adequately addressed cognitive difference and alternative rationalities – the subject of queer theory is, to a greater degree, predicated on a knowing subject. Does that invalidate what I have been arguing? I do not think it does if queer theory begins to take on a more explicit focus on the politicisation of disability and how cognitive differences are manifested.

Jasbir Puar's book *The Right to Maim: Debility, Capacity, Disability* (2017) extends her queer theoretical work to consider how disability is deliberately constructed under conditions of neo-liberalism in ways that can be used to create and extract value. In a blistering critique of a whole range of institutions, states and forms of identity politics, Puar defines this process as one in which 'bodies... are sustained in a perpetual state of debilitation precisely through foreclosing the social, cultural, and political translation to disability' (2017, p. xiv).

Within this constellation of theoretical concepts and ideas, Puar offers critical dementia studies and queer theory itself a renewed focus on the practices of actual and symbolic violence that operate when certain people, certain bodies and certain selves are identified and governed as pathological but controllable through the institutions of the modern state. I opened this chapter with the suggestion that dementia is one of the 'major causes of disability and dependency among older people worldwide [with] physical, psychological, social and economic impacts' (World Health Organization, 2021). This indicates to me why queer theory and its insights are useful in challenging biomedical definitions, but also why incorporating insights from crip/queer/trans studies has much to offer critical studies of dementia as well (Baril and Silverman, 2022; Johnson, 2015; Silverman and Baril, 2021).

Conclusion

This chapter has examined the usefulness and indeed some of the problems of taking a queer theoretical approach towards studies of dementia. I have argued that through several turns, queer theory has much to offer critical dementia studies. This is not to say that there are no problems with doing this important theoretical and conceptual work and I have highlighted points where this is the case. Overall, however, the deconstructive, denaturalised and anti-foundational approach of queer theory provides an important source of critique to the highly biomedical framing of dementia and as such, I think that it adds to approaches from across the social sciences and humanities in seeking to redress this framing.

References

Baldwin, C. and Capstick, A. (2007) *Tom Kitwood on Dementia*. Maidenhead: Open University Press.
Baril, A. and Silverman, M. (2022) 'Forgotten Lives: Trans Older Adults Living with Dementia at the Intersection of Cisgenderism, Ableism/Cogniticism and Ageism'. *Sexualities* 25(1–2): 117–131.
Bartlett, R. and O'Connor, D. (2007) 'From Personhood to Citizenship: Broadening the Lens for Dementia Practice and Research'. *Journal of Aging Studies* 21(2): 107–118.
Butler, J. (1990) *Gender Trouble*. London: Routledge.
Butler, J. (1993) *Bodies that Matter: On the Discursive Limits of Sex*. New York: Routledge.

Butler, J. (2004) *Precarious Life*. London: Verso.

Butler, J. (2010) *Frames of War: When Is Life Grievable?* London: Verso.

Choo, H.Y. and Ferree, M.M. (2010) 'Practicing Intersectionality in Sociological Research: A Critical Analysis of Inclusions, Interactions, and Institutions in the Study of Inequalities*'. *Sociological Theory* 28(2): 129–149.

Davis, D.H.J. (2004) 'Dementia: Sociological and Philosophical Constructions'. *Social Science & Medicine* 58(2): 369–378.

Edelman, L. (2004) *No Future: Queer Theory and the Death Drive*. Durham, NC: Duke University Press.

Ferguson, R.A. (2019) *One-dimensional Queer*. Cambridge: Polity Press.

Foucault, M. (1978) *The Will to Knowledge - The History of Sexuality Volume 1*. London: Penguin.

Freeman, E. (2010) *Time Binds: Queer Temporalities, Queer Histories*. Durham, NC: Duke University Press.

Fuss, D. (1991) 'Inside/Out'. In: Fuss, D. (ed.), *Inside/Out: Lesbian Theories, Gay Theories*. London: Routledge, 1–10.

Gjødsbøl, I.M. and Svendsen, M.N. (2019) 'Time and Personhood across Early and Late-Stage Dementia'. *Medical Anthropology* 38(1): 44–58.

Green, A.I. (2007) 'Queer Theory and Sociology: Locating the Subject and the Self in Sexuality Studies'. *Sociological Theory* 25(1): 26–45.

Haeusermann, T. (2019) 'Forced Continuity: Explorations of Biographical Narratives in Dementia Care'. *Journal of Aging Studies* 49: 1–8.

Halberstam, J. (2005) *In a Queer Time and Place: Transgender Bodies, Subcultural Lives*. New York: NYU Press.

Halberstam, J. (2011) *The Queer Art of Failure*. Durham, NC: Duke University Press.

Harding, N. and Palfrey, C. (1997) *The Social Construction of Dementia: Confused Professionals?* London: Jessica Kingsley Publishing Ltd.

Hennessy, R. (2000) *Profit and Pleasure: Sexual Identities in Late Capitalism*. London: Routledge.

Hulko, W. (2004) 'Social Science Perspectives on Dementia Research: Intersectionality'. In: Innes, A., Archibold, C. and Murphy, C. (eds.), *Dementia and Social Inclusion: Marginalised Groups and Marginalised Areas of Dementia Research, Care and Practice*. London: Jessica Kingsley Publishers Ltd, 237–254.

Hulko, W. (2009) 'The Time- and Context-Contingent Nature of Intersectionality and Interlocking Oppressions'. *Affilia* 24(1): 44–55.

Johnson, M.L. (2015) 'Bad Romance: A Crip Feminist Critique of Queer Failure'. *Hypatia* 30(1): 251–267.

King, A. (2016) 'Queer(y)ing Dementia – Bringing Queer Theory and Studies of Dementia into Dialogue'. In: Price, E. and Westwood, S. (eds.), *Lesbian, Gay, Bisexual and Transgender (LGBT) Individuals Living with Dementia*. London: Routledge, 71–84.

King, A. (2021) 'Queer Futures? Forget It! Dementia, Queer Theory and the Limits of Normativity'. *Journal of Aging Studies*. https://doi.org/10.1016/j.jaging.2021.100993.

Kirsch, M.H. (2000) *Queer Theory and Social Change*. London: Routledge.

Kitwood, T. (1997) *Dementia Reconsidered: When the Person Comes First*. Buckingham: Open University Press.

Kontos, P., Radnofsky, M.L., Fehr, P., Belleville, M.R., et al. (2021) 'Separate and Unequal: A Time to Reimagine Dementia'. *Journal of Alzheimer's Disease* 80(4): 1395–1399.

Lindeza, P., Rodrigues, M., Costa, J., Guerreiro, M., et al. (2020) 'Impact of Dementia on Informal Care: A Systematic Review of Family Caregivers' Perceptions'. *BMJ Supportive & Palliative Care.* https://spcare.bmj.com/content/early/2022/08/21/bmjspcare-2020-002242

McCann, H. and Monaghan, W. (2020) *Queer Theory Now: From Foundations to Futures.* London: Red Globe Press.

Moussawi, G. and Vidal-Ortiz, S. (2020) 'A Queer Sociology: On Power, Race, and Decentering Whiteness'. *Sociological Forum* 35(4): 1272–1289.

Muñoz, J.E. (1999) *Disidentifications: Queers of Color and the Performance of Politics.* Minneapolis: University of Minnesota Press.

Odzakovic, E., Kullberg, A., Hellström, I., Clark, A., et al. (2021) '"It's Our Pleasure, We Count Cars Here": An Exploration of the 'Neighbourhood-Based Connections' for People Living alone with Dementia'. *Ageing and Society* 41(3): 645–670.

Puar, J. (2017) *The Right to Maim: Debility, Capacity, Disability.* Durham, NC: Duke University Press.

Sandberg, L. (2018) 'Dementia and the Gender Trouble?: Theorising Dementia, Gendered Subjectivity and Embodiment'. *Journal of Aging Studies* 45: 25–31.

Sandberg, L. and King, A. (2019) Queering Gerontology. In: Gu, D. and Dupre, M. E. (eds.), *Encyclopedia of Gerontology and Population Aging (Living Edition).* Cham: Springer, 273–271.

Sandberg, L. and Marshall, B. (2017) 'Queering Aging Futures'. *Societies* 7(21): 1–11.

Silverman, M. and Baril, A. (2021) 'Transing Dementia: Rethinking Compulsory Biographical Continuity through the Theorization of Cisism and Cisnormativity'. *Journal of Aging Studies* 58. https://doi.org/10.1016/j.jaging.2021.100956.

Sullivan, N. (2003) *A Critical Introduction to Queer Theory.* Edinburgh: Edinburgh University Press.

Ward, R., Clark, A., Campbell, S., Graham, B., et al. (2018) 'The Lived Neighborhood: Understanding How People with Dementia Engage with their Local Environment'. *International Psychogeriatrics* 30(6): 867–880.

Warner, D.F. and Brown, T.H. (2011) 'Understanding How Race/Ethnicity and Gender Define Age-Trajectories of Disability: An Intersectionality Approach'. *Social Science & Medicine* 72(8): 1236–1248.

Westwood, S. (2016) 'LGBT* Ageing in the UK: Spatial Inequalities in Older Age Housing/Care Provision'. *Journal of Poverty and Social Justice* 24(1): 63–76.

World Health Organization. (2021) *Dementia.* https://www.who.int/news-room/fact-sheets/detail/dementia.

18 Neurodiversity and dementia

Pitfalls, possibilities and some personal notes

Linda Örulv

Introduction

Following in the footsteps of the disability movement, a citizenship perspective for dementia is increasingly gaining ground. People with dementia are recognised as active agents, albeit within the boundaries of their condition and with a certain amount of vulnerability to marginalisation (Bartlett and O'Connor, 2007, 2010). The time has now come for dementia research to learn from critical perspectives and analytical tools within the disability movement(s) to investigate the relationship between the boundaries of the condition and the process of marginalisation. This chapter tentatively outlines how the concept of neurodiversity and (selectively) the neurodiversity paradigm can contribute to critical dementia studies, including both pitfalls and possibilities. As we shall see, it comes with some urgent caveats to avoid inviting harmful inferences and comparisons.

Now, first I need to say something about my own relationship to the topic. As a communication ethnographer in the field of dementia, my research interest has been centred around the perspectives of people with dementia as they develop and take shape in social interaction, especially among peers. As a contrast to the 'personal tragedy' discourse that often accompanies a one-sidedly medical model for understanding the condition(s), I have emphasised how residents in dementia residential care actively used their remaining linguistic and cognitive resources to make sense of their situations, their surroundings and their lives. I have also for seven years worked closely together with a group of people with early-stage dementia engaged in mutual support and self-advocacy. I'm currently writing a book on mutual support among people with dementia, highlighting among other things how the participants create a space together that allows them to interact in ways better adapted to their current functioning. This is all very much in line with what the neurodiversity paradigm is about. However, the self-advocates in the group have fought hard to have their symptoms taken seriously without any trivialisation and recognised as something distinctly different from 'normal' (or expected) ageing or the regular ups and downs of human life. While positioning themselves as agentive and resourceful, the medical

DOI: 10.4324/9781003221982-23

diagnosis has been of utmost importance to them – for sense-making purposes, as a tool to manage and negotiate social interactions and expectations and eliciting understanding and support, and as a foundation on which they base claims to specific rights warranted by impairment. They would most definitely welcome a cure to what they experience as a disruption to their previous functioning and as a source of distressing symptoms intruding into their lives. To the extent that a neurodiversity paradigm opposes pathologising varieties of cognitive functioning in general – something that is under debate among proponents – the dementia self-advocates that I know would find that it is against their interests and even harmful. Therefore, I cannot vouch for such an application of the paradigm with regard to dementia.

However, I am 'neurodivergent' myself, or part of a neurominority[1] – I am autistic, and I have ADHD and Tourette's syndrome. While I medicate to alleviate some difficulties that come together with my ADHD in this society, I generally subscribe to a conviction that variation of neuro-functioning is valuable to humankind. While I certainly wish to cure my depressions as needed, I find attempts at 'curing autism' deeply worrying to say the least. Quite frankly, I consider it to be eugenics, and I know I am far from alone in that, even though I cannot speak for everyone. So, you see, this is a sensitive topic, and a complex one. It is deeply existential and political and a potential minefield when we dig deeper into the implications of specific ontological claims if taken far enough. Hence the need to untangle such claims from 'epistemically useful' concepts and analytical tools (Chapman, 2020b). If we accept that they fulfil different purposes we can apply a 'no harm' approach that is sensitive to the lived experiences of people with different conditions or neuro-configurations. I do not believe in a 'one size fits all' principle as to what neurodiversity means ontologically. There is a place for ontological claims as an important part of a political struggle for social change, and researchers can support that as allies (while making clear whether something is an assumption or empirically based), but claims may need to differ between different groups (and within groups as well, depending on how groups are delineated).

Neurodiversity as a concept refers to variations in cognitive, affectual and sensory functioning, including both the predominant neurotype – the neurological wiring of the so-called neurotypical population – and divergences from it, as it is a quality pertaining to a group and not to individuals (Bertilsdotter Rosqvist et al., 2020). So far, we are talking about an ontological fact about human biology. As a group, human beings are diverse when it comes to functioning, and neurodiversity pertains to specific modalities of variation, namely cognitive, affectual and sensory functioning. When people talk about a neurodiversity *perspective* or *paradigm*, they usually mean something beyond that mere fact (Walker, 2014). A major component is that of challenging normative models of functioning (Bertilsson Rosqvist et al., 2020). I can see how this could be applied to dementia insofar as it points to how those norms limit our possibilities to act and interact in society, thereby alienating and marginalising minorities that diverge from them. In other words, it would highlight mechanisms of 'cognitive othering' (ibid., p. 2, see also Chapter 14 in this volume).

However, the paradigm is also associated with a political struggle to de-pathologise neurodivergence (Chapman, 2020a, 2020b; Walker, 2014) and even question the use of a 'species norm for assessing (and valuing) our functional abilities at all, in favour of the notion that diversity itself is normal' (Chapman, 2020b). This is where it gets complicated. The very strength of the idea is also what makes it sensitive.

It has been argued that neurodiversity is a 'moving target' insofar as it will continue to change depending on interactions between different groups of people and different societal institutions, entangled in complex ways. A singular definition may not be possible (Chapman, 2020b). Bertilsdotter Rosqvist et al. (2020) conclude that the scoping of neurodiversity (in the sense of a movement or paradigm, I would presume) needs further reflection insofar as it is an empirical question whether medical conditions perceived as 'interruptions' coincide with subjectively experienced differences and identities. Boundaries between normality and otherness are 'always subject to cultural and ideological pressures' (Bertilsdotter Rosqvist et al., 2020, p. 2). The authors mention the possibility that dementia may be recognised as part of a 'broader continuum of sensory, affectual, and cognitive processing' (ibid.) while also clarifying that 'this still requires the recognition that particular configurations of human minds come with particular challenges within different stages of our lives, including those that are considered impairments by the individual' (ibid.).

In the following, I will discuss the pitfalls of relativising increasingly disruptive difficulties among people with dementia diseases on the one hand, and on the other hand undermining the struggle in some groups (autistic self-advocates and others) to de-pathologise their functioning. I will then reflect on the possibilities for new knowledge production in terms of elucidating and deconstructing taken-for-granted assumptions about cognitive, affectual and sensory functioning.

The pitfall of relativising disruptive difficulties

In the field of critical autism studies, the book corresponding to this one (Bertilsdotter Rosqvist et al., 2020) leads with the following quotation:

> My [autistic] personhood is intact. My selfhood is undamaged. I find great value in my life, and I have no wish to be cured of being myself.
> (Sinclar, 1992, p. 302, quoted in Bertilsdotter Rosqvist et al., 2020, p. v)

Leading with a similar quote as a pamphlet for critical dementia studies would possibly be seen as provocative, perhaps even disrespectful, to the experiences that many people with dementia do express of having their

sense of self challenged by acquired brain damage, not to mention the identification with the condition as one's very being.[2]

Thankfully, the earlier one-sidedly deficit-oriented discourse on dementia as entirely robbing the individual of their self (see Ballenger, 2006;
Downs, 2000; Herskovits, 1995; and Lyman, 1989, for overviews) has
over time met extensive criticism and had to give way to more nuanced
approaches such as the personhood perspective (Kitwood, 1988, 1993,
1997a, 1997b; Kitwood and Bredin, 1992) and later also the citizenship
perspective (Bartlett and O'Connor, 2007, 2010) and other agency-based
perspectives (Hydén and Antelius, 2017; see also Chapter 6). Over the last
two decades, an increasing body of research has demonstrated how people
with dementia actively use remaining resources to maintain their social
identity, how they continue to honour their values, and so forth (e.g. Hydén
and Örulv, 2009; Örulv, 2014a; Örulv and Hydén, 2006), and how they can
also remain agentive in everyday interactions and in society (e.g. Örulv,
2012). Thus, the notion of undamaged selfhood and intact personhood is
not that far-fetched when it comes to dementia, apart from the difficulties
that make them fragile. Yet, the quotation seems to imply something else –
the context is that of de-pathologising the condition and reclaiming it as a
minority identity.

If we compare the cases of dementia and autism, there are crucial differences to how they manifest. While dementia sets in as a disruption to the
functioning that was already in place, autism is often likened to functioning from a different 'operative system' altogether and is described by self-
advocates as something that is deeply integrated into the very core of one's
personality. Somehow, I doubt that we will ever see an identity-first declaration from dementia self-advocates, protesting the phrasing 'person with',
whereas this is central for the majority of autistic self-advocates. A scenario
where people living with dementia oppose the idea of a possible cure seems
even more far-fetched.

There are occasional (rare) examples of individuals with dementia framing their condition mainly as an asset rather than a disorder. A case study on
dementia at the intersections (O'Connor et al., 2010) describes a woman with
indigenous descent who found that the unfolding of dementia brought her
closer to her spiritual roots and helped her develop as an artist. The notion
of dementia as coming home spiritually would certainly be interesting to
explore further if empirical data allow it. An interesting note here is that
when people with dementia do report not being bothered by difficulties, it
is commonly seen as being in denial, so it might be the case that positive
aspects of dementia are overlooked.

However, I believe it is fair to say that most people who develop dementia,
at least in societies with high demands on intellectual skills and independence in daily life, would welcome a cure as long as they are able to understand the implications of it. While people with dementia can develop coping
strategies (e.g. Pearce et al., 2002) and (contrary to common belief) are still

able to learn new skills (Ingebrand et al., 2021) and solve problems together (Örulv, 2019), let alone actively use their remaining resources in productive and creative ways (Hydén et al., 2013; Hydén and Örulv, 2009, 2010; Örulv, 2008, 2010, 2014a; Örulv and Hydén, 2006), there is no denying that disruptive changes occur, especially at later stages. Conditions such as Alzheimer's disease and vascular dementia are progressive, unlike autism, which means that over time the need for support in daily life tends to increase, and eventually they may even lead to death. As Sandberg argues in Chapter 15 on feminism and dementia, getting caught up in the dichotomy of negativity and decline versus the positive, productive and agentic is an all too common trap, and we tend to be invested in the latter. We need to get beyond that to see the nuances.

People with dementia who are engaged in activism and/or mutual support tend to choose not to downplay their difficulties, but rather to emphasise them and thereby claim their right to support and understanding (Bartlett, 2014; Beard and Fox, 2008; Örulv, 2017a). In doing so, they accentuate experiences and needs that are shared among the group members and affirmed in solidarity (Bartlett, 2014). However, they do not internalise the tragedy discourse that is so often put forward in the public discourse, perhaps especially in fund-raising, portraying them as victims and burdens.

In a long-term ethnographic study of a dementia self-help and self-advocacy group (Örulv, 2012, 2014b, 2017b, 2019), I found that the participants were involved in complex balancing acts, manoeuvring artfully between two evils, or navigating between the proverbial Scylla and Charybdis:[3] trivialisation and dismissal. While putting forward their difficulties in advocacy work, fighting to have their support needs be taken seriously, they at the same time put forward their mutual experiential knowledge as a major source of authority, which demonstrated competency. They fought a two-front battle facing both trivialisations of symptoms and dismissal due to stereotypical assumptions (Örulv, 2012); this has been referred to as dealing with double stigmatisation (Ohlsson, 2009). The complexity of navigating in-between trivialisation and negative categorisations was reflected in the group sharing as well. Participants skilfully and with great finesse drew on rather contrasting storylines to balance reports on increasing difficulties and support needs with more agentive images and other attributes supporting a positive sense of self – both for themselves and for their friends (Örulv, 2012, 2014b, 2017b). The intricacy of the 'footwork' and positioning involved deserves a book on its own (which is why I am also currently writing one).

Additionally, the participants brought forward a social perspective of being interrelated with others and with society, as agents depending on other agents, in line with a social model of disability (Örulv, 2012). They were able to do that without relativising the disruptive difficulties that they were experiencing, even though their audience and the people around them weren't always able to appreciate those nuances. It is my hope that in bringing the concept of neurodiversity into the field of dementia studies, we too, as well as our readers, will find ways to hold more than one thought simultaneously and thus avoid throwing out the baby with the bathwater. After all, it is possible to critically discuss norms around cognitive, affectual and sensory functioning and to acknowledge and respectfully meet the great variety of needs within the human population without adhering to full-on relativism or denying any hardship that might be inherent to a condition even with full support from society.

The pitfall of pathologising neurodiversity (or undermining de-pathologisation)

In bringing the concept of neurodiversity into the field of dementia, we are also bringing dementia into the discourse on neurodiversity. Let us say that we manage to avoid the pitfall of trivialising disruptive difficulties associated with dementia by way of maintaining the disease/disorder status. If so, we are instead facing the risk of undermining the political struggle within neurodiversity movements to de-pathologise diagnoses such as autism, unless we can successfully explain why medical diagnoses are warranted in some cases and not in others.

Chapman (2020a) delves into why a biostatistical species norm with regard to neuro-functioning is untenable. A biostatistical species norm is based on the idea that we can measure whether or not any given subsystem is functioning correctly by comparing it to the standard (average) functioning within a so-called reference class that is supposedly homogenous. This might include, for instance, same species, age and sex – criteria that are for some reason deemed naturally uniform. The assumption here is that health is the same thing as what is statistically normal. The problem is that it is far from self-evident what criteria should be included in the reference class. It turns out that any such categorisation involves normative assumptions. Who is to say that Down Syndrome or some other neurotype is any less 'naturally uniform' than sex? As Chapman (2020a, p. 61) points out, 'depending on what we decided to include or not, the outcome in terms of who is considered pathological or not will shift'. A neurodiversity paradigm contests the very notion that the neurocognitive functioning of our species is uniform enough for a statistical average to be considered the healthy or correct functioning. Using a biostatistical species norm of normal neurocognitive functioning to distinguish dementia from other conditions would thus ignore this important critique of the medical model, which would undermine one of the strongest arguments that the neurodiversity paradigm presents.

Furthermore, Walz (2020) presents a historical development that clearly illustrates the danger of normative assumptions about neurocognitive functioning. She argues that the pathologisation of neurodivergence has a painful history which is in many respects still ongoing, especially when we take other intersections and socioeconomic processes into account on top of it. Chown (2020) elucidates how the use of pathologising language not only legitimates striving for an eradication of divergent ways of functioning, such as autism, but even hides the fact that there is an ethical issue there to discuss and to assess in research ethics committees, as used to be the case with homosexuality.[4]

Using a biostatistical species norm for what is healthy neurocognitive functioning to distinguish dementia from other conditions to avoid trivialising disruptive experiences would ignore the methodological issues associated with the construction of such a norm. It would also probably not be the best move ethically, as accepting such a norm is the basis for pathologising neurodivergence in general which I – and many with me – would argue is harmful. As Chown (2020, p. 31) puts it,

> [m]any autistic scholars believe that no researcher should ever assume that it is appropriate to seek to destroy any aspect of humanity without societal acceptance of the justification of their work, an acceptance that must be based on the most thorough of investigations and debates because the very survival of a category of people depends on it.

The difference would have to have a firm basis in lived experiences from the inside (cf Borkman, 1976 and 1999, on experiential knowledge), and be focused on well-being (Chapman, 2020a) rather than some neuronormative generalised pseudo-scientific ideal regarding functioning.

The neurodiversity paradigm as an explorative stance

Above I have briefly outlined some of the political terrain that critical dementia studies need to navigate with regard to a neurodiversity paradigm. Admittedly, a question that has been running at the back of my mind is whether it is such a good idea to fit a condition (or group of conditions) such as dementia into a paradigm which not only focuses on the agentic aspects of lived experience (which has been at the heart of my own research) but is also associated with celebrating the diversity that it would be part of. Are the differences in lived experiences in-between groups too vast? Are the goals of self-advocacy in conflict between the groups? Do the benefits make up for the risks? I came to the conclusion that those are empirical questions, not something that I can take it upon myself to assess prematurely, and that exploring both the differences and the similarities would add to the knowledge base of what it is like to be human under different conditions. After all, it would be highly ironic to reserve the discourse of neurodiversity for a homogenous group.

Hart (2020), seeking an alliance between the neurodiversity movement and the hearing voices movement, sees neurodiversity as something that is flexible enough to bridge between conflicting discourses and move beyond unhelpful polarisations. A similar bridging function has been noted by Graby (2015) for the disability movement in relation to the mental health system survivors' movement. Perhaps we can also see echoes here of Kafer's (2013) emphasis on affinities in the crip movement as potential grounds for political coalitions.

For those theoretically inclined who wish to delve into ontological questions about the nature of neurodiversity, Chapman (2020a) proposes distinguishing between what is inherently good or bad versus what is good or bad in a specific context (of both external conditions and other individual traits). He argues that in terms of well-being, neurodiversity is value neutral when it comes to inherent qualities. Applying this to dementia would mean that there might be circumstances under which dementia might not have a negative effect on well-being and could even be considered to have positive effects. Apart from a supportive environment, such circumstances might include a combination of personal conditions that would help frame the changes in functioning in a positive way, such as a propensity for optimism and valuing other qualities than the intellect.

This seems to resonate with the experience of the case study mentioned earlier (O'Connor et al., 2010), the artist with indigenous descent who found that dementia helped her to reconnect with her spiritual roots. The conditions seemed to be just right for her to have a positive experience, at least at that point in the development. Bartlett (2014) mentions a window of opportunities for activism in the early stages, not only because such engagement is still possible within that time frame but also because aspects of the development seem to provide conditions for the kind of bravery that activism demands. Some of my informants have similarly mentioned that since the onset of dementia, they have been less prone to forsake their own needs and well-being and bend over backwards to accommodate others as they were previously inclined to do because of normative expectations.

Empirically, it might turn out that there are aspects of the neuro-functioning in dementia that are not inherently bad whereas others are. Following Chapman (2020a), it could thus be argued that aspects that turn out to be inherently bad in terms of well-being would fall outside the scope of the neurodiversity paradigm and instead be seen as medical issues. With a progressive development, the configuration of specific ways of functioning changes over time, wherefore the applicability of different frameworks might change too. While avoiding hardship-denying claims, this opens up interesting research questions. Under what specific conditions might aspects of dementia stand out as positive developments? Are there ways to cultivate such conditions to make those aspects of neuro-functioning flourish, and what would that look like at different stages of the development?[5]

Since human experience is always situated, it may not be possible to tease out once and for all what 'bads' are inherently bad and which ones are dependent on external circumstances that could be changed, such as normative expectations. Whereas dementia self-advocates tend to use the disease label as a resource, as mentioned earlier, it has also been argued by some researchers (for instance Ballenger, 2006; Herskovits, 1995) that the pathologisation transforming senility to Alzheimer's disease has increased the stigma rather than the opposite. People with dementia have become the 'unsuccessful others' to notions of successful ageing (Sandberg and Marshall, 2017).

I have suggested elsewhere (Örulv, 2008) that medical approaches to dementia are not problematic per se, although arguably quite deficit oriented. The problem is due to the lack of pervasive alternative resources for making sense of dementia in our everyday world outside of the medical territory – which is why critical dementia studies is needed. With a neurodiversity paradigm in mind, I will have to admit that I do not actually know exactly where the medical territory begins and ends. I would be cautious about making judgements as to whether specific traits of neuro-functioning associated with dementia are aspects of 'natural' variation or 'naturally' pathological. As an ethnographer, instead I would stay true to empirical data and depict the meaning-making processes of groups as they organically develop, elucidating the grounds for their own preferred positioning. There are always political aspects to what questions we ask in our research, or even to what questions we can come up with depending on our own biases, which is why we need critical lenses in the first place.

As researchers it is not our role to outline which groups are allowed to identify as neurominorities and on what grounds. Our role is to use concepts tentatively, exploratively, to see what kinds of new knowledge it produces and how it resonates with lived experiences. Slicing and dicing things along different axes makes it possible to investigate dimensions that are otherwise neglected. Chapman (2020b, p. 219) proposes that neurodiversity is 'more of an epistemically useful concept than anything else' insofar as it 'helps us imagine the world differently to how it currently is'. He further suggests that 'by adopting a neurodiversity perspective, we can alter actual relations; all the way from how we empathize with neurological others on a personal level, to how we design scientific experiments or public spaces' (p. 220), something that may eventually change our shared world for the better. In the meantime, we can develop shared vocabularies and other tools for our shared sense-making and for knowledge production. I do believe that this is the way forward.

Approaching dementia without a neurotypical gaze

On a personal note, I cannot ignore the affiliation I have felt with my research participants on the very ground that they were neurodivergent too, and the recognition that exists between us in some respects even though there have also been great differences. I would say that my most important contributions to the field of dementia research are due to being part of a neurominority on my own part, or due to the lack of a neurotypical gaze (Bertilsdotter Rosqvist, Örulv et al., 2020; Stenning, 2020). For instance, I was able to see the active meaning-making that was going on in a long sequence of confabulation.[6] I tuned into the narrative logic, the integration of interactional and environmental clues, the identity work that was going on, with moral agency as a key component, and the logical adaptation of the storyline to better fit with new clues. All this while staying true to the original moral of what was being said (Örulv and Hydén, 2006). Similarly, I was able to see previously neglected dimensions of disorientation, with regard to both social and moral understandings of places as they manifest from moment to moment in social interaction and available frameworks (Örulv, 2010, 2014a). From a somewhat reductionist angle, I could say that it was thanks to my own experiences of having to do constant detective work in order to fit into neurotypical practices – a difficulty associated with being a minority that turned out to be a condition for a fresh perspective (cf Stenning, 2020, on Greta Thunberg's life writing). However, that does not entirely cover it.

My lack of neurotypical gaze made me less prone to generalise in accordance with common neurotypical categorisations of social situations. This impacted how I collected my data. Rather than recording pre-defined activities within fixed timeslots, I chose to record fewer but longer periods of times. This enabled me to record in full spontaneously arising episodes which were meaningful from the perspectives of the participants with dementia, regardless of how they fitted into the overall planning of activities. The recording was done in an improvising mode sensitive to the action and the drama that I was able to perceive at the time. In contrast to common neuronormative[7] assumptions that being autistic would make it difficult for me to tune into the perspectives of other people, I would argue that the opposite was the case. Not only could I easily relate to navigating a confusing environment adapted for a different cognitive, affective and sensory functioning than mine; I could viscerally sense it in my own body as it happened. The kind of step-by-step meaning-making that one adheres to when being alienated by the social environment – that navigational stance is embodied. In mirroring it, there was an embodied knowing that alerted me and informed my ethnographic intuition. Correspondingly, the research participants seemed to share a similar alert system, recognising me as a 'fellow alien', which made them comfortable enough to share glimpses of their inside experience that would otherwise have remained backstage. This tells me that there is something important to be gained from reaching out to each other and reinforces the argument for why a neurodiversity paradigm is so valuable to our understanding of dementia.

In my later research with the mutual support and advocacy group for people with dementia, my own neurodivergence enabled me to take part in the sharing and exchange of strategies of dealing with daily life in a way that neurotypical people could not do without violating boundaries. We shared solidarity, and the group participants did not feel that my recognising myself in them was trivialising their difficulties.

Some implications for research design – *What if?*

In the field of dementia research, the urgency of 'bringing the social back in' was emphasised more than three decades ago as a criticism of the bio-medicalisation of dementia in everyday life (Lyman, 1989), and that position has become more and more influential since then. There is thus already an alignment between dementia research in the social sciences and what Jurgens (2020) calls an 'enactivist' framework within neurodiversity studies, pointing to the need for research to be firmly rooted in its intersubjective social context. For instance, the following quote on understanding autistic individuals should ring a bell:

> [O]nce we stop thinking of the main action of social cognition as happening in the heads of individuals and put it back in the space of interactions themselves it becomes clear that successful social engagement is a joint responsibility. It is best conceived of as a shared endeavour in which adjustments need to be made by all parties involved to ensure successful outcomes.
>
> (Hipólito et al., 2020, p. 206)

The same point has been argued with regard to dementia by researchers such as Kitwood (1988, 1993, 1997a, 1997b; Kitwood and Bredin, 1992) and Sabat (1994a, 1994b, 2001, 2006; Sabat and Harré, 1994), among many others, during the last few decades. Yet, a significant aspect of the social interaction has been overlooked in dementia research, namely the neuro-typical gaze or positionality. What if the adjustments needed for successful interaction – along with the very understanding of what it is like to live with dementia – can only be fully understood by way of venturing beyond that gaze? What if the neurotypical positionality of researchers, which has so rarely been problematised within dementia research, renders invisible the most urgent questions by neglecting neurominority perspectives that could possibly envision alternative ways of living well?

More recently, in proposing a citizenship perspective for dementia, Bartlett and O'Connor (2007, 2010) have paved the way for structural analyses and opened up the field to empirical research on self-advocacy and activism, thus acknowledging dementia as disability and as a political issue. A neurodiversity lens might provide a useful tool for exploring *how* it is a political issue and thereby generate new knowledge.

Jurgens (2020) argues that an enactive (intersubjectivity-focused) framework is especially well suited for neurodiversity studies. In emphasising the importance of social practices and institutions, it can elucidate 'the ways in which neurotypical social practices and institutions can harm autistic individuals' social cognitive skills, identity, and wellbeing' (Jurgens, 2020, p. 86). Applied to the field of dementia, this is basically Kitwood's malignant social positioning with a political twist and with the addition of being informed by the specificities of cognitive, affectual and sensory functioning, not as faults but as facts.

Following Kafer's (2013) ideas of forming affinities and affiliations to extend and challenge the parameters of disability theory, a cross-pollination between neurodiversity studies and critical dementia studies has the potential to bring forth new alliances, new ideas and new angles in both fields. This assumes an open explorative and tentative use of the neurodiversity lens, as a curious 'what if' and 'why this now' rather than a locked-in or fixed position. It also presupposes a focus on well-being rather than normality, opening up for alternative forms of well-being, while staying true to all the nuances – all the colours of the rainbow and of the dark clouds, depending on circumstances.

Rather than just exchanging theoretical concepts and comparing empirical data, as intellectual exercises, I see a potential in taking the enactive approach a step further by creating arenas for people with dementia to get together with and exchange experiences with different kinds of neurominority groups, preferably on their own. It would enable something different from the usual 'norm meets other' exchange, with the neurotypical gaze as the taken-for-granted default perspective against which the cognitive other is measured. In the absence of the neurotypical gaze, (current) normative assumptions just might collapse, as the norm around which they are centred is no longer present as their anchor. I am curious as to what might develop in their place as a new shared space organically comes into being, especially over time, based on the embodied knowing and mutual recognition that are made relevant in the interaction.

Notes

1 Divergence presupposes a norm from which an individual can diverge, and any basis for such a norm would have to be a construct. Furthermore, the more one investigates the process of establishing such norms, the more arbitrary it seems. See Chapman (2020a)·

2 With some imagination I can see how a similar quote could function as PR for some private residential care facility, accompanied with idyllic pictures of laughing residents being cared for by radiantly smiling nurses in perfectly clean and yet homelike settings.

3 Sea monsters between which Odysseus had to navigate according to Homer, or possibly other maritime hazards, located so close to each other that they posed an almost inescapable threat to passing sailors.

4 There is even social acceptance today of so-called therapies for (or rather against) autism that correspond to the conversion therapies that gay people have been subjected to, resulting in severe traumas.

5 As a bitter side note, with an increasing degree of austerity politics, it might not be realistic to expect anyone to articulate positive neurodiverse experiences. Given a development with less and less support for people with disabilities (or people who are disabled by society), there might be a need to articulate only the suffering and impairing aspects – or else risk not being admitted support. As researchers we need to be cautious about expressing ourselves in ways that could be used to legitimise dismantling of the social welfare systems.

6 In the broad sense, confabulations are usually defined as false narratives or statements about the world and/or self due to some pathological mechanisms or factors, and with no intention of lying.

7 Please note that the double empathy hypothesis (Milton, 2012a, 2012b) states that neurotypical people have just as much difficulty taking the perspectives of autistic people as the other way around – it's a mutual problem between two groups with inherently different cognitive styles in communication.

References

Ballenger, J.F. (2006) 'The Biomedical Deconstruction of Senility and the Persistent Stigmatization of Old Age in the United States', in Leibing, A. and Cohen, L. (eds.), *Thinking about Dementia. Culture, Loss, and the Anthropology of Senility.* New Brunswick, NJ and London: Ruthers University Press, pp. 106–120.

Bartlett, R. (2014) 'The Emergent Modes of Dementia Activism', *Ageing and Society*, 34, pp. 623–644.

Bartlett, R. and O'Connor, D. (2007) 'From Personhood to Citizenship: Broadening the Lens for Dementia Practice and Research', *Journal of Aging Studies*, 21, pp. 107–118.

Bartlett R. and O'Connor, D. (2010) *Broadening the Dementia Debate: Towards Social Citizenship.* Bristol: Policy Press.

Beard, R.L. and Fox, P.J. (2008) 'Resisting Social Disenfranchisement: Negotiating Collective Identities and Everyday Life with Memory Loss', *Social Science and Medicine*, 66, pp. 1509–1520.

Bertilsdotter Rosqvist, H., Chown, N. and Stenning, A. (eds.) (2020) *Neurodiversity Studies. A New Critical Paradigm.* London and New York: Routledge.

Bertilsdotter Rosqvist, H., Örulv, L., Hasselblad, S., Hansson, D., Nilsson, K. and Seng, H. (2020) 'Designing an Autistic Space for Research: Exploring the Impact of Context, Space, and Sociality in Autistic Writing Processes', in Bertilsdotter Rosqvist, H., Chown, N. and Stenning, A. (eds.), *Neurodiversity Studies. A New Critical Paradigm.* London and New York: Routledge, pp. 156–171.

Bertilsdotter Rosqvist, H., Stenning, A. and Chown, N. (2020) 'Introduction', in Bertilsdotter Rosqvist, H., Chown, N. and Stenning, A. (eds.), *Neurodiversity Studies. A New Critical Paradigm.* London and New York: Routledge, pp. 1–11.

Borkman, T. (1976) 'Experiential Knowledge: A New Concept for the Analysis of Self-help Groups', *The Social Service Review*, 50, pp. 445–456.

Borkman, T. (1999) *Understanding Self-help/Mutual Aid: Experiential Learning in the Commons.* New Brunswick, NJ and London: Rutgers University Press.

Chapman, R. (2020a) 'Neurodiversity, Disability, Wellbeing', in Bertilsdotter Rosqvist, H., Chown, N. and Stenning, A. (eds.), *Neurodiversity Studies. A New Critical Paradigm.* London and New York: Routledge, pp. 57–72.

Chapman, R. (2020b) 'Defining Neurodiversity for Research and Practice', in Bertilsdotter Rosqvist, H., Chown, N. and Stenning, A. (eds.) *Neurodiversity Studies. A New Critical Paradigm.* London and New York: Routledge, pp. 218–220.

Chown, N. (2020) 'Language Games Used to Construct Autism as Pathology', in Bertilsdotter Rosqvist, H., Chown, N. and Stenning, A. (eds.), *Neurodiversity Studies. A New Critical Paradigm.* London and New York: Routledge, pp. 27–38.

Downs, M. (2000) 'Ageing Update. Dementia in a Socio-Cultural Context: An Idea Whose Time Has Come', *Ageing and Society*, 20, pp. 369–375.

Graby, S. (2015) 'Neurodiversity: Bridging the Gap between the Diabled People's Movement and the Mental Health System Survivors' Movement?', in Spandler, H., Anderson, J. and Sapey, B. (eds.), *Madness, Distress and the Politics of Disablement*. Bristol: Policy Press, pp. 231–244.

Hart, A. (2020) 'A New Alliance? The Hearing Voices Movement and Neurodiversity', in Bertilsdotter Rosqvist, H., Chown, N. and Stenning, A. (eds.), *Neurodiversity Studies. A New Critical Paradigm*. London and New York: Routledge, pp. 221–225.

Herskovits, E. (1995) 'Struggling Over Subjectivity: Debates about the "Self" and Alzheimer's Disease', *Medical Anthropology Quarterly, New Series*, 9(2), pp. 146–164.

Hipólito, I., Hutto, D.D. and Chown, N. (2020) 'Understanding Autistic Individuals: Cognitive Diversity Not Theoretical Deficit', in Bertilsdotter Rosqvist, H., Chown, N. and Stenning, A. (eds.), *Neurodiversity Studies. A New Critical Paradigm*. London and New York: Routledge, pp. 193–209.

Hydén, L.C. and Antelius, E. (2017) 'Introduction: From Empty Vessels to Active Agents', in Hydén, L.C. and Antelius, E. (eds.), *Living with Dementia: Relations, Responses and Agency in Everyday Life*. London: Palgrave, pp. 1–13.

Hydén, L.C. and Örulv, L. (2009) 'Narrative and Identity in Alzheimer's Disease: A Case Study', *Journal of Aging Studies*, 23(4), pp. 205–214.

Hydén, L.C. and Örulv, L. (2010) 'Interaction and Narrative Structure in Dementia', in Schiffrin, D., De Fina, A. and Nylund, A. (eds.), *Telling Stories: Language, Narrative, and Social Life*. Washington, DC: Georgetown University Press, pp. 149–160.

Hydén, L.C., Örulv, L., Samuelsson, C. and Plejert, C. (2013) 'Feedback and Common Ground in Conversational Storytelling Involving People with Alzheimer's Disease', *Journal of Interactional Research in Communication Disorders*, 4, pp. 211–247.

Ingebrand, E., Samuelsson, C. and Hydén, L.C. (2021) 'People with Dementia Positioning Themselves as Learners', *Educational Gerontology*, 47(2), pp. 47–62.

Jurgens, A. (2020) 'Neurodiversity in a Neurotypical World: An Enactive Framework for Investigating Autism and Social Institutions', in Bertilsdotter Rosqvist, H., Chown, N. and Stenning, A. (eds.), *Neurodiversity Studies. A New Critical Paradigm*. London and New York: Routledge, pp. 73–88.

Kafer, A. (2013) *Feminist, Queer, Crip*. Bloomingdale and Indianapolis: Indiana University Press.

Kitwood, T. (1988) 'The Technical, the Personal, and the Framing of Dementia', *Social Behaviour*, 3, pp. 161–179.

Kitwood, T. (1993) 'Towards a Theory of Dementia Care: The Interpersonal Process', *Ageing and Society*, 13, pp. 51–67.

Kitwood, T. (1997a) 'Cultures of Care: Tradition and Change', in Kitwood, T. and Benson, S. (eds.), *The New Culture of Dementia Care*. London: Hawker Publications in association with Bradford Dementia Group, pp. 7–11.

Kitwood, T. (1997b) *Dementia Reconsidered. The Person Comes First*. Buckingham and Philadelphia, PA: Open University Press.

Kitwood, T. and Bredin, K. (1992) 'Towards a Theory of Dementia Care: Personhood and Well-Being', *Ageing and Society*, 12, pp. 269–287.

Lyman, K.A. (1989) 'Bringing the Social Back In: A Critique of the Biomedicalization of Dementia', *The Gerontologist*, 229, pp. 597–605.

Milton, D.E. (2012a) *So What Exactly Is Autism?* Autism Education Trust. http://capacity-resource.middletownautism.com/wp-content/uploads/sites/6/2017/03/damian-milton.pdf (Accessed 13 January 2023).

Milton, D.E. (2012b) 'On the Ontological Status of Autism: The Double Empathy Problem', *Disability and Society*, 27(6), pp. 883–887.

O'Connor, D., Phinney, A. and Hulko, W. (2010) 'Dementia at the Intersections: A Unique Case Study Exploring Social Locations', *Journal of Aging Studies*, 24(1), pp. 30–39.

Ohlsson, R. (2009) *Representationer av ohälsa: Egna erfarenheter och dialogiskt meningsskapande i fokusgruppssamtal* [Representations of Mental Illness: Illness Experience and the Dialogical Construction of Meaning in Focus Group Discourse]. PhD dissertation, Department of Education, Stockholm University, Stockholm.

Örulv, L. (2008) *Fragile Identities, Patched-up Worlds. Dementia and Meaning-Making in Social Interaction.* Linköping: Linköpings universitet. Linköping Studies in Arts and Sciences, ISSN 0282-9800; No 428. Linköping Dissertations on Health and Society, ISSN 1651-1646; No 12.

Örulv, L. (2010) 'Placing the Place, and Placing Oneself within It: (Dis)orientation and (Dis)continuity in Dementia', *Dementia: The International Journal of Social Research and Practice*, 9, pp. 21–44.

Örulv, L. (2012) 'Reframing Dementia in Swedish Self-help Group Conversations: Constructing Citizenship', *International Journal of Self Help and Self Care*, 6(1), pp. 9–41.

Örulv, L. (2014a) 'The Subjectivity of Disorientation: Moral Stakes and Concerns', in Hydén, L.C., Lindemann, H. and Brockmeier, J. (eds.), *Beyond Loss. Dementia, Identity, Personhood.* New York: Oxford University Press, pp. 191–207.

Örulv, L. (2014b) *Dependence, Resistance, Control, and Agency in the Face of Evolving Dementia: Constructing Selves in Group Talk on Support* [PowerPoint presentation]. Life With Dementia 2014: Relations, October 15th, 20014, Linköping University (Center for Dementia research), Linköping.

Örulv, L. (2017a) 'Self-help, Mutual Support and Advocacy: Peers Getting Together', in Hydén, L.C. and Antelius, E. (eds.), *Living with Dementia: Relations, Responses and Agency in Everyday Life.* London: Palgrave, pp. 168–187.

Örulv, L. (2017b) *Self-help Groups for People with Dementia: Peers Managing Group Processes Together* [PowerPoint presentation in P2 Post-diagnostic support]. 27th Alzheimer Europe Conference: Care Today, Cure Tomorrow, October 3rd, 2017, Berlin.

Örulv, L. (2019) *Solving Everyday Problems Together in Group Conversation: Peer Support and Maintaining Involvement In Dementia* [Poster Presentation PO.F:01]. International Association of Gerontology and Geriatrics European Region (IAGG-ER) Congress, May 24th, 2019, Gothenburg.

Örulv, L. and Hydén, L.C. (2006). 'Confabulation: Sense-making, Self-making and Worldmaking in Dementia', *Discourse Studies*, 8(5), pp. 647–673.

Pearce, A., Clare, L. and Pistrang, N. (2002) 'Managing Sense of Self. Coping in the Early Stages of Alzheimer's Disease', *Dementia*, 1(2), pp. 173–192.

Sabat, S.R. (1994a) 'Excess Disability and Malignant Social Psychology: A Case Study of Alzheimer's Disease', *Journal of Community & Applied Social Psychology*, 4, pp. 157–166.

Sabat, S.R. (1994b) 'Language Function in Alzheimer's Disease: A Critical Review of Selected Literature', *Language & Communication*, 14(4), pp. 331–351.

Sabat, S.R. (2001) *The Experience of Alzheimer's Disease. Life through a Tangled Veil*. Oxford and Malden, MA: Blackwell.

Sabat, S.R. (2006) 'Mind, Meaning, and Personhood in Dementia: The Effects of Positioning', in Hughes, J.C., Louw, S.J. and Sabat S.R. (eds.), *Dementia: Mind, Meaning, and the Person*. New York: Oxford University Press, pp. 287–302.

Sabat, S.R. and Harré, R. (1994) 'The Alzheimer's Disease Sufferer as a Semiotic Subject', *Philosophy, Psychiatry, & Psychology*, 1(3), pp. 145–160.

Sandberg, L.J. and Marshall, B.L. (2017) 'Queering Aging Futures', *Societies*, 7(3), article number 21, 11 pages; https://doi.org./10.3390/soc7030021.

Sinclair, J. (1992) 'Bridging the gaps: An inside-out view of autism', in Shopler, E. and Mesibov, G.B. (eds.), *High-functioning individuals with autism*. Boston, MA: Springer, pp. 294-302.

Stenning, A. (2020) 'Understanding Empathy through a Study of Autistic Life Writing: On the Importance of Neurodivergent Morality', in Bertilsdotter Rosqvist, H., Chown, N. and Stenning, A. (eds.), *Neurodiversity Studies. A New Critical Paradigm*. London and New York: Routledge, pp. 108–124.

Walker, N. (2014) 'Neurodiversity: Some Basic Terms & Definitions', *Neurocosmopolitanism, 27*. https://neuroqueer.com/neurodiversity-terms-and-definitions/ (Accessed 28 September 2022).

Walz, M. (2020) 'The Production of the "Normal" Child: Neurodiversity and the Commodification of Parenting', in Bertilsdotter Rosqvist, H., Chown, N. and Stenning, A. (eds.), *Neurodiversity Studies. A New Critical Paradigm*. London and New York: Routledge, pp. 15–26.

19 Thinking back and looking ahead

Co-ordinates for critical methodologies in dementia studies

Richard Ward and Linn J. Sandberg

Introduction

In her chapter in this book, Hailee Yoshizaki-Gibbons points to arguments in the related field of critical disability studies for moving away from approaches that treat disability as an object of study and towards thinking of a critical approach as primarily a question of methodology (see, for example, Minich, 2016; Schalk, 2017). We admit a certain hesitance here, wondering, for instance, whether this would mean abandoning to a biomedical domain any effort to explain and define dementia, given what we know of the material consequences this has had for people's lives in the past. But also, as we come on to argue, because object/subject and methodology are in continual dialogue – arguably even co-constitutive. Nonetheless, there is real merit in thinking through this question of critical dementia studies as heralding a distinctive methodology or at least causing us to re-work existing methodologies – de-familiarising what has become routine, habitual and assumed. Such a move could help shift the locus of dementia research from a politically insulated concern with the person and their experience of the condition to an outward vista where dementia (or as Linn suggests earlier, a 'demented standpoint') becomes a basis on which to analyse broader social and political conditions. Indeed, we suggest this could be a key objective for critical dementia studies and as Richard has argued elsewhere:

> Such a development could mark the opening of a radical critique of 'able-mindedness' as an organising principle and normative influence upon the social, political and material environments inhabited by us all.
> (Ward, 2016, p. 227)

With this in mind, we want to use this final chapter to consider the co-ordinates that might guide emerging critical methodologies for dementia research and/or disrupt established methodologies in the field. With a particular focus on ethnographic approaches, we draw on the work of feminist ethnographer Patti Lather (2007), who has called for an academic form of getting lost as the basis for a new kind of methodology – one that

DOI: 10.4324/9781003221982-24

embraces uncertainty, not knowing and a loss of confidence as methodological strengths.

Our aim is to consider Lather's arguments hand-in-hand with Alison Kafer's (2013) proposal for a political-relational approach to illness and disability and to draw out the implications for dementia research. Kafer outlines the transformative potential of a critical lens by opening to question the (biomedicalised) constitution of discrete categories of illness and disability. She argues that deconstructing such categories can aid in the identification of 'collective affinities' between previously sub-divided groups and that this can lead to forging 'strategic alliances' as the basis of a new coalitional politics. Kafer targets the de-politicisation of illness and disability and the way that structural conditions are so often framed as matters of interpersonal cruelty or insensitivity. We might argue such of the enduring focus upon stigma as an explanatory framework for the social exclusion experienced by people living with dementia. For Kafer, a shift in thinking entails less of a focus upon the individual experience of disability and more on the political experience of disablement, an agenda that is intimately caught up with questions of methodology. Bringing Kafer into dialogue with Lather offers a useful pathway to rethinking how we engage with dementia through research. In part, this entails questioning what we have been taught to value and prioritise and what so often gets overlooked or side-lined.

The double(d) practice of critical methodology

While the origins of critical theory can be traced back (at least) to Kant (Simons, 2002), Lather (2007) offers a chronology of a more recent 'critical turn'. Her account opens with Marcus and Fischer's (1986) efforts to shed light on a mounting crisis of representation in the field of anthropology. Drawing upon an emergent post-colonial critique of anthropology for framing other cultures according to a Western lens (e.g. Said's Orientalism, 1979), the crisis of representation threw into question the very foundations of anthropology and the grand narratives around which it was organised. This included the many Western-centric assumptions and unexamined power differentials embedded within ethnographic practice. As Lather observes, the shockwaves of this disciplinary implosion rippled outwards with implications for the many different fields of scholarship that had adopted ethnographic practices as method and/or methodology. As part of the impact upon feminist ethnography, the crisis of representation fostered interrogation of a universalising category of 'woman' that elided differences of race, class, sexuality and disability (e.g. as noted by Morris, 1993) most often from an unmarked white, middle-class standpoint (see Chapter 8 for how dementia functions as a similarly elisional construct).

Lather's response was to propose a methodology organised around the challenge of abandoning the certainties of our discipline(s) by relinquishing a degree of control and shedding the familiar, comfortable and routine ways of doing research. Her argument is for a methodology that can work in the 'ruins' of a once confident social science, one that might lead not only to new knowledge but to new ways of knowing. Lather outlines two guiding concerns for the formulation of this methodology that she describes as the double(d) practice necessary to research.

The first concerns the need for researchers to negotiate the tension between what she describes as 'emancipation' and 'usurpation'. This means being conscious of an enduring conflict between the power of research to shed light on experiences of exclusion and disenfranchisement and the potential for such experiences to be exploited and appropriated through research. Interlocking with the emancipation-usurpation tension is the need to acknowledge and be guided by what she calls the 'non-innocence of representation'. Think, for example, of the many different social, moral and cultural beliefs and expectations that shape the way a person describes their experiences and the power relations in which those accounts are produced. This includes how the research encounter itself may influence what a person says and how they say it. Influenced by Derridean deconstructive thinking (that also informed the emergence of queer theory that Andrew King describes in Chapter 17), Lather suggests that any critical methodology that seeks to engage with the experience of others needs to be alive to the constructedness of the accounts and stories elicited and the processes and influences by which they are produced. She challenges the way in which the storying of people's lives is assumed to unproblematically convey lived experience and where gathering such narratives is too often considered an end in itself.

Making the difference in dementia studies

In this section, we consider what Lather's methodological proposals might mean for dementia scholarship given that the field has increasingly come to embrace ethnographic methods and approaches (see, for example, Keady et al., 2017). In part, our argument is a call, if not for greater honesty, then for increased transparency as a tenet of critical methodology. We echo here and build upon Linn's argument earlier in this book for re-casting difference as a generative and potentially transformative basis from which to understand and make sense of the social and political significance of dementia. Such a perspective draws upon Kafer's (2013) integrative treatise that combines feminist, queer and crip arguments in making the case for a political-relational approach to illness and disability.

Emancipation/usurpation

Critically driven methodologies open to question that which often remains unsaid and unacknowledged in the research process. This includes exposing to scrutiny the privilege that researchers enjoy, relative to those with whom they conduct research. Lather is thereby keen to inspire a healthy mistrust of research where routine claims are made for empowering or 'giving voice' to oppressed and precarious groups, speaking on behalf of collectives to which the researcher does not belong. As Lather argues, too often in emancipatory research, it is researchers themselves who somehow emerge as the heroes of their own story, where 'narratives of salvage and redemption' can serve as ever deeper places for privilege to hide.

Building on Lather's work, our understanding of usurpation encompasses those diverse occasions when researchers extract information, learning and experience for purposes that do not necessarily benefit the participant or the wider collective to which they belong (and of course we need to be mindful of what we assume 'benefit' to mean). There are various ways in which researchers, individually and collectively, draw advantage from research with disempowered groups that have become normalised and thereby pass largely unquestioned and remain unacknowledged. Richard was reminded of this in the context of an interview aimed at exploring experiences of living with early-onset dementia with Claire (a pseudonym), who commented:

> And so many people do take our words and use them and go up the career ladder and we're saying, hang on a minute, we're perfectly able to articulate what it's like having this [condition]. And there's a limit to how many times you can actually tell this story, but we have got a voice. We are the experts because none of you know what it's like to be in our heads.

By making explicit something that would routinely have remained unsaid, Claire's comments worked to shift the footing of the interview, making visible the usurpatory potential of the research encounter.

Lather describes usurpation as often driven by the researcher's assumed 'right to know' – a pre-given even before we engage with participants. We would venture to suggest that right to know underpins much dementia care practice too. There is a tacit transactional expectation that prospective service users, often repeatedly, surrender all manner of personal information (relational, biographical, health and, of course, financial). In return, they may be considered for support, but with little control over how those details are subsequently used. In the case of research, the right to know similarly feeds a right to use and own data. Think, for example, of data archiving practices, whereby first-hand expertise/experiences become the property of researchers who then relinquish them to funders. Future analytical opportunities are created for researchers who are entirely divorced from the conditions in which the data were produced.

Instead, Lather argues that as researchers we need to consider the value of 'not knowing' and, of course, in a dementia context, not assume that what there is to know is tellable in the first place. We suggest that a considered and strategic use of 'not knowing' alongside respect for the right not to tell could be invaluable to dementia research. Not least, it might under-cut the latent belief that as researchers we are better able to tell the stories of other people's lives – which is what Claire seems to be pushing back at in her comments above. There is a mounting argument within dementia studies for leaving some aspects of knowledge production to the person who owns it or has lived the experience from which it originates. Even in a context where knowledge is understood as co-created, we need to recognise, as Lather acknowledges, the potential for its distortion and political usage.

Likely many of us would sign up to an emancipatory agenda through our work but how well do we own the potentially usurpatory effects of what we do? Scholarship in related fields of disability and mental health has often been spearheaded by those with lived experience whose affinity with research participants augments their understanding and analysis. Yet, despite participatory and co-productive methods taking hold in countries such as the UK, it remains the case that universities simply do not offer tenured posts to those in the role of experts by experience. Nor does the higher education sector pay an hourly or daily rate to such experts at a level commensurate with an academic salary. There is a built-in inequity surrounding how we value different types of knowledge and different ways of knowing.

Consequently, we need to explicitly theorise the relationship of the researcher to the researched, both collectively and by giving an account of ourselves individually. Rather than this leading to what Folkes (2022) describes as 'shopping list positionality' (i.e. a tick-box approach to reflexivity), our argument is for bringing our own 'social location' (O'Connor et al., 2010) into dialogue with a situated engagement with dementia. This could entail asking in what way (if at all) are we allies/accomplices in the manner that Wendy Hulko outlines in Chapter 16. For instance, how do we better account for the hidden but controlling hand of the researcher (or practitioner), often as an arbiter of broader cultural and moral expectations, as the words of people with dementia are crafted into 'voice'? The challenge is to look more closely at the way this is done, the purposes it serves and the outcomes it leads to.

Research with oppressed and precarious groups can also feed into broader sets of interests and relations of power, reinforcing (biomedically constituted) categories and facilitating what Grenier and Phillipson refer to (in Chapter 10) as 'dividing practices'. Indeed, Grant (2016) makes the salient point that research which only works within diagnostic categories ultimately restores power to biomedical science where such categories are presented as value-free, apolitical and ahistorical. Yoshizaki-Gibbons (Chapter 14) notes the continued authority of a 'prevent-care-cure' framing of research into disability and dementia. This foregrounds an ambition to contain and ultimately eradicate conditions rather than learn from them, let alone recognise their socially and politically transformative potential.

In this context, usurpation also potentially manifests as methods are mobilised and travel between contexts and platforms. Let us take the now well-established body of work in dementia studies that draws upon narrative and storytelling as a focus for consideration. We refer here specifically to research that employs oral methods of knowledge production, rather than emerging work on more embodied and multi-sensory approaches. Oral traditions have long informed therapeutic interventions in dementia care and have been central to a dialogue between research and practice.

Increasingly, dementia-related storytelling has become woven into the public face of corporate and charitable service provider organisations. They are frequently presented online, through promotional material or service evaluations to anchor claims to 'allyship' and to signal an authenticated epistemology that draws upon lived experience. Many such organisations are in receipt of public funding. Yet, in countries such as the UK, over the last decade these same organisations have been tasked with rationing and even withdrawing support as funding cuts impact the care system. There is a hidden curatorial hand at work here, where individualised (arguably depoliticised) stories of personal struggle, resilience and self-realisation take prominence over collective accounts of the impact of over a decade of incremental defunding of social care.

Talking of illness narratives in general, Kafer (2021) has registered her unease with their uniformity, including a linear chronological temporality and sequential ordering. Their focus favours and foregrounds continuity, conveying a belief in selfhood as uniformly persisting in continuous time despite the disruptive potential of illness (see Chapter 17 and Haeusermann, 2019 for a critique). Furthermore, where dementia narratives are collaboratively produced in research and practice contexts, they are often notable for an absence of those interludes of unknowing, confusion or disorientation, and altered relationships to time and place so common to dementia (see Changfoot et al., 2022, for further discussion). Instead, stories are pieced together that bypass such dimensions to people's lives. Writing in 2006, Williams and Keady noted: 'Arguably, the dementia field has, to date, attempted to bring "order" to the apparent "chaos" of the lived lives of people with dementia by providing narratives that "turned on" but did not "tune in" to what was being storied' (2006, p. 164). Such work suggests that researchers and practitioners have interpreted their own role as imposing order, adopting a kind of narrative hygiene whereby fragmenting, disorderliness, gaps and messiness are treated as an unwanted intrusion upon the person. Any hint of chaos is approached as something to be contained, and through narrative it is erased in favour of an ordered sense of self.

Our aim here is not to critique the storying of experience per se. Indeed, as Linn reminds us in her chapter, shared narratives can provide the spark for consciousness-raising and resistance. The point we are making concerns the way that articulating the experience of dementia is so often funnelled into carefully curated and narrowly defined cultural modes of expression. These are notable for being individualising and biographically oriented and are often politically insulated (Grant, 2016). It seems that experts by experience are authorised to speak about dementia as long as they stick to the script. Where were the political spaces for people with dementia to speak out (and be listened to) about the impact of austerity policies upon care or to have influenced decision-making during the COVID pandemic?

Perhaps then, we can understand usurpation politically as a way of asserting control over the public narrative of dementia, conveying it as an individualised challenge of upholding biographical continuity and the rehabilitation of an essentialised selfhood – rather than one of disrupting inequitable and unjust conditions. Critical methodologies thus have a particular contribution to make to dementia scholarship and practice. They can be a vehicle to illuminate the ever-present tension between emancipation and usurpation, while tracing the contribution of research to a broader political narrative of dementia.

The non-innocence of representation

In this section, we continue our interest in that body of dementia research that has focused upon the spoken word and the question of how words become voice and how voice comes to stand for something more than words, even for more than a single speaker, but for an entire category of people, becoming a 'voice for all' (Cayton, 2004). Our argument is that much qualitative research in dementia studies still operates under the shadow of positivism. It is shaped by a set of assumptions that have paradoxically muted the very perspectives it supposedly sought to amplify.

Lather (2007) points out that critical scholars face a tension between making experience visible and seeking to question the status of that experience and its relationship to 'voice'. Such tension is particularly sensitive within dementia studies because people living with dementia have a long history of epistemic injustice (Jongsma et al., 2017, Price and Hill, 2021) marked by active exclusion from research, policymaking and even the planning and provision of dementia care. The capacity to offer testimony to the conditions of their own lives has been largely denied through positivist approaches, which have treated the person with dementia as an unreliable witness, lacking competence to convey the truth of their situation. In the wake of this injustice and political silencing, subsequent efforts to hear the voice (singular) of people (plural) with dementia (Goldsmith, 1996) and to 'give' people a voice (e.g. Moore and Hollett, 2003) have tended to treat that voice as sacrosanct. This means that narratives of experience have arguably been invested with an 'excessive evidentiary weight' that reifies the spoken word by lifting it out of the context of its production (Mazzei and Jackson, 2009).

A liberal-humanist approach begins with the person, and, as MacLure (2009) points out, is characterised by an assumption that the person always means what they say and knows what they mean. In this context, research participants are often seen as conveying insights into an already existing set of experiences while researchers are there to record and report on this. Lather is critical of the supposedly 'innocent' researcher, who appears to write from a neutral stance or perspective that is free of political entanglements. This has particular resonance for the therapeutically-driven nature of much humanist dementia research where (empowered) practitioner-researchers have largely failed to account for their own positioning or to make visible the differentials that frame their relations with the person with dementia as research subject. Instead, the emphasis in much of this work has been upon an assumed consensus, and an unquestioned belief that the practitioner and/or researcher is working in the interests of the person with dementia with common goals and objectives (Ward and River, 2011).

By contrast, a political-relational lens considers meaning not only as co-produced through a research encounter but as imbued with relations of power, and where the storying of experience is always partial and contingent (for researchers as well as the researched). This implies the need to re-examine the assumed status and routine handling of data. On this basis, St Pierre and Jackson (2014) question the ways in which research lifts the spoken word out of context, treating words as 'brute data' akin to quantitative data handling within positivistic research. They argue that coding of spoken data can constitute a distancing practice, involving the production of discrete categories of experience as 'countable items' that rely upon notions of a stable and continuous identity. In this way, they argue, narratives of experience are cumulative and homogenising, becoming the basis for generalising across a category of people, while reinforcing the boundaries of that category.

Notions of a fixed and essentialised identity assume that certain practices are intrinsic to these stable identities. As a result, dementia has become reified through research, disentangled from its intersections with different forms of identification and social location (Hulko, 2009). This has led to reliance within policy and practice upon what Jackson (2013) describes as 'single liberatory strategies'. Externally derived 'solutions' to the challenges people face are repeatedly proposed which ignore the emergent and politically complex nature of social experience. Through such an approach, social experience is set apart from context, implying a narrow deterministic belief in a causal relationship between dementia-related interventions and certain pre-determined outcomes (Ceci et al., 2020). Writing more broadly about mental health nursing research, Grant (2014) highlights the way in which narrative research de-emphasises the context of its own production. He argues that clinical and healthcare settings are unquestioningly assumed to offer a benign backdrop. The way that healthcare functions as a political regime that positions people accessing support is overlooked. Consequently, narratives of experience are insulated from wider systems of power that inscribe people's lives. It is precisely this active depoliticising of the experience of illness and disability that Kafer seeks to address through arguments for a political-relational approach.

We also need to consider the largely hidden and unacknowledged ways in which 'voice' is produced through a process of sifting and selection as a routine aspect of analysis and writing up research. Mazzei (2009) points out that researchers habitually favour the most easily understood, friendly and 'tame' voices in aid of packaging their research for mass consumption. The more slippery, less easily comprehended and potentially transgressive voices too often end up 'lying on the cutting room floor' (p. 59). Yet, this familiar process into which we are encultured as researchers has particular implications for dementia research. The faltering voice of certain participants, prolonged silences, uncertainty, the struggle with word-finding and narrative detours are all inherent to dementia. They constitute instances of what Schillmeier (2014) might describe as 'dementing moments' and yet are frequently deselected in favour of the clear competent voice that is more easily made sense of.

In this way, we suggest, much existing research has collectively and cumulatively erased certain voices (and dimensions of voice) from the research canon. Perhaps then we should understand these commonplace 'sense-making' research practices as political choices that reinforce an appearance of sameness. Our argument is for the need to resist the impulse to deliver what Lather calls a 'tidy text' – 'that maps easily onto our usual ways of sense-making' (2007, p. 87). Not only should we hold on to the messiness, uncertainty and hard-to-decipher encounters in our research, but treat these as potentially illuminating. Why is it commonly assumed that the dissonant, disordered and chaotic need cleaning up or correcting? Whose interests are being served when we do this?

Allied to this is the question of how research that prioritises explicit expression (i.e. the spoken word) renders the absence of such expression meaning-less. MacLure et al. (2010) have sought to question assumptions about what is prioritised and privileged and what is treated as an annoyance or interference in encounters with research data. They highlight the potential for silence to signal refusal and everyday modes of resistance (see Chapter 13 for further such examples) and ultimately its resistance to analysis. We argue that such questions lie at the heart of critical dementia studies, and open into a critique of far broader assumptions about what is valued and what is discarded or dismissed by research. Critical methodologies recognise the implication of disagreement over consensus, and could fruitfully orient towards ambiguity, uncertainty, contradictions and incoherencies as productive foci for analysis. Such attributes closely resonate with and reflect experiences of dementia and yet seem to be readily underplayed by the sense-making practices of dementia scholars.

Bringing ourselves closer in

In developing a political-relational framework, Kafer argues for making situated knowledge and ways of knowing central while throwing into question supposedly stable categories of difference. Indeed, she advocates 'refusing' fixed definitions of disability. Rather than being corralled under a particular diagnosis, Kafer argues that what matters is recognising the ethical, epistemic and political responsibilities associated with illness and disability. On this basis, she calls for '*more* attention to how different bodies/minds are treated differently, not less' (p. 13). In many ways, this can be interpreted as a call to action for critical research and for researchers, collectively and individually. As a first step, we would point to the vast numbers of us who occupy the hinterland of illness and disability, who live with and manage all manner of health issues without necessarily identifying as disabled or sick. There are many who could loosely be defined as 'academics (and practitioners) *with conditions*'.

Lather has warned of how guilt at an almost voyeuristic dimension to social research can lead to researchers turning in on themselves, such that their research takes a detour into self-analysis and where reflexivity merely becomes a means of self-authorisation for an existing set of practices. Mindful of this advice, we argue nonetheless for redefining the relationship of the researcher to the researched by bringing ourselves closer in. *Academics-with-conditions* is a collective that doesn't (yet) see itself as such, made up of those who routinely bracket off or even actively conceal from their workplace a vast array of both chronic and acute illnesses, conditions or disorders. We do this every day, as a response to increasingly neoliberal conditions of governance and the construct of the hyper-able academic/practitioner that we are required to emulate (Lau, 2019, Price, 2021). Our workplace treats illness as weakness and as detrimental to our status as worthy professionals. Indeed, for this reason there may well be challenges associated with collectives that are founded upon shared vulnerability in such neoliberal times. Yet, how can we dislocate ourselves from our own lived experience while claiming the capacity to empower or 'give voice' to oppressed and precarious groups such as those living with dementia?

Outside of dementia studies, there is mounting interest in the way that crip epistemologies can bridge the researcher-researched divide by beginning to identify collective affinities. An apposite example is offered by Mel Y. Chen (2014) as she reflects on the experience of brain fog, using this to question what Andrew King (2016, Chapter 17) describes as the 'cognonormativity' of academia. Chen's reflections are driven by a 'wish for shared epistemologies that can be developed together among differently cognating beings' (2014, p. 172). She identifies a series of experiences that might draw the 'differently cognating' together, including that of chronicity and the way it requires us to 'renavigate standard timeliness'. Chen points to shared experiences of cognitive change that stem from shifts due to age, illness, disability or other bodily transitions (we might add here the effects of Long COVID) over the life course and asks how 'profiles of race, gender, and labour produce variable "body"-"mind" distributions' (p. 176). How, for example, are cognitive lapses deemed more 'forgivable' within certain privileged groups than for others?

At the heart of Chen's argument is a call to recognise the way in which academic institutions produce 'disciplined cognators'. She asks: 'Our disciplining [as academics] goes much further than disciplinarity. We know this, but to what degree have we explored its consequences for our production of epistemologies?' (p. 178). In our struggle to live up to what is expected of the disciplined cognator, we need to ask what kinds of knowledge and ways of knowing get ruled in – and what gets ruled out? Ultimately, this is a question of how our own experience might be allowed to bring us closer to people with dementia, outside of conventional treatment, therapy and even emancipatory frameworks that have dominated the field of dementia studies to date.

Linda Örulv's contribution to this book shows what is possible when we bring ourselves closer in, using our own experience of difference as a point of connection with the experiences of people living with dementia. Her chapter provides a poignant illustration of what can be achieved by working with and across difference as a route to making visible what Kafer (2013) describes as 'collective affinities'. As Örulv's chapter demonstrates, difference is productive to understanding and a foundation to transformative action. Rather than appealing to an inevitably normative and exclusionary emphasis upon sameness, Örulv works with neurodiversity in ways that show how it can shape methodology, relationships in the field and subsequent sense-making practices.

Örulv's chapter stands out, in our opinion, as an exemplar of critical methodology in action. She hints at the power and potential of disrupting and de-familiarising conventional research practices and of exposing the unmarked and privileged standpoint from which analyses of dementia are so frequently framed. Her work demonstrates the value of critical research as provocation, and of adopting a contestatory stance in respect to more mainstream dementia studies. Critical dementia studies may then lead to better understanding of the affinities and challenges that are shared along different lines. This includes common experiences of a particular brand of neoliberal ableism/cognonormativity that is as active in contemporary academia (Brown and Leigh, 2020) as it has been in the political framing of health and social care services and support.

Beyond words... beyond dementia

In drawing together the strands of our argument, we end by advocating a paradoxical stance for critical methodology – of needing to move closer to dementia by shifting farther away. By this we mean finding new and innovative ways of engaging more directly with situated and emergent experiences of dementia and disablement, while looking beyond dementia as a discrete and stable category.

An evolving methodological challenge for dementia scholarship is that of how to account for the non-representational. Researchers are grappling with how to engage with and capture the processual nature of embodiment and practice. Increasingly, our everyday multi-sensory experience, corporeality and bodily movement are understood as tangled up with material, immaterial, temporal and ephemeral dimensions to the empirical world (Sumartojo and Pink, 2019). There is growing awareness of the value of this unspoken world to the lives of people with dementia (as Chapters 6 and 7 discuss) but also of how this sphere of experience for people with dementia might enable us to reflect critically upon the limits of our understanding of the world. Growing attention to the situatedness of dementia and the significance of context has thus begun to throw into question conventional methods defined by decontextualising data, as outlined earlier. Work in areas such as dementia, affect and atmosphere (Campbell, 2019, Hatton, 2014) as well as temporality (see Chapter 6, and Changfoot et al., 2022) holds out much potential for a deeper and diversified understanding of what dementia can teach us. These lines of investigation reach beyond the 'constructedness' of narrative and the storying of experience, which invariably position the person at the centre of events. Yet, this emerging field of study is no less subject to tensions between emancipation and usurpation. The often diffuse, nebulous and (by definition) non-representational nature of this domain of experience is arguably even more vulnerable to distortion through the sense-making practices of researchers. Moving forward, much then can be drawn from Lather's call for a less confident, less certain methodology that embraces unknowing.

Efforts to look beyond language and the constructedness of representation open into questions of the performativity of knowledge, and more affective and sensorial ways of knowing (Schillmeier, 2014). These provide a basis for approaching dementia differently, and, as Örulv points out in Chapter 18, of viewing it along different lines that do not necessarily correspond with neurotypical or other privileged research priorities and preoccupations. In this context, we suggest the challenge lies in drawing out the no less political dimension of such experience. Indeed, we need to ask how engaging with less mediated aspects of experience may enhance an emancipatory endeavour. In what ways can such a focus open up new kinds of political space for understanding and learning from dementia?

In his chapter for this book, Jenkins (Chapter 7) argues that establishing critical dementia studies requires the pursuit of a 'more radical ontological-epistemological-ethical project'. In this final chapter, we've argued that critical methodologies are integral to such an endeavour. Drawing on Lather's proposals, we have made the case for a kind of research that is capable of being uncertain and unconfident and at times that embraces unknowing and that sees the strength and potential in such an approach. It is a way of doing and feeling about research that reflects and learns from ways of doing and feeling with dementia. We have argued that this could provide a basis for bringing ourselves, as researchers and practitioners, closer into the lives of people with dementia. Ultimately, we hope that critical dementia studies will provide a basis for forging alliances currently untapped that may even take us beyond dementia to spark a coalitional politics that helps to reimagine our collective futures.

References

Brown, N. and Leigh, J. (2020) *Ableism in Academia: Theorising Experiences of Disabilities and Chronic Illnesses in Higher Education*. London: UCL Press.

Campbell, S. (2019) *Atmospheres of Dementia Care: Stories Told through the Bodies of Men*, PhD Thesis, University of Manchester. https://www.proquest.com/openview/b42c84d7f440a4f63aef7fba882696ff/1?cbl=51922&diss=y&pq-origsite=gscholar [Accessed 10th March 2022].

Cayton, H. (2004) Telling Stories: Choices and Challenges on the Journey of Dementia. *Dementia*, 3(1), pp. 9–17.

Ceci, C., Symonds Brown, H. and Judge, H. (2020) Rethinking the Assumptions of Intervention Research Concerned with Care at Home for People with Dementia. *Dementia*, 19(3), pp. 861–877.

Changfoot, N., Rice, C., Chivers, S., Williams, A.O., Connors, A., Barrett, A., Gordon, M. and Lalonde, G. (2022) Revisioning Aging: Indigenous, Crip and Queer Renderings. *Journal of Aging Studies*, 63, 100930.

Chen, M.Y. (2014) Brain Fog: The Race for Cripistemology. *Journal of Literary & Cultural Disability Studies*, 8(2), pp. 171–184.

Folkes, L. (2022) Moving beyond 'Shopping List' Positionality: Using Kitchen Table Reflexivity and In/Visible Tools to Develop Reflexive Qualitative Research. *Qualitative Research*, 0(0), p. 14687941221098922

Goldsmith, M. (1996) *Hearing the Voice of People with Dementia: Opportunities and Obstacles*. Bristol: Jessica Kingsley Publishers.

Grant, A. (2014) Troubling 'Lived Experience': A Post-Structural Critique of Mental Health Nursing Qualitative Research Assumptions. *Journal of Psychiatric and Mental Health Nursing*, 21(6), pp. 544–549.

Grant, A.J. (2016) Storying the World: A Posthumanist Critique of Phenomenological-Humanist Representational Practices in Mental Health Nurse Qualitative Inquiry. *Nursing Philosophy*, 17(4), pp. 290–297.

Haeusermann, T. (2019) Forced Continuity: Explorations of Biographical Narratives in Dementia Care. *Journal of Aging Studies*, 49, pp. 1–8.

Hatton, N. (2014) Re-imagining the Care Home: A Spatially Responsive Approach to Arts Practice with Older People in Residential Care. *Research in Drama Education: The Journal of Applied Theatre and Performance*, 19(4), pp. 355–365.

Hulko, W. (2009) From 'Not a Big Deal' to 'Hellish': Experiences of Older People with Dementia. *Journal of Aging Studies*, 23(3), pp. 131–144.

Jackson, A.Y. (2013) Spaces of Power/Knowledge: A Foucauldian Methodology for Qualitative Inquiry. *Qualitative Inquiry*, 19(10), pp. 839–847.

Jongsma, K., Spaeth, E. and Schicktanz, S. (2017) Epistemic Injustice in Dementia and Autism Patient Organizations: An Empirical Analysis. *AJOB Empirical Bioethics*, 8(4), pp. 221–233.

Kafer, A. (2013) *Feminist, Queer, Crip*. Bloomington: Indiana University Press.

Kafer, A. (2021) After Crip, Crip Afters. *South Atlantic Quarterly*, 120(2), pp. 415–434.

Keady, J., Hydén, L.C., Johnson, A. and Swarbrick, C. (eds.) (2017) *Social Research Methods in Dementia Studies: Inclusion and Innovation*. London: Routledge.

King, A. (2016) 'Queer(y)ing Dementia – Bringing Queer Theory and Studies of Dementia into Dialogue', In S. Westwood and E. Price (eds.), *Lesbian, Gay, Bisexual and Trans* Individuals Living with Dementia: Concepts, Practice and Rights*. London: Routledge, pp. 71–84.

Lather P. (2007) *Getting Lost: Feminist Efforts toward a Double(d) Science*. New York: SUNY Press.

Lau, T.C.W. (2019) 'Slowness, Disability, and Academic Productivity: The Need to Rethink Academic Culture', In C. McMaster and B. Whitburn (eds.), *Disability at the University: A Disabled Students' Manifesto*. New York: Peter Lang, pp. 11–19.

MacLure, M. (2009) 'Broken Voices, Dirty Words: On the Productive Insufficiency of Voice', in L.A. Mazzei and A.Y. Jackson (eds.), *Voice in Qualitative Inquiry: Challenging Conventional, Interpretive and Critical Conceptions in Qualitative Research*. London: Routledge, pp. 109–126.

MacLure, M., Holmes, R., Jones, L. and MacRae, C. (2010) Silence as Resistance to Analysis: Or, on Not Opening One's Mouth Properly. *Qualitative Inquiry*, 16(6), pp. 492–500.

Marcus, G. and Fisher, R. (1986) *Anthropology as Cultural Critique: An Experimental Moment in the Human Sciences*. Chicago, IL and London: Chicago University Press.

Mazzei, L.A. (2009) 'An Impossibly Full Voice', in L.A. Mazzei and A.Y. Jackson (eds.), *Voice in Qualitative Inquiry: Challenging Conventional, Interpretive and Critical Conceptions in Qualitative Research*. London: Routledge, pp. 57–74.

Mazzei, L.A. and Jackson, A.Y. (2009) 'Introduction: The Limit of Voice', in L.A. Mazzei and A.Y. Jackson (eds.), *Voice in Qualitative Inquiry: Challenging Conventional, Interpretive and Critical Conceptions in Qualitative Research*. London: Routledge, pp. 1–14.

Minich, J.A. (2016) Enabling Whom? Critical Disability Studies Now. *Lateral* [online], 5(1). https://csalateral.org/issue/5-1/forum-alt-humanities-critical-disability-studies-now-minich/.

Moore, T.F. and Hollett, J. (2003) Giving Voice to Persons Living with Dementia: The Researcher's Opportunities and Challenges. *Nursing Science Quarterly*, 16(2), pp. 163–167.

Morris, J. (1993) Feminism and Disability. *Feminist Review*, 43(1), pp. 57–70.

O'Connor, D., Phinney, A. and Hulko, W. (2010) Dementia at the Intersections: A Unique Case Study Exploring Social Location. *Journal of Aging Studies*, 24(1), pp. 30–39.

Price, K.A. and Hill, M.R. (2021) The Silence of Alzheimer's Disease: Stigma, Epistemic Injustice, and the Inequity of Those with Progressive Cognitive Impairment. *Communication Research and Practice*, 7(4), pp. 326–343.

Price, M. (2021) Time Harms: Disabled Faculty Navigating the Accommodations Loop. *South Atlantic Quarterly*, 120(2), pp. 257–277.

Said, E. (1979) *Orientalism*. New York: Random House.

Schalk S. (2017) Critical Disability Studies as Methodology. *Lateral* [online], 6(1). https://csalateral.org/issue/6-1/forum-alt-humanities-critical-disability-studies-methodology-schalk/.

Schillmeier, M. (2014) *Eventful Bodies: The Cosmopolitics of Illness*. London: Routledge.

Simons, J. (ed.) (2002) *From Kant to Lévi-Strauss: The Background to Contemporary Critical Theory*. Edinburgh, UK: Edinburgh University Press.

St Pierre, E.A. and Jackson, A.Y. (2014) Qualitative Data Analysis after Coding. *Qualitative Inquiry*, 20(6), pp. 715–719.

Sumartojo, S. and Pink, S. (2019) *Atmospheres and the Experiential World: Theory and Methods*. London: Routledge.

Ward, R. (2016) 'To Equality and Beyond? Queer Reflections on an Emerging Rights-Based Approach to Dementia in Scotland', in S. Westwood and E. Price (eds.), *Lesbian, Gay, Bisexual and Trans* Individuals Living with Dementia: Concepts, Practice and Rights*. London: Routledge, pp. 237–249.

Ward, R. and River, L. (2011) 'Between Participation and Practice: Inclusive User Participation and the Role of Practitioners', in J. Keady and S. Watts (eds.), *Mental Health and Later Life: Delivering an Holistic Model for Practice*. Abingdon, Oxon: Routledge, pp. 9–21.

Williams, S. and Keady J. (2006) The Narrative Voice of People with Dementia. *Dementia*, 5(2), pp. 163–166.

Index

Note: *Italic* page numbers refer to figures and page numbers followed by "n" denote endnotes.

For Product Safety Concerns and Information please contact our EU
representative GPSR@taylorandfrancis.com
Taylor & Francis Verlag GmbH, Kaufingerstraße 24, 80331 München, Germany

www.ingramcontent.com/pod-product-compliance
Lightning Source LLC
Chambersburg PA
CBHW052120230326
41598CB00080B/3895